Topics in Transplantation Imaging

Editors

PUNEET BHARGAVA
MATTHEW T. HELLER

RADIOLOGIC CLINICS OF NORTH AMERICA

www.radiologic.theclinics.com

Consulting Editor
FRANK H. MILLER

March 2016 • Volume 54 • Number 2

ELSEVIER

1600 John F. Kennedy Boulevard • Suite 1800 • Philadelphia, Pennsylvania, 19103-2899

http://www.theclinics.com

RADIOLOGIC CLINICS OF NORTH AMERICA Volume 54, Number 2
March 2016 ISSN 0033-8389, ISBN 13: 978-0-323-41663-4

Editor: John Vassallo (j.vassallo@elsevier.com)
Developmental Editor: Donald Mumford

Radiologic Clinics of North America (ISSN 0033-8389) is published bimonthly by Elsevier Inc., 360 Park Avenue South, New York, NY 10010-1710. Months of issue are January, March, May, July, September, and November. Periodicals postage paid at New York, NY and additional mailing offices. Subscription prices are USD 460 per year for US individuals, USD 784 per year for US institutions, USD 100 per year for US students and residents, USD 535 per year for Canadian individuals, USD 1002 per year for Canadian institutions, USD 660 per year for international individuals, USD 1002 per year for international institutions, and USD 315 per year for Canadian and foreign students/residents. To receive student and resident rate, orders must be accompanied by name of affiliated institution, date of term and the signature of program/residency coordinatior on institution letterhead. Orders will be billed at individual rate until proof of status is received. Foreign air speed delivery is included in all *Clinics* subscription prices. All prices are subject to change without notice. **POSTMASTER:** Send address changes to *Radiologic Clinics of North America*, Elsevier Health Sciences Division, Subscription Customer Service, 3251 Riverport Lane, Maryland Heights, MO63043. **Customer Service: Telephone: 1-800-654-2452** (U.S. and Canada); **1-314-447-8871** (outside U.S. and Canada). **Fax: 1-314-447-8029. E-mail:** journalscustomerservice-usa@elsevier.com **(for print support);** journalsonlinesupport-usa@elsevier.com **(for online support).**

Reprints. For copies of 100 or more of articles in this publication, please contact the Commercial Reprints Department, Elsevier Inc., 360 Park Avenue South, New York, New York 10010-1710. Tel.: +1-212-633-3874; Fax: +1-212-633-3820; E-mail: reprints@elsevier.com.

Radiologic Clinics of North America also published in Greek Paschalidis Medical Publications, Athens, Greece.

Radiologic Clinics of North America is covered in *MEDLINE/PubMed (Index Medicus), EMBASE/Excerpta Medica, Current Contents/Life Sciences, Current Contents/Clinical Medicine, RSNA Index to Imaging Literature, BIOSIS, Science Citation Index,* and *ISI/BIOMED.*

Printed in the United States of America.

Contributors

CONSULTING EDITOR

FRANK H. MILLER, MD
Chief, Body Imaging Section and Fellowship
Program; Medical Director of MRI; Professor,
Department of Radiology, Northwestern
University Feinberg School of Medicine,
Chicago, Illinois

EDITORS

MATTHEW T. HELLER, MD, FSAR
Director, Radiology Residency Program;
Associate Professor, Division of Abdominal
Imaging, Department of Radiology, University
of Pittsburgh Medical Center, University of
Pittsburgh School of Medicine, Pittsburgh,
Pennsylvania

PUNEET BHARGAVA, MD
Associate Professor, Body Imaging,
Department of Radiology, VA Puget Sound
Health Care System, University of Washington
School of Medicine, Seattle, Washington

AUTHORS

LEAH M. BACKHUS, MD, MPH, FACS
Associate Professor, Department of
Cardiothoracic Surgery, Stanford University,
Stanford, California

AKSHAY D. BAHETI, MD
Body Imaging Fellow, University of
Washington, Seattle, Washington

SENTA M. BERGGRUEN, MD
Assistant Professor of Radiology,
Northwestern University Feinberg School
of Medicine, Chicago, Illinois

PUNEET BHARGAVA, MD
Associate Professor, Body Imaging,
Department of Radiology, VA Puget Sound
Health Care System, University of Washington
Medical Center, University of Washington
School of Medicine, Seattle, Washington

KRISTINE S. BURK, MD
Resident Physician, Department of Radiology,
Massachusetts General Hospital, Boston,
Massachusetts

PATRICIA T. CHANG, MD
Instructor, Department of Radiology, Boston
Children's Hospital, Harvard Medical School,
Boston, Massachusetts

JAMIE FROST, DO
Instructor, Department of Radiology, Boston
Children's Hospital, Harvard Medical School,
Boston, Massachusetts

NITIN P. GHONGE, MD
Consultant Radiologist and Academic
Coordinator, Department of Radiology,
Indraprastha Apollo Hospitals, New Delhi,
India

RICHARD HA, MD
Clinical Assistant Professor, Department of
Cardiothoracic Surgery, Stanford University,
Stanford, California

CARLA B. HARMATH, MD
Assistant Professor of Radiology,
Northwestern University Feinberg School of
Medicine, Chicago, Illinois

MATTHEW T. HELLER, MD, FSAR
Director, Radiology Residency Program;
Associate Professor, Division of Abdominal
Imaging, Department of Radiology, University
of Pittsburgh Medical Center, University of
Pittsburgh School of Medicine, Pittsburgh,
Pennsylvania

ANASTASIA L. HRYHORCZUK, MD
Assistant Professor, Department of Radiology,
Floating Hospital for Children, Tufts Medical
Center, Boston, Massachusetts

CHRISTOPHER R. INGRAHAM, MD
Assistant Professor, Interventional Radiology
Division, Department of Interventional Radiology,
University of Washington, Seattle, Washington

CLINTON JOKERST, MD
Assistant Professor, Department of Radiology,
Mayo Clinic Arizona, Scottsdale, Arizona

VENKATA KATABATHINA, MD
Associate Professor, Department of Radiology,
University of Texas Health Science Center,
San Antonio, Texas

DOUGLAS S. KATZ, MD
Professor and Vice Chairman, Department of
Radiology, Winthrop University Hospital,
Mineola, New York

EDWARD Y. LEE, MD, MPH
Chief, Division of Thoracic Imaging; Associate
Professor of Radiology, Departments of
Radiology and Medicine, Pulmonary Division,
Boston Children's Hospital, Harvard Medical
School, Boston, Massachusetts

MEGHAN LUBNER, MD
Associate Professor, Department of Radiology,
University of Wisconsin, Madison, Wisconsin

CHRISTINE O. MENIAS, MD
Professor, Department of Radiology, Mayo
Clinic, Scottsdale, Arizona

PARDEEP K. MITTAL, MD
Director of Body MRI; Associate Professor,
Department of Radiology and Imaging
Sciences, Emory University School of
Medicine, Atlanta, Georgia

TAN-LUCIEN H. MOHAMMED, MD, FCCP
Associate Professor, Department of Radiology,
University of Florida College of Medicine,
Gainesville, Florida

MARTIN MONTENOVO, MD
Assistant Professor, Division of Transplant
Surgery, Department of Surgery, University of
Washington, Seattle, Washington

COURTNEY COURSEY MORENO, MD
Assistant Professor, Department of
Radiology and Imaging Sciences, Emory
University School of Medicine, Atlanta,
Georgia

MARIAM MOSHIRI, MD
Associate Professor, Department of Radiology,
University of Washington Medical Center,
Seattle, Washington

MICHAEL S. MULLIGAN, MD
Professor, Division of Cardiothoracic
Surgery, Department of Surgery, University
of Washington, Seattle, Washington

RYAN B. O'MALLEY, MD
Assistant Professor, Department of Radiology,
University of Washington Medical Center,
Seattle, Washington

SHERIF OSMAN, MD
Department of Radiology, University of
Washington Medical Center, Seattle,
Washington

TARUN PANDEY, MD, FRCR
Associate Professor of Radiology,
MSK/Body-MRI and Cardiac Imaging
Fellowship Director, University of Arkansas
for Medical Sciences, Little Rock, Arkansas

GRACE S. PHILLIPS, MD
Associate Professor, Department of Radiology,
Seattle Children's Hospital, University of
Washington School of Medicine, Seattle,
Washington

PERRY PICKHARDT, MD
Professor, Department of Radiology, University
of Wisconsin, Madison, Wisconsin

SRINIVASA R. PRASAD, MD
Professor, Department of Radiology, University
of Texas MD Anderson Cancer Center,
Houston, Texas

DUSHYANT SAHANI, MD
Associate Professor, Department of Radiology,
Massachusetts General Hospital, Boston,
Massachusetts

RUPAN SANYAL, MD
Associate Professor, Body Imaging,
Department of Radiology, University of
Alabama, Birmingham, Alabama

JABI E. SHRIKI, MD
Associate Professor, Department of Radiology,
University of Washington; Diagnostic Imaging
Service, VA Puget Sound Health Care System,
Seattle, Washington

AJAY K. SINGH, MD
Assistant Professor, Department of Radiology,
Massachusetts General Hospital, Boston,
Massachusetts

ARLENE SIRAJUDDIN, MD
Assistant Professor, Department of Medical
Imaging, University of Arizona, College of
Medicine, Tucson, Arizona

A. LUANA STANESCU, MD
Assistant Professor, Department of Radiology,
Seattle Children's Hospital, University of
Washington School of Medicine, Seattle,
Washington

EKAMOL TANTISATTAMO, MD, FASN
Transplant Nephrology Fellow, Division
of Nephrology, Department of Medicine,
Comprehensive Transplant Center,
Northwestern University Feinberg School
of Medicine, Chicago, Illinois

STEPHEN THOMAS, MD
Assistant Professor of Radiology, University of
Chicago, Chicago, Illinois

PARSIA A. VAGEFI, MD
Assistant Professor of Surgery, Department of
Radiology, Massachusetts General Hospital,
Boston, Massachusetts

CECIL G. WOOD III, MD
Clinical Instructor of Radiology, Northwestern
University Feinberg School of Medicine,
Chicago, Illinois

Contents

renal transplant complications are diagnosed with imaging. Medical complications including rejection, acute tubular necrosis, and drug toxicity also can impair renal function. These medical complications are typically indistinguishable at imaging, and biopsy may be performed to establish a diagnosis. Normal transplant anatomy, imaging techniques, and the appearances of renal transplant complications at ultrasound, computed tomography, and MR imaging are reviewed.

Whole pancreas transplantation is an effective treatment for obtaining euglycemic status in patients with insulin-dependent diabetes mellitus, and is usually performed concurrent with renal transplantation in the affected patient. This article discusses complex surgical anatomical details of pancreas transplantation including surgical options for endocrine and exocrine drainage pathways. It then describes several possible complications related to surgical factors in the immediate post operative period followed by other complications related to systemic issues, vasculature, and the pancreatic parenchyma.

Liver, kidney, and pancreas transplants are complex procedures that have evolved over the past several decades from pioneering, experimental procedures into well-developed, refined procedures that have saved countless lives. Previously encountered technical, immunologic, and perioperative obstacles have now been overcome and improved upon, allowing for the success of these procedures today. This article reviews the basic surgical techniques used for solid organ transplantation that are relevant to, and are currently encountered by radiologists. This article also reviews commonly encountered postoperative complications, and the techniques and strategies that have evolved in interventional radiology to overcome these complications.

The anatomy, normal postoperative radiological appearance, and imaging features of common postoperative complications of pediatric abdominal transplants are reviewed, including renal, liver, and intestinal transplants. Doppler ultrasound is the mainstay of imaging after transplantation. Computed tomography (CT) and CT angiography, MR imaging and magnetic resonance (MR) angiography, MR cholangiopancreatography, conventional angiography, and nuclear medicine imaging may be used for problem-solving in pediatric transplant patients. Accurate and timely radiological diagnosis of transplant complications facilitates appropriate treatment and minimizes morbidity and mortality.

Availability of novel immunosuppressive drugs is the most important factor responsible for significant improvement in long-term graft survival rates after solid organ transplantation. However, chronic immunosuppression predisposes patients to a myriad of potentially life-threatening complications. In addition to drug-related adverse effects, transplant recipients are at increased risk of developing opportunistic microbial infections and a spectrum of unique cancers, many of which are caused by oncogenic viruses. Cross-sectional imaging studies play a crucial role in the timely diagnosis and management of post-transplant infections and malignancies.

In the past decade, with improved surgical technique and knowledge of immunosuppression, pediatric lung and heart transplantation have been established as viable therapeutic interventions for pediatric patients with end-stage cardiopulmonary disease from various underlying congenital and acquired disorders. Although outcomes for pediatric patients are similar to those for adult patients, thoracic organ transplantation in this special age group carries unique challenges for preoperative and postoperative imaging evaluation. This article provides an up-to-date review of the postoperative transplant anatomy, imaging techniques, and complications of pediatric lung and heart transplantation.

Modifications in recipient and donor criteria and innovations in donor management hold promise for increasing rates of lung transplantation, yet availability of donors remains a limiting resource. Imaging is critical in the work-up of donor and recipient including identification of conditions that may portend to poor posttransplant outcomes or necessitate modifications in surgical technique. This article describes the radiologic principles that guide selection of patients and surgical procedures in lung transplantation.

Imaging plays a key role in the diagnosis and management of complications following lung transplantation. This article outlines the imaging modalities available for evaluation of posttransplant complications with a focus on major indications and key strengths and weaknesses of each modality. A brief description of surgical technique and relevant anatomy is included. Descriptions of some of the more commonly encountered complications are outlined with a focus on imaging findings. Complications are grouped by anatomic or imaging-based findings and subcategorized chronologically to help order the differential diagnosis.

The role of stem cell therapy in the treatment of hematologic and nonhematologic conditions is ever increasing. A thorough knowledge of the applications of stem cells and transplant physiology is essential for understanding the imaging manifestations.

Stem cell imaging includes molecular imaging, and diagnostic and interventional radiology. It is possible to make a diagnosis of various complications and diseases associated with stem cell transplant. This article presents a simplified overview of stem cell applications and techniques with focus on hematopoietic stem cell transplant imaging.

PROGRAM OBJECTIVE
The objective of the *Radiologic Clinics of North America* is to keep practicing radiologists and radiology residents up to date with current clinical practice in radiology by providing timely articles reviewing the state of the art in patient care.

TARGET AUDIENCE
Practicing radiologists, radiology residents, and other health care professionals who provide patient care utilizing radiologic findings.

LEARNING OBJECTIVES
Upon completion of this activity, participants will be able to:
1. Review pre-surgical imaging techniques for patients undergoing transplantation.
2. Discuss interventional and surgical techniques using transplantation imaging.
3. Recognize possible imaging complications in liver, renal, pancreas, and lung transplantation.

ACCREDITATION
The Elsevier Office of Continuing Medical Education (EOCME) is accredited by the Accreditation Council for Continuing Medical Education (ACCME) to provide continuing medical education for physicians.

The EOCME designates this enduring material for a maximum of 15 *AMA PRA Category 1 Credit*(s)™. Physicians should claim only the credit commensurate with the extent of their participation in the activity.

All other health care professionals requesting continuing education credit for this enduring material will be issued a certificate of participation.

DISCLOSURE OF CONFLICTS OF INTEREST
The EOCME assesses conflict of interest with its instructors, faculty, planners, and other individuals who are in a position to control the content of CME activities. All relevant conflicts of interest that are identified are thoroughly vetted by EOCME for fair balance, scientific objectivity, and patient care recommendations. EOCME is committed to providing its learners with CME activities that promote improvements or quality in healthcare and not a specific proprietary business or a commercial interest.

The planning committee, staff, authors and editors listed below have identified no financial relationships or relationships to products or devices they or their spouse/life partner have with commercial interest related to the content of this CME activity:
Leah M. Backhus, MD, MPH, FACS; Akshay D. Baheti, MD; Senta M. Berggruen, MD; Kristine S. Burk, MD; Patricia T. Chang, MD; Anjali Fortna; Jamie Frost, DO; Nitin P. Ghonge, MD; Richard Ha, MD; Carla B. Harmath, MD; Anastasia L. Hryhorczuk, MD; Christopher R. Ingraham, MD; Clinton Jokerst, MD; Venkata Katabathina, MD; Douglas S. Katz, MD; Edward Y. Lee, MD, MPH; Christine O. Menias, MD; Frank H. Miller, MD; Pardeep K. Mittal, MD; Tan-Lucien H. Mohammed, MD; Martin Montenovo, MD; Courtney Coursey Moreno, MD; Mariam Moshiri, MD; Michael S. Mulligan, MD; Ryan B. O'Malley, MD; Sherif Osman, MD; Tarun Pandey, MD, FRCR; Grace S. Phillips, MD; Perry Pickhardt, MD; Dushyant Sahani, MD; Erin Scheckenbach; Jabi E. Shriki, MD; Ajay K. Singh, MD; Arlene Sirajuddin, MD; A. Luana Stanescu, MD; Karthik Subramaniam; Ekamol Tantisattamo, MD, FASN; Stephen Thomas, MD; Parsia A. Vagefi, MD; John Vassallo; Cecil G. Wood III, MD.

The planning committee, staff, authors and editors listed below have identified financial relationships or relationships to products or devices they or their spouse/life partner have with commercial interest related to the content of this CME activity:
Puneet Bhargava, MD has an employment affiliation with Elsevier B.V.
Matthew T. Heller, MD, FSAR is a consultant/advisor for, with royalties/patents from Amirsys, Inc.
Meghan Lubner, MD has research support from NeuWave Medical, Inc.; Koninklijke Philips N.V.; and General Electric Company.
Srinivasa R. Prasad, MD is a consultant/advisor for Virtuo CTC, LLC and Bracco, has stock ownership in Cellectar BioSciences, and has research support from Koninklijke Philips N.V.
Rupan Sanyal, MD receives roylaties/patents from Oxford University Press.

UNAPPROVED/OFF-LABEL USE DISCLOSURE
The EOCME requires CME faculty to disclose to the participants:
1. When products or procedures being discussed are off-label, unlabelled, experimental, and/or investigational (not US Food and Drug Administration [FDA] approved); and
2. Any limitations on the information presented, such as data that are preliminary or that represent ongoing research, interim analyses, and/or unsupported opinions. Faculty may discuss information about pharmaceutical agents that is outside of FDA-approved labelling. This information is intended solely for CME and is not intended to promote off-label use of these medications. If you have any questions, contact the medical affairs department of the manufacturer for the most recent prescribing information.

TO ENROLL

To enroll in the *Radiologic Clinics of North America* Continuing Medical Education program, call customer service at 1-800-654-2452 or sign up online at http://www.theclinics.com/home/cme. The CME program is available to subscribers for an additional annual fee of USD 315.

METHOD OF PARTICIPATION

In order to claim credit, participants must complete the following:
1. Complete enrolment as indicated above.
2. Read the activity.
3. Complete the CME Test and Evaluation. Participants must achieve a score of 70% on the test. All CME Tests and Evaluations must be completed online.

CME INQUIRIES/SPECIAL NEEDS

For all CME inquiries or special needs, please contact elsevierCME@elsevier.com.

RADIOLOGIC CLINICS OF NORTH AMERICA

ISSUE OF RELATED INTEREST

Magnetic Resonance Imaging Clinics, February 2016 (Vol. 24, Issue 1)
Functional and Molecular Imaging in Oncology
Antonio Luna, *Editor*
Available at: http://www.mri.theclinics.com

THE CLINICS ARE AVAILABLE ONLINE!
Access your subscription at:
www.theclinics.com

Preface
Transplant Imaging— Focusing on a Systematic Approach

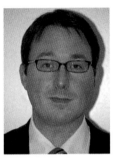 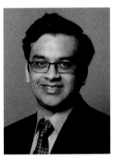

Matthew T. Heller, MD, FSAR   Puneet Bhargava, MD

Editors

Following the world's first successful liver transplantation in the 1960s, the field of transplantation has exploded and rapidly evolved. Pancreas, kidney, small bowel, multivisceral, and stem cell transplants are now commonplace. The success of transplantation has been largely due to improvements in immunosuppression and surgical technique. In addition, imaging has evolved to play a significant role in the care of the transplant patient. Both donors and recipients are often evaluated with advanced cross-sectional imaging techniques during the initial workup and preoperative planning. Ultrasound has emerged as the primary imaging modality for intraoperative consultation and in guiding perioperative management. Surveillance imaging has become a mainstay of the long-term follow-up for transplant patients.

Imaging of the transplant patient can seem formidable to those outside of a major transplant center. The altered anatomy, variable surgical techniques, and imaging protocols and optimization can present challenges to the interpreting radiologist. In addition, the effects of immunosuppression create an environment with a unique gamut of complications that can affect almost any organ system.

However, these challenges can be met through use of a systemic approach to imaging studies of the transplant patient. First, a thorough understanding of the pretransplant and posttransplant anatomy is essential to properly performing and interpreting an imaging examination. This is achieved through familiarity with the typical orientation of the transplanted organs and the common surgical techniques. We have found it extremely helpful to frequently engage the transplant surgical team in a discussion during interpretation of the imaging examination. This may allow recognition of an alternative surgical technique or sequela of an intraoperative complication. Alternatively, a thorough review of the operative note may also provide insight to the findings on the imaging examination. Recognizing that most transplant complications involve the anastomoses will allow the interpreting radiologist to focus the majority of the imaging time at these sites. Certainly, as perfusion of the transplanted organ is of paramount importance, a concerted effort should always be made to clearly identify the vascular anastomoses and to promptly communicate any findings of altered or compromised blood flow. Vascular complications are a leading cause of graft compromise and are often readily treatable if diagnosis is facilitated. Similarly, perigraft fluid collections are usually quite amenable to diagnosis and percutaneous intervention. The diagnosis and management of perigraft fluid collections are important to allow optimal graft function and to treat potential infection. In the absence of complications identified at imaging, the information contained in the imaging report contains critical information for the

Radiol Clin N Am 54 (2016) xv–xvi
http://dx.doi.org/10.1016/j.rcl.2015.11.001
0033-8389/16/$ – see front matter © 2016 Published by Elsevier Inc.

transplant team. The absence of a mechanical complication will allow exclusion of several differential diagnoses and may prompt image-guided percutaneous biopsy to assess the parenchyma for changes of rejection. This plus knowledge of the common manifestations of disease states associated with immunosuppression will facilitate titrating of immunosuppressive agents.

This issue of *Radiologic Clinics of North America* organizes transplantation imaging into organ system and focuses on the essential anatomy, most common surgical techniques, and key points for aiding patient management. Despite the many complexities involved in transplant imaging, the ability to follow a standard approach for each patient will allow the radiologist to triage transplant patients into those who may most benefit from immediate surgical or angiographic intervention, adjustment of immunosuppression, or continued imaging and clinical surveillance.

Matthew T. Heller, MD, FSAR
University of Pittsburgh
School of Medicine and Medical Center
200 Lothrop Street
Suite 201 East Wing
Pittsburgh, PA 15213, USA

Puneet Bhargava, MD
University of Washington School of Medicine
1959 Northeast Pacific Street
Room BB308, Box 357115
Seattle, WA 98195-7115, USA

E-mail addresses:
hellermt@upmc.edu (M.T. Heller)
bhargp@uw.edu (P. Bhargava)

Pretransplantation Imaging Workup of the Liver Donor and Recipient

Kristine S. Burk, MD[a], Ajay K. Singh, MD[b],
Parsia A. Vagefi, MD[c], Dushyant Sahani, MD[b],*

KEYWORDS

- Liver transplantation • Preliving donor liver transplant imaging • Hepatic artery anatomy and variants
- Portal vein anatomy and variants • Hepatic vein anatomy and variants • Biliary anatomy and variants

KEY POINTS

- Preoperative evaluation of the hepatic vasculature, parenchyma, and biliary system with computed tomography (CT) and MR imaging/magnetic resonance cholangiopancreatography (MRCP) allows for improved candidate selection and a reduction in transplant operative complication rates.
- Use of low-dose CT protocols, contrast-enhanced MRCP, and image postprocessing (3-dimensional, maximal intensity projection [MIP], and volume rendering) maximizes preoperative planning while minimizing the risk of imaging to the donor.
- The purpose of preoperative recipient imaging is to define vascular inflow and outflow, and to determine the extent of tumor burden in Hepatocellular Carcinoma (HCC) patients awaiting transplant.
- Preoperative living donor liver transplantation donor imaging involves assessment of the vascular and biliary anatomy; evaluation of the hepatic parenchyma for steatosis, iron, and focal lesions; and calculation of liver volumes.
- Surgically relevant vascular and biliary anatomic variants are common, but most remain eligible for donation because of prospective identification with imaging and advances in microvascular surgical technique.

INTRODUCTION

Liver transplantation has become the accepted treatment for patients with end stage liver disease, with 15,294 candidates currently on the waiting list.[1] In 2013 alone, 5921 liver transplants were performed. Unfortunately, the availability of organs remains inadequate to keep up with demands; by the end of 2013, 12,407 candidates remained on the transplant list, with 1767 patients dying while on the waiting list, and 1223 being removed as they became too sick to qualify for transplant.[2]

Because of the shortage of cadaveric liver grafts, transplantation of partial grafts from both living and deceased donors has developed as a method for expansion of the potential donor pool. Although these operations pose a substantial technical challenge, they do allow a portion of the waitlisted candidate population to achieve transplantation, often in an expedited fashion.[3] Concomitant with the technical refinements in partial liver transplantation has been the increased use of imaging techniques to allow for a precise

Disclosure Statement: The authors have nothing to disclose.
[a] Department of Radiology, Massachusetts General Hospital, Radiology Founders 205, 55 Fruit Street, Boston, MA 02114, USA; [b] Department of Radiology, Massachusetts General Hospital, Radiology WHT-270, 55 Fruit Street, Boston, MA 02114, USA; [c] Department of Radiology, Massachusetts General Hospital, White 521c, 55 Fruit Street, Boston, MA 02114, USA
* Corresponding author.
E-mail address: dsahani@partners.org

Radiol Clin N Am 54 (2016) 185–197
http://dx.doi.org/10.1016/j.rcl.2015.09.010
0033-8389/16/$ – see front matter © 2016 Elsevier Inc. All rights reserved.

understanding of donor and recipient anatomy prior to surgery. This has allowed for improved candidate selection and a reduction in operative complication rates.

TRANSPLANT OPERATION
Cadaveric Liver Transplant

There are 3 types of liver transplants performed today: whole-liver cadaveric transplant, split-liver cadaveric transplant, and living donor liver transplant. The most common type is a complete cadaveric liver transplant, wherein the entire donor liver is transplanted into the recipient. This has the advantage of being the most technically straightforward operation, although organ availability is limited.[4]

Split-Liver Cadaveric Transplant

Least common is a split-liver cadaveric transplant, which accounted for only 1.2% of transplants in 2013.[2] Cadaveric split liver can be performed in situ (in the donor prior to organ retrieval), or ex vivo (on the back table following liver retrieval) (**Fig. 1**).[5,6] The most common cadaveric splitting technique involves a transection plane to the right of the falciform ligament, resulting in a right triesegment graft (segments I and IV–VIII) for an adult recipient, and a left lateral graft (segments II–III) for a pediatric recipient. More rarely, a true right–left split technique can be utilized for 2 adult recipients, and involves a transection plane to the right of the middle hepatic vein (MHV) to create a right hemi-liver graft (segments V-VIII +/− I) and a left hemi-liver graft (segments II-IV +/− I).[7-9] Split-liver transplantation helps mitigate the shortage of donor livers available, but is a technically demanding operation and poses an increased risk of complications for the graft recipient.[10-12]

Living Donor Liver Transplant

Living donor liver transplant accounted for 4.0% of the liver transplants performed in the last 10 years (**Fig. 2**).[13] The decision of which lobe is transplanted is based on donor anatomic considerations and the anticipated residual liver and graft sizes. The residual donor liver must be greater than 30% of the total donor hepatic volume to ensure adequate postoperative liver function, and the graft-to-recipient body weight ratio must be greater than 0.8 to minimize the risk of small-for-size syndrome in the recipient.[4]

A left lateral segmentectomy technique is typically used for a pediatric recipient. In this operation, the transection plane runs just to the right of the falciform ligament (**Fig. 3**A). If a larger-volume graft is required, then a full left hepatic lobectomy with inclusion of the MHV can be performed, with or without the caudate lobe.

For an adult recipient, either a full-right or full-left hepatic graft can be used. Historically, the right lateral hepatectomy technique has been most commonly performed. In this operation, the liver is split approximately 1 cm to the right of the MHV, close to Cantlie line that connects the inferior vena cava (IVC) to the gallbladder fossa (**Fig. 3**B). Variations in anatomy of the MHV are critically important to the success of this

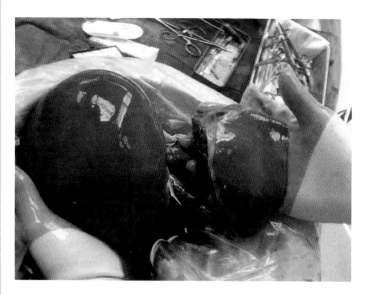

Fig. 1. Ex vivo split-liver cadaveric transplant—the right tri-segment graft was transplanted into an adult recipient with HCC, while the left lateral segment graft went to an infant with fulminant hepatic failure.

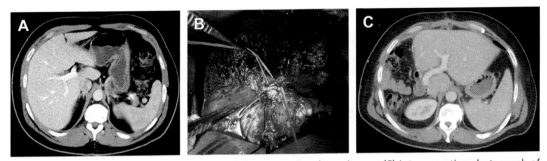

Fig. 2. Right lobe living donor liver transplant. (*A*) Preoperative donor image. (*B*) Intraoperative photograph after liver parenchymal division but prior to vascular division. (*C*) Postoperative donor image showing growth in the remnant left hepatic lobe.

operation, and are discussed in subsequent sections of this review.[14] More recently, there has been a rise in popularity of left hepatic graft transplantation. As it represents less volume removed for the donor, and accordingly, less volume transplanted to the recipient, the latter procedure is thought to shift the risk of postoperative complications from the living donor to the recipient.[15]

Overall, the mortality risk to a living donor is 0.15% to 0.20%, and the risk of postoperative complication is 40%. Approximately 95% of these complications are classified as Clavien grade I or II, requiring at most a percutaneous intervention.[16,17] Recipients of living donor liver grafts also experience a higher rate of complications postoperatively when compared to recipients of whole-liver grafts. However, this increased risk is felt to be offset by the ability to achieve liver transplant with a high-quality liver allograft.[18]

IMAGING TECHNIQUES

With the advent of biliary contrast agents and imaging postprocessing techniques, CT and MR imaging have replaced conventional angiography, endoscopic retrograde cholangiopancreatography (ERCP), and intraoperative cholangiography as the workhorses of pretransplant imaging. Although MR imaging can be used as a sole imaging modality for this purpose, CT and MR imaging are more often used together due to their complimentary strengths.[19]

Computed Tomography/Computed Tomography Angiography

At the authors' institution, potential donors are first imaged with dual-energy CT/CT angiography (CTA). With its superior spatial resolution, CTA better delineates the small segmental hepatic arteries and accessory hepatic veins. It is also utilized as an initial screen for parenchymal abnormalities that would be contraindications for donation.[20] In the past, CT had also been used to evaluate the biliary anatomy with the use of iodinated contrast agents excreted in the bile (**Fig. 4**). However, these agents were taken off the US market a few years ago, and as a result, CT cholangiography is no longer performed. Efforts are being made to reduce the radiation dose of the examination as much as possible, as donors are often young and healthy. Methods to accomplish this and other details of the authors' preoperative CT protocol are described in **Table 1**.

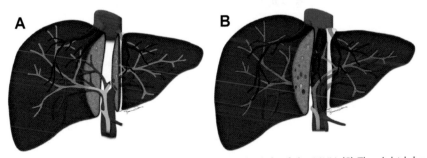

Fig. 3. (*A*) The left lateral segmentectomy LDLT plane runs to the left of the MHV. (*B*) The right lobe LDLT plane connects the gallbladder fossa and IVC and runs 1 cm to the right of the MHV.

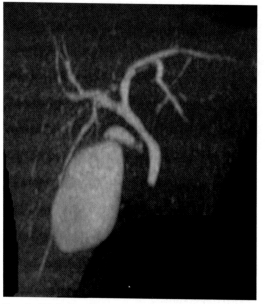

Fig. 4. CT cholangiogram showing the common bile duct and intrahepatic biliary ducts. (*From* Singh AK, Cronin CG, Verma HA, et al. Imaging of preoperative liver transplantation in adults: what radiologists should know. Radiographics 2011;31:1029; with permission.)

MR Imaging/Magnetic Resonance Cholangiopancreatography

Next, an MR imaging/ magnetic resonance cholangiopancreatography (MRCP) is performed using a hepatobiliary contrast agent. Fast spoiled gradient echo sequences are utilized to decrease image acquisition time and minimize motion artifacts. Parenchymal evaluation involves characterizing incidental focal lesions and determining the degree of hepatic steatosis.[21] Biliary system evaluation involves a traditional T2 weighted noncontrast MRCP in addition to a T1 weighted contrast-enhanced MRCP utilizing Gd-BOPTA (Multihance, Bracco Diagnostics Inc. Princeton, NJ) or Gd-EOB-DTPA (Eovist, Bayer Whippany, NJ).[22] These MRCP images supplement the intraoperative cholangiogram routinely performed at the time of surgery. Further technical aspects of the authors' preoperative MR imaging protocol can be found in **Table 1**.

Image Postprocessing

Postprocessing of the CT and MRI images is routinely performed. This includes multiplanar reformations, 3-dimensional reconstruction with

Table 1
Technical details of pretransplant imaging by computed tomography and MR imaging

Sequence	Sequence Details	Structures Evaluated
CT		
Non-contrast	2–4 thick slices through the liver at 140 and 80 kVp	Parenchyma (steatosis)
Arterial phase	Limit field of view (FOV) to abdomen Iterative reconstruction Low kVp	Arterial anatomy Parenchyma (focal lesions)
Combined Portal venous/ Hepatic venous phase	Limit FOV to abdomen Iterative reconstruction Weight-based kVp (80 kVp if <150 lbs, 100 kVp if 150–200 lbs, 120 kVp if >200 lbs)	Portal and hepatic venous anatomy Parenchyma (focal lesions)
MR imaging		
T1 Pre-contrast	Chemical shift imaging Dixon method imaging	Parenchyma (steatosis and iron quantification)
T2 SSFSE	Coronal and axial planes	Biliary system
T2 3-dimensional MRCP	—	Biliary system
TI Postcontrast 2-dimensional or 3-dimensional GRE gradient echo (GRE)	Coronal and axial planes Arterial, portal venous, delayed phases	Arterial, portal venous, and hepatic venous anatomy parenchyma (focal lesions)
TI Post-contrast MRCP	20 min delayed phase	Biliary system

maximal intensity projection (MIP) images, and volume rendering. This image processing allows for optimal evaluation of the anatomy in the ideal planes—the hepatic arteries on 3-dimensional or axial MIPs, the hepatic veins on axial MIPs, the portal veins on coronal MIPs, and the biliary tree on 3-dimensional T2-weighted or 3-dimensional T1-weighted, postcontrast coronal oblique images. Liver volume rendering is performed by manually tracing the margins of the hepatic parenchyma on each axial section, then summing them up into a 3-dimensional model; this can be done for the entire liver, or can be used to isolate individual liver segments or hepatic lobes.[23] The volume renderings, vascular models, and biliary models can be superimposed on one another for further delineation of the anatomy.

PREOPERATIVE IMAGING OF THE RECIPIENT
Model for End-Stage Liver Disease Score and Candidate Eligibility

Candidate eligibility is determined by the patient's model for end-stage liver disease (MELD) score. This 6–40 scoring system—based on the patient's bilirubin, international normalized ratio (INR), and creatinine—was initially created to predict the 3-month mortality for patients with nonHCC end-stage liver disease (ESLD) undergoing a Transjugular Intrahepatic Portosystemic Shunt (TIPS) procedure. It was later applied to transplant allocation in order to allow for candidate list prioritization based upon medical need.[24,25] The MELD score replaced the Child-Turcotte-Pugh score as the major determinant of waitlist rank order in 2002.

Those candidates with a diagnosis of unresectable HCC for whom liver transplantation is the appropriate treatment often have preserved hepatic function. As a result, their calculated MELD score often predicts a lower risk of death than is appropriate. In order to provide HCC candidates access to liver transplantation, MELD exception points were created. This exception score starts with a MELD score of 22, with additional exception points awarded every 3 months if the HCC candidate remains within Milan criteria.

The primary purpose of recipient imaging in the preoperative setting is to (1) define arterial and portal vascular inflow and venous outflow in select cases (ie, Budd Chiari disease), and (2) to determine the extent of tumor burden in HCC patients awaiting transplant. The former is extremely useful in the candidate undergoing retransplantation. Contraindications to transplant that need to be excluded by imaging include extrahepatic malignancy, complete thrombosis of the entire portal venous system, and stage 3 or 4 primary HCC. Other critical imaging findings in the transplant recipient are discussed in **Table 2.**

Table 2
Critical findings in recipient pretransplant imaging

Relevant Anatomy	Surgical Implication
Arterial anatomy	
Accessory or replaced left or right hepatic artery	Additional surgical step during anastomosis
Celiac artery stenosis or median arcuate ligament syndrome (MALS)	May require vascular reconstruction due to increased risk for biliary complications and graft infarction
Splenic artery aneurysm	Must be surgically treated to prevent rupture after transplant
Hepatic venous	
Assessment of thrombus extent in patients with Budd Chiari	May require an operative thorombectomy
Location of stent in patients with TIPS	Clamp location is influenced location of proximal portion of stent in the hepatic vein
Portal venous	
Acute portal venous thrombosis	Must perform intraoperative thrombectomy
Chronic portal venous thrombosis	Attempt intraoperative thrombectomy or use donor iliac vein interposition graft for inflow.

HCC Nodule Characterization and Transplant Criteria

For patients with HCC, the Organ Procurement and Transplantation Network (OPTN) or Liver Imaging Reporting and Data System (LI-RADS) criteria are used to characterize liver lesions as benign, suspicious for HCC, or definitely HCC (**Table 3**). These classification systems rely on nodule characteristics including intrinsic signal intensity and enhancement pattern, washout pattern, capsule appearance, and nodule architecture to determine the likelihood that a nodule is HCC.[26,27] Once the liver nodules are characterized, the Milan criteria are used to determine transplant candidacy. According to these, in order for a patient to qualify for a transplant, there must be either a single tumor less than 5 cm, or less than 3 tumors that are each less than 3 cm but greater than 1 cm, without extrahepatic malignancy or macrovascular invasion.[28] The University of California San Francisco (UCSF) criteria have been proposed as an expansion of the previously defined Milan Criteria and have shown similar post-transplant outcomes to the Milan criteria. According to these, there must be either: a single tumor less than 6.5 cm, or less than 3 tumors that are each less than 4.5 cm, with the total sum of tumor diameters being less than 8 cm.[29]

Bridging and Down-Staging HCC with Locoregional Therapy

Patients with HCC whose tumors are growing at a significant rate or who are expected to wait more than 6 months on the transplant list may be offered locoregional therapy to prevent tumor expansion beyond criteria. This practice, called "bridging to transplant," can be accomplished by multiple types of interventions including: alcohol injection, thermal ablation (including radiofrequency and microwave ablation), transarterial radioembolization (TARE), and most commonly transarterial chemoembolization (TACE).[30] The choice of which therapy to offer is typically guided by the Barcelona Clinic Liver Cancer Staging (BCLC) Criteria, which take into account the number and size of HCC nodules, the patient's Child-Pugh score, and the patient's Eastern Cooperative Oncology Group (ECOG) performance status.[31] In some regions, these methods can also be used to downstage a patient from a transplant-ineligible to transplant-eligible status.[32]

PREOPERATIVE IMAGING OF THE LIVING DONOR LIVER TRANSPLANTATION DONOR

During preoperative imaging of the living donor liver transplantation (LDLT) donor, several features are assessed including the vascular and biliary anatomy for relevant variants; the hepatic parenchyma for degree of fatty infiltration, iron content, and focal hepatic lesions; and the calculation of liver volumes. Although many potential donors are found to have surgically relevant vascular (44%) and/or biliary (48%) anatomic variants, most remain eligible for donation because of advances in microvascular surgical technique. Only 1.9% of these donors are excluded for these reasons (**Table 4**).[33,34]

Table 3
Organ Procurement and Transplantation Network and Liver Imaging Reporting and Data System liver nodule classification systems

Nodule Description	OPTN Classification	LI-RADS Classification
Incomplete or technically inadequate study	Class 0	—
Definitely benign	Class 1	LR-1
Probably benign	Class 2	LR-2
Indeterminate probability for HCC	Class 3	LR-3
Probably but not definitely HCC	Class 4	LR-4
Definitively HCC	Class 5A: = or >1 cm but <2 cm Class 5B: = or >2 cm but <5 cm Class 5X: = or >5 cm	LR-5 LR-SV: with HCC invading vein —
HCC status after local therapy	Class 5T	LR-Treated
Probably malignant, but not specific for HCC	—	LR-M

Table 4
Contraindications for transplant donors

Anatomic Contraindications	Frequency of Exclusion (%)
>30% Fatty infiltration	10.4
Inadequate remnant liver volume	21.6
Small for size graft	3.4
Vascular variants	1.9
Biliary variants	1.9

Table 5
Michel classification of hepatic artery anatomy

Type	Frequency of Occurrence (%)	Description
I	55	Standard anatomy – RHA, MHA, LHA from CHA
II	10	Replaced LHA from LGA
III	11	Replaced RHA from SMA
IV	1	Replaced RHA from SMA and LHA from LGA
V	8	Accessory LHA from LGA
VI	7	Accessory RHA from SMA
VII	1	Accessory RHA from SMA and LHA from LGA
VIII	4	Replaced RHA and accessory LHA or Replaced LHA and accessory RHA
IX	4.5	CHA replaced to SMA
X	0.5	CHA replaced to LGA

Abbreviations: CHA, common hepatic artery; LGA, left gastric artery; LHA, left hepatic artery; MHA, middle hepatic artery; RHA, right hepatic artery; SMA, superior mesenteric artery.

Hepatic Arteries

Normal hepatic arterial anatomy (Michel Type I) is found in only 55% of the population.[35] This is a result of the complex pruning and fusion that must take place in utero to convert from the embryogenic hepatic perfusion pattern (left lateral segment by the left gastric artery, paramedian segment by the common hepatic artery, right lateral segment by the superior mesenteric artery) to the normal hepatic perfusion pattern.[21,35] Variant arteries that substitute the normal artery are termed "aberrant" or "replaced," and variant arteries that persist in addition to the normal artery are termed "accessory." These variants are further described in **Table 5**.[35] Only some of these variant anatomies are surgically relevant, and their relevance depends on the type of LDLT being performed. A description of the relevant hepatic arterial variants is found in **Table 6 (Fig. 5)**.[19]

Table 6
Critical findings in donor pretransplant imaging: hepatic arteries

Description	Surgery Affected	Surgical Implications
Replaced or accessory RHA	Right LDLT	Different or extra step during arterial ligation
Replaced or accessory LHA (see **Fig. 5**)	Full Left or Left lateral segment LDLT	Different or extra step during arterial ligation
MHA anatomy	Both	Must be preserved in the donor to prevent hepatic failure
RHA or LHA <2 mm	Both	May contraindicate donation since anastomosis is difficult

Abbreviations: LDLT, living donor liver transplant; LHA, left hepatic artery; MHA, middle hepatic artery; RHA, right hepatic artery.

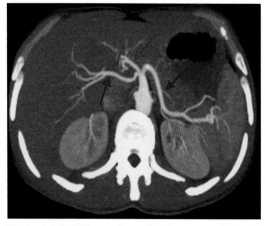

Fig. 5. Axial MIP image from CTA demonstrating early branching of the celiac artery into the left hepatic artery (*red arrow*), right hepatic artery (*purple arrow*), and splenic artery (*blue arrow*).

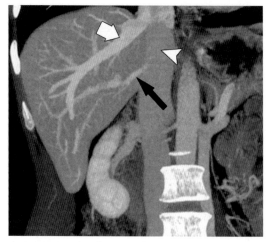

Fig. 6. Coronal reformatted image from a contrast enhanced CT demonstrating an accessory right hepatic vein (RHV) (*black arrow*) draining into the IVC (*white arrowhead*), separate from the RHV (*white arrow*). This was separately anastomosed in the recipient. (*Adapted from* Sahani D, Mehta A, Blake M, et al. Preoperative hepatic vascular evaluation with CT and MR Angiography: implications for surgery. Radiographics 2004;24:1374; with permission.)

Hepatic Veins

Hepatic venous variants are seen in 16% to 33% of the population and comprise 30% of the surgically relevant anatomic variants (**Figs. 6** and **7**).[36–38] If not dealt with intraoperatively, these can lead to hepatic insufficiency in the donor or recipient if drainage to a liver segment is compromised.[34] Genetic predisposition for hepatic venous variants has been described; if these are noted in the donor, special attention should be paid to the anatomy in a related recipient and vice versa.[36] As with the hepatic arteries, the surgical relevance of these variants depends on the type of LDLT being performed (**Table 7**).[19]

Portal Veins

Portal venous anatomic variants are less common, although a few surgically relevant variations exist (**Fig. 8, Table 8**). Preoperative imaging of the portal veins also involves measuring the vein diameter at the site of the proposed anastomosis, since anastomosis of veins of a similar size decreases the risk of thrombosis or stenosis. This is one of the most common portal venous complications of liver transplantation.[39] A statistically significant association between portal venous and biliary system variants has been described. Thus, if portal venous

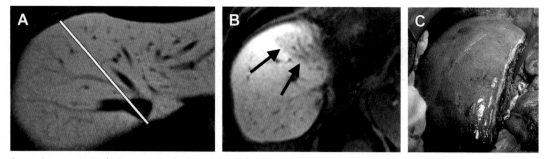

Fig. 7. Segment VIII drainage into the MHV. (*A*) Axial T1-weighted preoperative image of a living donor shows a tributary vein draining segment VIII into the MHV. The hemi-hepatectomy plane transects this accessory vein. (*B*) Postoperative axial T1-weighted MR image of the recipient shows atrophy (*arrows*) of segment VIII caused by inadequate drainage. (*C*) Corresponding intraoperative photograph shows congestion of segment VIII. (*Adapted from* Catalano OA, Singh AH, Uppot RN, et al. Vascular and biliary variants in the liver: implications for liver surgery. Radiographics 2008;28:369; with permission.)

Table 7
Critical findings in donor pretransplant imaging: hepatic veins

Description	Surgery Affected	Surgical Implications
Accessory RHV(s) draining VI, VII, V (see **Fig. 6**)	Right LDLT	Separate anastomosis needed to preserve drainage of the segment
Right lobe segment veins draining into MHV (see **Fig. 7**)	Right LDLT	Separate anastomosis needed to preserve drainage of the segment
Segment IV draining into LHV	Right LDLT	Move hepatectomy plane to the left of the MHV since it is not required for remnant liver drainage
Common trunk of MHV and LHV	Left lateral segment LDLT	Ensure MHV remains intact for preservation of remnant liver drainage
Small RHV with MHV draining a significant portion of the right hepatic lobe	Full Left LDLT	Switch from a full left LDLT to a left lateral segment LDLT if possible
Early confluence of the hepatic veins	Both	Increases surgical complexity. May be a contraindication to donation if the graft will be too small

Abbreviations: LDLT, living donor liver transplant; LHV, left hepatic vein; MHV, middle hepatic vein; RHV, right hepatic vein.

variants are identified, attention should be paid to the associated biliary tree.[40]

Biliary System

Biliary system anatomic variations are seen in up to 33% of the population and have differing implications based on the type of surgery being performed (**Fig. 9, Table 9**).[4] A detailed understanding of the biliary anatomy is critical, since biliary complications are the most common cause for morbidity after transplant, occurring in up to 40% of patients.[39] The most common types of biliary complications are bile duct stricture and

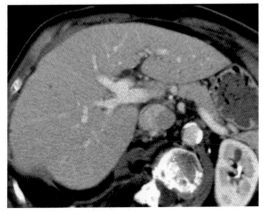

Fig. 8. Axial CT scan in the portal venous phase demonstrates trifurcation of the portal veins.

bile leak, either from branches to the caudate, the hepatic duct stump, or from the parenchymal transection surface.[19] Understanding the donor biliary anatomy through the use of preoperative MRCP has been shown to prevent these types of complications.[22,41]

Liver Parenchyma

The final step of preoperative donor imaging is evaluation of the hepatic parenchyma. This involves 3 steps: the detection and characterization of focal liver lesions, evaluation for hepatic steatosis, and measurement of liver volumes. Focal liver lesions are seen in up to 18% of donors but do not necessarily contraindicate transplant. Depending on lesion etiology (eg, cyst, focal nodular hyperplasia (FNH), adenoma, hemangioma), size, and location, focal lesions may or may not disqualify a donor.[39]

The degree of hepatic steatosis must also be determined, as greater than 30% fatty infiltration will overestimate the predicted liver function in both the donor and recipient. This can result in hepatic failure after transplant. Therefore, 30% steatosis is the upper limit tolerated for donation.[42] CT findings consistent with this degree of steatosis include: hepatic density more than 10 hounsfield units (HU) lower than the spleen, hepatic density less than 40 HU on noncontrast CT, and a hepatic-to-splenic density ratio of less than 0.8 on noncontrast CT.[43–45] MR imaging findings consistent with this degree of

Table 8
Critical findings in donor pretransplant imaging: portal veins

Description	Surgery Affected	Surgical Implications
LPV from RAPV	Right LDLT	Relative contraindication to donation
RAPV from LPV	Left LDLT	Relative contraindication to donation
Trifurcation into RPPV, RAPV, and LPV (see Fig. 8)	Both	Right: must clamp and anastomose these separately Left: ensure you exclude RAPV from graft

Abbreviations: LDLT, living donor liver transplant; LPV, left portal vein; RAPV, right posterior portal vein; RPPV, right anterior portal vein.

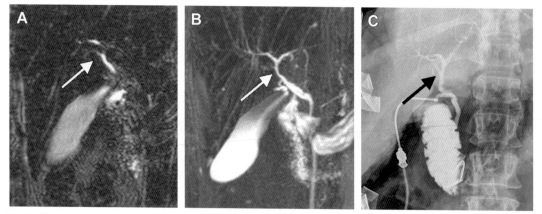

Fig. 9. An accessory right posterior hepatic duct (*arrow*) drains into the proximal common hepatic duct. Additionally, a segment 4 duct drains into right anterior hepatic duct. This right LDLT donation was aborted due to these anatomic variants. (*A*) Source coronal T2 image showing the accessory right posterior hepatic duct draining into the Common Hepatic Duct (CHD). (*B*) MIP coronal T2 MRCP image shows this duct proximal to the bifurcation. (*C*) intraoperative cholangiogram confirmed the findings.

Table 9
Critical findings in donor pretransplant imaging: biliary system

Description	Surgery Affected	Surgical Implications
RPHD or RAHD draining into LHD	Both	Contraindication to left lobe donation Increases complexity of right lobe donation
LHD draining into RAHD or RPHD	Both	Contraindication to right lobe donation Increases surgical complexity of left lobe donation
Trifurcation of RAHD, RPHD, LHD	Both	Increases surgical complexity
Accessory hepatic duct (see Fig. 9)	Both	Increases surgical complexity. May be a contraindication to donation.
Segment IV hepatic duct	Right LDLT	Must be preserved in the donor to prevent biliary complications and hepatic failure

Abbreviations: LHD, left hepatic duct; LDLT, living donor liver transplant; RAHD, right anterior hepatic duct; RPHD, right posterior hepatic duct.

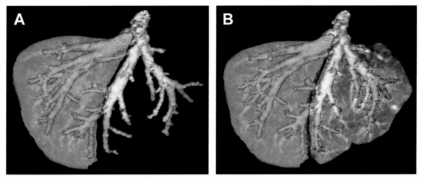

Fig. 10. Liver volume imaging and virtual hepatectomy. (*A*) Axial 3-dimensional reconstructed CT images demonstrating the proposed residual donor liver. (*B*) Virtual hepatectomy plane running through the donor liver. (*From* Singh AK, Cronin CG, Verma HA, et al. Imaging of preoperative liver transplantation in adults: what radiologists should know. Radiographics 2011;31:1029; with permission.)

steatosis include 30% signal dropout on Dixon-type chemical shift in and out-of-phase imaging, with liver parenchymal signal drop-out normalized to the spleen (SI inphase-SI outphase/SI inphase $\times 100$ where SI = average liver intensity/ average spleen intensity).[46]

Finally, liver volumes are calculated to ensure there will be adequate hepatic volume transplanted into the recipient and an adequate remnant volume in the donor. In order to perform this accurately, single breath hold images with minimal motion artifact on both CT and MR imaging are critical (**Fig. 10**). The critical report components for LDLT donor pretransplant imaging are listed in **Table 10**.

SUMMARY

Preoperative imaging with CT and MR imaging/ MRCP is important for transplant donor and recipient candidate selection and for preoperative planning. A complete understanding of the indications and contraindications to transplant, the indications and post-treatment appearance of bridging/downstaging procedures for patients with HCC, and the steps of the transplant operation help the radiologist craft a succinct and meaningful report. Respectively, a full understanding of the vascular, biliary, and parenchymal anatomy helps the surgeon perform liver transplant in as safe a manner as possible.

Table 10
Preliving donor liver transplant donor imaging report components

Structure Evaluated	Components of Report
Liver parenchyma	Description of fatty/iron infiltration Characterization of focal lesions
Liver volume	Total liver volume = X Left lobe volume = Y Right lobe volume = Z
Hepatic artery anatomy	Description of normal anatomy or accessory/replaced hepatic arteries The segment 4 artery is a branch of X
Portal venous anatomy	Description of bifurcation/trifurcation
Hepatic venous anatomy	Description of three hepatic veins and common trunk Description of any accessory hepatic veins
Biliary anatomy	Description of bile duct bifurcation/trifurcation Description of any accessory or anomalous ducts

REFERENCES

1. Available at: optn.transplant.hrsa.gov. Accessed April 25, 2015.

2. Kim WR, Lake JR, Smit JM, et al. OPTN/SRTR 2013 Annual dada report: liver. Am J Transplant 2015; 15(Suppl 2):1–28.

3. Vagefi PA, Ascher NL, Freise CE, et al. Use of living donor liver transplantation varies with the availability of deceased donor liver transplantation. Liver Transpl 2012;18(2):160–5.

4. Singh A, Cronin CG, Verma HA, et al. Imaging of preoperative liver transplantation in adults: what radiologists should know. Radiographics 2011;31: 1017–30.

5. Vagefi PA, Parekh J, Ascher NL, et al. Outcomes with split liver transplantation in 106 recipients: the University of California, San Francisco, experience from 1993 to 2010. Arch Surg 2011;146(9):1052–9.

6. Yersiz H, Renz JF, Farmer DG, et al. One hundred in situ split-liver transplantations: a single-center experience. Ann Surg 2003;238(4):496–505 [discussion: 506–7].

7. Humar A, Ramcharan T, Sielaff TD, et al. Split liver transplantation for two adult recipients: an initial experience. Am J Transplant 2001;1(4):366–72.

8. Vagefi PA, Parekh J, Ascher NL, et al. Ex vivo split-liver transplantation: the true right/left split. HPB (Oxford) 2014;16(3):267–74.

9. Azoulay D, Castaing D, Adam R, et al. Split-liver transplantation for two adult recipients: feasibility and long-term outcomes. Ann Surg 2001;233(4): 565–74.

10. Foster R, Zimmerman M, Trotter JF. Expanding donor options: marginal, living, and split donors. Clin Liver Dis 2007;11(2):417–29.

11. Broering DC, Wilms C, Lenk C, et al. Technical refinements and results in full-right full-left splitting of the deceased donor liver. Ann Surg 2005;242(6): 802–12 [discussion: 812–3].

12. Wilms C, Walter J, Kaptein M, et al. Long-term outcome of split liver transplantation using right extended grafts in adulthood: a matched pair analysis. Ann Surg 2006; 244(6):865–72 [discussion: 872–3].

13. OPTN National Data Report. Transplants by Donor type 1/1/1988-1/31/2015". Available at: http://optn. transplant.hrsa.gov/converge/latestData/rptData.asp. Accessed April 25, 2015.

14. Guiney MJ, Kruskal JB, Sosna J, et al. Multi– detector row CT of relevant vascular anatomy of the surgical plane in split-liver transplantation. Radiology 2003;229(2):401–7.

15. Roll GR, Parekh JR, Parker WF, et al. Left hepatectomy versus right hepatectomy for living donor liver transplantation: shifting the risk from the donor to the recipient. Liver Transpl 2013;19(5): 472–81.

16. Abecassis MM, Fisher RA, Olthoff KM, et al, A2ALL Study Group. Complications of living donor hepatic lobectomy–a comprehensive report. Am J Transplant 2012;12(5):1208–17.

17. Clavien PA, Camargo CA, Croxford R, et al. Definition and classification of negative outcomes in solid organ transplantation: application in liver transplantation. Ann Surg 1994;220:109–20.

18. Freise CE, Gillespie BW, Koffron AJ, et al, A2ALL Study Group. Recipient morbidity after living and deceased donor liver transplantation: findings from the A2ALL Retrospective Cohort Study. Am J Transplant 2008;8(12):2569–79.

19. Catalano OA, Singh AH, Uppot RN, et al. Vascular and biliary variants in the liver: implications for liver surgery. Radiographics 2008;28:359–78.

20. Schroeder T, Malagó M, Debatin JF, et al. "All-in-one" imaging protocols for the evaluation of potential living liver donors: comparison of magnetic resonance imaging and multidetector computed tomography. Liver Transpl 2005;11:776–87.

21. Hennedige T, Anil G, Madhavan K. Expectations from imaging for pre-transplant evaluation of living donor liver transplantation. World J Radiol 2014; 6(9):693–707.

22. Goldman J, Florman S, Varotti G, et al. Non-invasive preoperative evaluation of biliary anatomy in right-lobe living donors with mangafodipir trisodium-enhanced MR cholangiography. Transplant Proc 2003;35(4):1421–2.

23. Kazemier G, Hesselink EJ, Lange JF, et al. Dividing the liver for the purpose of split grafting or living related grafting: a search for the best cutting plane. Transplant Proc 1991;23(1 pt 2): 1545–6.

24. Kamath PS, Wiesner RH, Malinchoc M, et al. A model to predict survival in patients with end-stage liver disease. Hepatology 2001;33(2):464–70.

25. Cholongitas E, Marelli L, Shusang V, et al. A systematic review of the performance of the model for end-stage liver disease (MELD) in the setting of liver transplantation. Liver Transpl 2006; 12(7):1049–61.

26. Rosenkrantz AB, Campbell N, Wehrli N, et al. New OPTN/UNOS classification system for nodules in cirrhotic livers detected with MR Imaging: Effect on hepatocellular carcinoma detection and transplant allocation. Radiology 2015;274(2):426–33.

27. Liver imaging reporting and data system. Available at: http://www.acr.org/quality-safety/resources/LIRADS. Accessed May 24, 2015.

28. Koffron A, Stein JA. Liver transplantation: indications, pretransplant evaluation, surgery, and post-transplant complications. Med Clin North Am 2008; 92(4):861–88, ix.

29. Yao FY, Ferrell L, Bass NM, et al. Liver transplantation for hepatocellular carcinoma: expansion of the

tumor size limits does not adversely impact survival. Hepatology 2001;33:1394–403.

30. Prasad MA, Kulik LM. The role of bridge therapy prior to orthotopic liver transplantation. J Natl Compr Canc Netw 2014;12:1183–91.

31. Forner A, Gilabert M, Gruix J, et al. Treatment of intermediate-stage hepatocellular carcinoma. Nat Rev Clin Oncol 2014;11:525–35.

32. Clavien PA, Lesurtel M, Bossuyt PMM, et al. Recommendations for liver transplantation for hepatocellular carcinoma: an international consensus conference report. Lancet Oncol 2012;13:e11–22.

33. Tsang LL, Chen CL, Huang TL, et al. Preoperative imaging evaluation of potential living liver donors: reasons for exclusion from donation in adult living donor liver transplantation. Transplant Proc 2008; 40(8):2460–2.

34. Sahani D, Mehta A, Blake M, et al. Preoperative hepatic vascular evaluation with CT and MR angiography: implications for surgery. Radiographics 2004; 24:1367–80.

35. Michel NA. Blood supply and anatomy of the upper abdominal organs with a descriptive atlas. Philadelphia: Lippincott; 1955. p. 64–9.

36. Fan ST, Lo CM, Liu CL. Technical refinement in adult-to-adult living donor liver transplantation using right lobe graft. Ann Surg 2000;231:126–31.

37. Kennedy PA. Surgical anatomy of the liver. Surg Clin North Am 1977;57(2):233–44.

38. Huguet C. Technique of hepatic vascular exclusion for extensive liver resection. Am J Surg 1992; 163(6):602–5.

39. Sahani D, D'souza R, Kadavigere R, et al. Evaluation of living liver transplant donors: method for precise anatomic definition by using a dedicated contrast-enhanced MR imaging protocol. Radiographics 2004;24:957–67.

40. Lee VS, Morgan GR, Lin JC, et al. Liver transplant donor candidates: associations between vascular and biliary anatomic variants. Liver Transpl 2004; 10(8):1049–54.

41. Itamoto T, Emoto K, Mitsuta H, et al. Safety of donor right hepatectomy for adult-to-adult living donor liver transplantation. Transpl Int 2006;19(3):177–83.

42. Piekarski J, Goldberg HI, Royal SA, et al. Difference between liver and spleen CT numbers in the normal adult: its usefulness in predicting the presence of diffuse liver disease. Radiology 1980;137:727–9.

43. Boll DT, Merkle EM. Diffuse liver disease: strategies for hepatic CT and MR imaging. Radiographics 2009;29:1591–614.

44. Kodama Y, Ng CS, Wu TT, et al. Comparison of CT methods for determining the fat content of the liver. AJR Am J Roentgenol 2007;188:1307–12.

45. Park SH, Kim PN, Kim KW, et al. Macrovesicular hepatic steatosis in living liver donors: use of CT for quantitative and qualitative assessment. Radiology 2006;239:105–12.

46. Kreft BP, Tanimoto A, Baba Y, et al. Diagnosis of fatty liver with MR imaging. J Magn Reson Imaging 1992; 2:463–71.

Surgical Techniques and Imaging Complications of Liver Transplant

Akshay D. Baheti, MD[a],*, Rupan Sanyal, MD[b],
Matthew T. Heller, MD[c], Puneet Bhargava, MD[a]

KEYWORDS

- Liver transplant • Complications • Imaging • CT • MR imaging • US

KEY POINTS

- Liver transplant is the treatment of choice for end-stage liver disease.
- Management of transplant patients requires a multidisciplinary approach, with radiologists playing a key role in identifying complications in both symptomatic and asymptomatic patients.
- Ultrasonography remains the investigation of choice for the initial evaluation of symptomatic patients. Depending on the clinical situation, further evaluation with CT, MRI or biopsy may be performed or clinical and imaging surveillance may be continued.

Liver transplant is the treatment of choice for end-stage liver disease. Management of transplant patients requires a multidisciplinary approach, with radiologists playing a key role in identifying complications in both symptomatic and asymptomatic patients. Liver transplantation has progressed greatly since the world's first liver transplant in 1963, and liver transplant is now the treatment of choice for patients with end-stage acute or chronic liver disease.[1–4] As per the Organ Procurement and Transplantation Network (OPTN) data, 6455 liver transplants were performed in the United States in 2013 and 3862 transplants in 2014 (up to July 31). However, this remains inadequate, with 16,269 patients on the wait list as of October 2014.[5] Advances in surgical techniques, immunosuppressive therapy, and the multidisciplinary team approach have led to improved survival, with the 1-year, 5-year, and 10-year survival for deceased donor transplant being 84.3%, 68.3%, and 53.7% as per the 2009 OPTN data.[5,6] The corresponding rates for live donor transplant were 86.6%, 73.1%, and 61.8% respectively.[5] Despite these impressive figures, liver transplant remains a complex procedure with significant morbidity and mortality. The chief causes of early mortality include surgical complications and acute rejection. The improved survival has led to the emergence of long-term complications caused by chronic immunosuppressive therapy.[6]

We discuss the short-term and long-term posttransplant complications and the role of diagnostic radiologists in their identification and management.

SURGICAL TECHNIQUES FOR LIVER TRANSPLANTATION

It is important to understand the surgical techniques related to liver transplantation to proficiently assess patients in a posttransplant setting.

Disclosures: P. Bhargava is Editor-in-chief of Current Problems in Diagnostic Radiology, Elsevier Inc. The authors have no other disclosures.
[a] University of Washington, 1959 Northeast Pacific Street, Room BB308, Box 357115, Seattle, WA 98195-7115, USA; [b] Body Imaging, Department of Radiology, University of Alabama, Birmingham, 619 19th Street South, JTN 314, Birmingham, AL 35249, USA; [c] Radiology Residency Program, University of Pittsburg Medical Center, University of Pittsburg School of Medicine, 200 Lothrop Street, Suite 3950 PST, Pittsburgh, PA 15213, USA
* Corresponding author.
E-mail address: akshaybaheti@gmail.com

ORTHOTOPIC LIVER TRANSPLANT

The major steps of orthotopic liver transplant surgery include donor and recipient hepatectomies; inferior vena cava (IVC), portal venous arterial, and hepatic arterial anastomosis; followed by cholecystectomy and biliary anastomosis.[1,7,8]

The sites of vascular and biliary anastomosis are important to note for radiologists because these are the most frequent sites of future complications like stenosis. IVC anastomosis is usually the first anastomosis performed. Two techniques are popularly used. In the standard technique, the recipient's IVC is removed along with the liver and a side-to-side anastomosis of the donor IVC is performed with the superior and inferior ends of the recipient IVC. In the newer piggyback technique, the recipient IVC is not removed along with the liver, and an end-to-side anastomosis is performed between the donor's suprahepatic IVC and recipient hepatic veins at the common stump.[1,9–11] This technique decreases operative time and reduces the risk of hemorrhage, because no surgical dissection is required around the recipient IVC. Furthermore, it is more favorable hemodynamically for the patient because normal IVC flow is maintained during the operation, thus avoiding the need for a venovenous bypass.[1,9,10] The piggyback technique is preferred at our institute for caval anastomosis.

The portal venous anastomosis is an end-to-end anastomosis performed between the donor and recipient portal veins. The extrahepatic portal vein needs to be at least 4 to 5 mm in diameter for a successful anastomosis.[1,3,8] The hepatic arterial anastomosis is usually performed with the recipient hepatic artery as a fish-mouth anastomosis at the site of the gastroduodenal artery origin.[1,3,8] Variant hepatic vascular anatomy (such as replaced or accessory right or left hepatic arteries) are commonly encountered in the recipient or the donor, being present in 39% to 48% of people in previous studies.[12,13] Preoperative knowledge regarding the presence of an anatomic variant is essential and various surgical techniques have been described to navigate the variant vessels. Certain studies have reported the presence of variant anatomy to be associated with increased complications, although this remains controversial.[14,15]

The biliary anastomosis is generally performed as an end-to-end anastomosis between the donor common hepatic duct and the recipient common bile duct (CBD), thus preserving the sphincter of Oddi and minimizing the risk of reflux. A biliary-enteric anastomosis (choledochojejunostomy) may be performed in patients with diseased CBDs (as in primary sclerosing cholangitis [PSC]) or in cases with a variant CBD that is too short.[1,3,8] Conventionally, a T tube is placed across the biliary anastomosis after the operation to support the anastomosis. A T tube also helps to monitor bile output and provides access for cholangiogram. However, many institutions do not follow this approach, because it leads to increased patient discomfort and a higher risk of biliary leak and late stricture.[1,3,8,11,16]

LIVING DONOR LIVER TRANSPLANT

Living donor liver transplant is less common in Western countries because of potential risks to the donor (risk of death is 1.7 per 1000 in the United States) and a higher posttransplant complication rate.[17] However, it confers significant advantages in the form of increased donor pool and timely transplants.[17] Adequate assessment (usually computed tomography [CT]) of the donor liver anatomy, including split liver volumes, vascular and biliary anatomy variations, and fatty infiltration, is important.[18–20] Right lobar transplant is usually performed. The donor's right hepatic lobe is first removed, preserving the middle hepatic vein in the donor.[18–20] This step is followed by recipient hepatectomy and implantation of the donor lobe. The operation is technically much more challenging because of the short donor vessels. End-to-end hepatic venous, portal venous, and hepatic arterial anastomosis is performed, followed by biliary reconstruction with an end-to-end anastomosis or a hepaticojejunostomy.[18–20]

NORMAL POSTOPERATIVE APPEARANCE OF THE LIVER

Knowledge of the expected postoperative findings after a liver transplant is essential to accurately identify complications. As is the norm with most operations, a certain amount of postoperative fluid and inflammation can be expected at the surgical bed. A small amount of ascites or fluid in the perihepatic space or along the hepatic hilum is normally seen, as is mild reactive right pleural effusion. These conditions usually resolve spontaneously within a few weeks.[3,21] Prominent reactive periportal and portacaval lymph nodes are also normally seen.[3,21]

An appearance of periportal edema (periportal hypoattenuation) may be visualized, and occurs because of lymphedema secondary to disruption of the normal lymphatic drainage by the transplant. This appearance may resolve in a few weeks or may persist for months, and should not be confused with biliary dilatation. Periportal edema is a normal finding and does not correlate with rejection, as was initially suspected.[3,21,22]

Reperfusion edema and stasis of fluid are common after transplant and give rise to a starry-sky appearance of the liver on ultrasonography (US) (described in hepatitis), with hypoechoic appearance of the liver parenchyma with relatively echogenic portal venous walls.[11,23]

Areas of increased echogenicity on US and altered attenuation on CT may be seen, representing intraparenchymal bleed/contusion during surgical manipulation.[11,23] Pneumobilia is a normal findings as well. Similarly, portal venous gas is normally seen for the first 2 weeks after the operation and does not necessarily portend a serious complication.[11,24]

The postoperative state is an abnormal state for the body's physiology, with various factors such as postsurgical inflammation and edema, hepatic engraftment, recovery from the operation, and reperfusion in interplay.[11] This state leads to various seemingly abnormal Doppler findings. The postoperative appearance of the vessels and bile ducts is discussed along with their respective complications.

SURVEILLANCE STRATEGY FOR COMPLICATIONS/RECURRENCE

Institutional protocols vary but, most commonly, a baseline postoperative Doppler study is performed in the first few days after an uncomplicated transplant, and another is obtained before discharge. A 2010 International Consensus Conference recommended surveillance cross-sectional imaging along with alpha fetoprotein levels every 6 to 12 months after transplant.[25]

COMPLICATIONS OF HEPATIC TRANSPLANT

The complications of hepatic transplant can be classified as vascular, biliary, and others for the purposes of discussion (Table 1).[2,4] Clinically, patients with complications present with increased live enzyme/bilirubin levels, and the role of the radiologist is to rule out any surgical/technical causes that can be treated to reverse the abnormality. In the absence of radiologic findings to explain the altered hepatic function, further clinicopathologic work-up is performed to rule out other causes, such as infection, graft

Table 1 Complications of liver transplant	
Vascular	
Hepatic arterial complications	Thrombosis, stenosis, pseudoaneurysm
Portal venous complications	Thrombosis, stenosis
Hepatic vein/IVC complications	Thrombosis, stenosis
Arterioportal fistula	—
Biliary	
Biliary leak	—
Biliary stricture	—
Others: sphincter of Oddi dysfunction, cyclosporine-induced stones, mucocele of cystic duct	—
Others	
Collections	Seroma, biloma, hematoma, abscess
Hepatic ischemia/infarction	—
Rejection	—
Infections	—
Neoplasms	—
Recurrent disease	—

dysfunction, graft rejection, drug toxicity, and recurrence of the underlying disease, with a liver biopsy being required in most cases.[1,6]

Vascular Complications

Hepatic arterial complications
Normal postoperative appearance US with Doppler is usually performed within the first 24 hours after the operation to evaluate the baseline postoperative status of the patient. The normal hepatic artery shows hepatopetal flow, a rapid upstroke with an acceleration time (AT) of less than 0.08 seconds, and a resistive index (RI) of 0.5 to 0.8 (Fig. 1).[1,2,4] Increased peak systolic velocities, RI greater than 0.8, or absent diastolic flow may be seen in the first 72 hours after the operation, but they return to normal within 1 to 2 weeks and are not associated with increased risk of complications.[1,2,4,26] Similarly, lower RI values and tardus-parvus waveform may be visualized as well, caused by postoperative edema along the anastomotic site.[11] However, it is important to document their resolution, because these can be harbingers for vascular complications

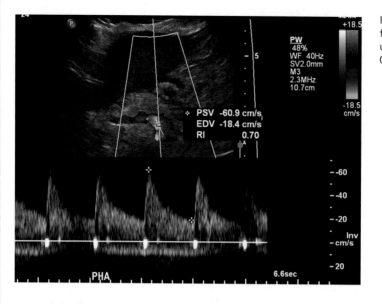

Fig. 1. Normal hepatic arterial waveform on Doppler with a rapid systolic upstroke, and an RI value between 0.5 and 0.8.

as well. Radiologists must also be familiar with the normal appearance of the fish-mouth anastomosis on CT (**Fig. 2**) to avoid misdiagnosing it as an aneurysm.

Hepatic artery thrombosis Hepatic artery thrombosis (HAT) is the most common vascular complication after transplant, occurring in 2% to 12% of patients (with a higher incidence in children), with mortalities of 20% to 60%.[1,4,23] Early HAT has been variably defined as occurring within 1 or 2 months of the operation, and is more severe than late HAT.[23,27,28] Late HAT can occur any time after this, with a median time interval of 6 months (range, 2–79 months) as per Gunsar and colleagues.[28] Although the transplanted liver has a dual blood supply, bile ducts are exclusively supplied by the hepatic artery, and thrombosis may cause biliary ischemia and necrosis. Complications of early HAT include hepatic necrosis, biliary leak and bilomas, bacteremia, sepsis, graft failure, and death.[27] Regular US monitoring has decreased the incidence of these complications by allowing early diagnosis and treatment.

Various risk factors that predispose to development of HAT include small caliber of the vessel (as in children), difference in calibers between the donor and recipient arteries, preexisting celiac trunk stenosis in the recipient, use of an interpositional conduit for the anastomosis, prolonged cold ischemia time for the donor liver, prolonged operative time, retransplant surgery, technical errors, variant arterial anatomy, and rejection.[2,27,29]

Doppler sonography has a high accuracy (85%–92%) in diagnosing HAT.[30,31] The diagnosis is based on the demonstration of absent flow in the hepatic artery proper or in the intrahepatic arteries on Doppler.[1,2,4] A syndrome of impending

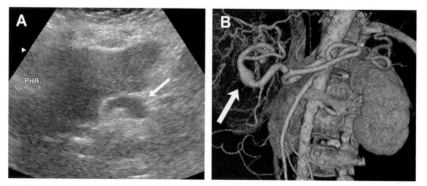

Fig. 2. Normal bulbous appearance of the fish-mouth anastomosis on US (*arrow* in *A*) and three-dimensional (3D) CT reconstruction of the arterial phase (*arrow* in *B*), which should not be mistaken for an aneurysm.

thrombosis has been described on Doppler US, characterized by progression of the hepatic arterial waveform from normal diastolic flow to absent diastolic flow to reduced systolic peaks to completely absent arterial flow.[31] False-positive Doppler findings can occur because of hepatic edema, severe hepatic artery stenosis (HAS), or systemic hypotension.[1,2,4] False-negative findings can occur in late HAT because of the presence of collaterals, which give rise to a tardus-parvus waveform in the intrahepatic arteries. Thus, presence of such a waveform should raise suspicion for HAT along with HAS.[1,2,4]

Contrast-enhanced US further improves the sensitivity of Doppler, if available, and can be used as a problem-solving tool to avoid the need for angiography.[32,33] CT angiography is an extremely sensitive and specific technique for evaluating for HAT and may be used in cases of an indeterminate US scan, and may show secondary hepatic infarcts or findings suggestive of biliary ischemia (Fig. 3). MR imaging is less commonly used because of longer examination time and need for breath holding.[1,2,4]

Treatment of HAT includes endovascular and surgical thrombectomy and surgical reconstruction. Retransplant is ultimately required in most cases.[1,2,4]

Hepatic artery stenosis HAS is the second most common vascular complication, occurring in 4% to 11% of patients.[1,2,34] It usually develops at the anastomotic site within 3 months of the operation, but can present even years after the operation.[2,3,35,36] The risk factors for HAS are similar to those for HAT, with an additional important factor being clamp injury. Patients may present with altered liver function tests or biliary stenosis, or may be asymptomatic, with progression to hepatic failure and sepsis if not corrected.[1,2,34]

Doppler US is again the investigation of choice to initially evaluate for HAS. Turbulence and focal area of increased peak systolic velocity (PSV) greater than 200 cm/s in the main hepatic artery are direct signs of HAS.[1,2,4] Demonstration of parvus-tardus waveform in the hepatic arteries distal to the stenosis is an important secondary sign (Fig. 4). This condition is visualized as delayed upstroke (AT >0.08 seconds) and increased diastolic flow (RI <0.5).[1,2,4] False-positives can occur because of HAT with collaterals (as previously discussed) and atherosclerotic aortic/celiac disease.[1,2,4] Doppler US has its limitations and can miss low-grade stenosis. Hence, multidetector CT or digital subtraction angiography should be performed in patients with high clinical suspicion and normal or indeterminate Doppler findings.[1,2,4]

Percutaneous balloon angioplasty or stenting are comparable treatments of choice for treating HAS. Since their advent, the need for revision surgery and retransplant has declined.[1,2,4,34]

Pseudoaneurysm Hepatic artery pseudoaneurysms are rare complications of liver transplant, with an incidence of 1% to 2%.[37] They are mycotic or secondary to interventional procedures like angioplasty. They can also arise in the small intrahepatic arteries secondary to a biopsy or a biliary procedure.[1,2,4,37] They can be asymptomatic, or can rupture into the bile ducts, gastrointestinal tract, or peritoneum to cause hemobilia, upper or lower gastrointestinal bleeding, or frank hemoperitoneum, respectively.[1,2,4,37]

Pseudoaneurysms appear as cystic structures along the course of the hepatic artery on US, with Doppler revealing internal turbulent flow with the characteristic yin-yang sign (Fig. 5). Doppler interrogation of any cystic-appearing structure in the hepatic hilum is important so

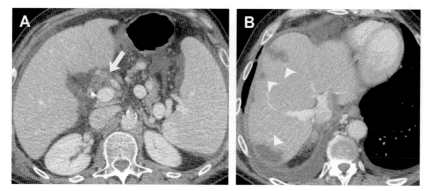

Fig. 3. A 64-year-old man at day 11 after liver transplant with altered liver function tests. US (not shown) showed lack of color flow in the hepatic artery. Axial contrast CT shows nonopacification of the hepatic artery (*arrow* in *A*) with wedge-shaped peripheral hypodensities (*arrowheads* in *B*), consistent with infarcts.

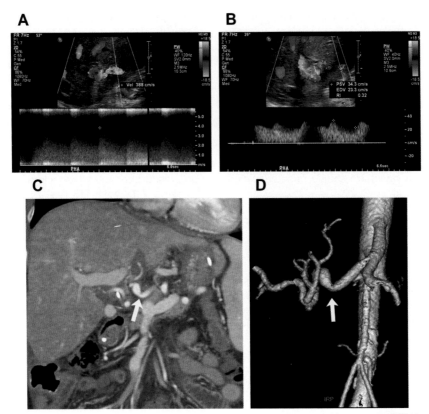

Fig. 4. A 47-year-old man 3 years after liver transplant, presenting with altered liver function tests. Doppler images show high PSV at the site of anastomosis in the proper hepatic artery (*A*) and parvus-tardus waveform distally (*B*), consistent with high-grade stenosis. CT angiography (*C*) with 3D reconstruction (*D*) confirmed the presence of stenosis with poststenotic dilatation (*arrows*), indicating a hemodynamically significant stenosis. Angioplasty with stenting was performed (images not shown) and the patient's liver function tests normalized subsequently.

as not to miss a pseudoaneurysm. CT and MR imaging clearly show the arterial enhancing pseudoaneurysm.[1,2,4,37]

Treatment options include surgical resection with arterial reconstruction, especially for mycotic pseudoaneurysms, for which endovascular treatment has the risk of serving as a nidus for infection. An actively bleeding pseudoaneurysm may require emergency occlusion of the hepatic artery for stabilization. Coil embolization for intrahepatic

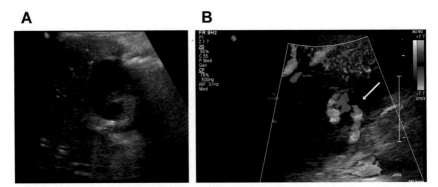

Fig. 5. A 47-year-old asymptomatic man 1 month after liver transplant. Gray-scale US shows an anechoic area (*A*) that shows color flow on Doppler with the classic yin-yang pattern (*B*, *arrow*), consistent with pseudoaneurysm. The pseudoaneurysm was successfully repaired surgically. This case shows the importance of applying Doppler on every anechoic area that otherwise appears like a collection to rule out a pseudoaneurysm.

pseudoaneurysms and stent-graft placement for extrahepatic pseudoaneurysms are the endovascular treatment options.[1,2,4,37]

Portal venous complications

Normal postoperative appearance A difference in caliber of up to 5 mm at the site of portal venous anastomosis may be seen without any clinical impact.[1,23] A normal Doppler study shows hepatopetal flow with mild phasicity and low velocity (16–40 cm/s) (**Fig. 6A**).[38] The normal postoperative portal venous flow is usually increased (PSV range, 15–400 cm/s) because of reactive increase in the splanchnic flow, as is transient portal vein compression by the postoperative edema, which decreases over time (**Fig. 6B**).[1,11,39] The high flow velocity may also cause turbulence, which should be considered normal in the postoperative setting and improves with time.[1,11]

Portal venous complications are rare and occur in approximately 1% to 2% of cases.[1,2,40] Chief causes include technical issues such as different calibers of the donor and recipient veins, prothrombotic states, and history of prior surgery.[1,3,4] Patients usually present with fulminant hepatic failure in the acute form and with progressive ascites and portal hypertension in the chronic form.[3,6]

Portal vein thrombosis Portal vein thrombosis usually presents within the first month after transplant, but can occur at any time.[41] The normal posttransplant portal vein shows an anechoic lumen and smooth, regular contour on gray-scale US. Acute portal vein thrombosis appears on US as an echogenic thrombus with no flow on Doppler (**Fig. 7**). Rarely, an acute thrombus appears anechoic, but Doppler still shows a lack of flow.[1–4] Power Doppler is useful to detect slow flow and distinguish between partial and complete thrombosis. A partial thrombus shows some flow, and may be managed medically, unlike complete thrombosis.[1–4] CT, MR imaging, and angiography all show filling defects in the portal vein. Chronic thrombosis may be associated with formation of a portal cavernoma.[1–4] Treatment options for portal thrombosis include thrombolysis, angioplasty, surgical thrombectomy, revision of anastomosis or venous jump graft, and retransplant.[1–4]

Portal vein stenosis Portal vein stenosis commonly involves the anastomotic site and is generally a late complication (mean time of presentation, >1 year).[41,42] A mild discrepancy in size is normally seen on imaging. Doppler plays a major role in the diagnosis, with aliasing and increased PSV visualized (**Fig. 8**).[1,2,4] A retrospective study of 94 transplants found PSV greater than 125 cm/s and an anastomotic/preanastomotic velocity ratio of 3:1 (normally 1.5:1) to be 73% sensitive and 95% to 100% specific for the diagnosis.[43] Secondary signs, such as increasing size of collaterals and splenomegaly, may be seen because of portal hypertension. A pressure gradient across the anastomosis of more than 5 mm Hg on direct transhepatic portography is considered diagnostic.[1,2,44] Angioplasty and stenting is the treatment of choice.[1,2,4]

Hepatic vein and inferior vena cava complications

Normal hepatic veins show a triphasic waveform caused by direct continuity with the right atrial pressure (**Fig. 9**).[38] Loss of phasicity, monophasic waveform, increased velocities, and turbulent flow may be seen in the early postoperative period caused by anastomotic edema or compression by an adjacent collection or hematoma. The prone position often helps in showing triphasic flow on follow-up.[1–4,11]

IVC and hepatic venous complications are uncommon (approximately 1%–2% of cases) and include thrombosis and stenosis.[1,2,40] Predisposing factors include discrepant sizes of the donor

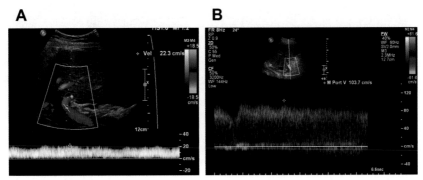

Fig. 6. Normal portal venous Doppler (*A*) showing hepatopetal flow with mild phasicity. Doppler study of a male patient on day 1 after liver transplant shows expected increased velocity (*B*), which should not be considered abnormal in this setting.

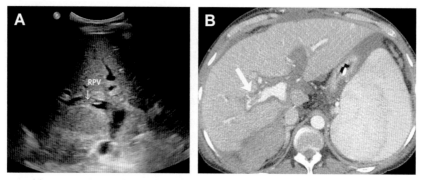

Fig. 7. A 32-year-old man on day 6 after liver transplant. Doppler shows an echogenic partial thrombus in the right portal vein (RPV; *A, arrow*), confirmed on CT (*B, arrow*). The patient was anticoagulated immediately and the thrombus resolved completely on the subsequent study (not shown).

and recipient vessels, pediatric transplant, and retransplant. The piggyback anastomosis is more prone to certain complications, including hemorrhage (which may be caused by hepatic injury during the operation or by anastomotic dehiscence) and development of Budd-Chiari syndrome.[1,2,45] Clinical manifestations include progressive abdominal distention caused by ascites and hepatomegaly.[1,2,45]

Hepatic vein/inferior vena cava thrombosis Thrombosis most commonly involves the excluded piggyback retrohepatic IVC stump, and does not involve the IVC directly.[46] US depicts an echogenic thrombus in the vessel with lack of flow on Doppler. CT/MR imaging shows the thrombosis and may also show secondary signs, such as mosaic perfusion **(Fig. 10)**.[1–3]

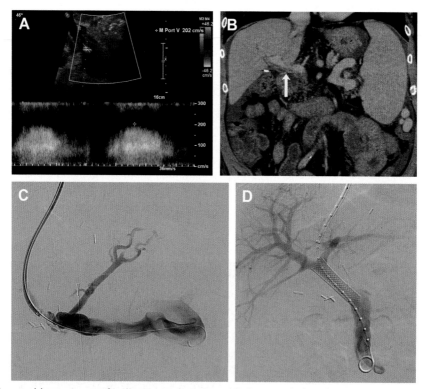

Fig. 8. A 54-year-old man 1 year after liver transplant. Doppler shows turbulent flow at the site of the portal vein anastomosis with a high PSV of 202 cm/s, suspicious for stenosis (*A*). The PSV in the preanastomotic segment (not shown) was 34 cm/s. Coronal venous-phase CT image (*B*) confirms the finding of portal vein stenosis (*arrow*). Endovascular portal venous stenting was performed. The prestenting portogram (*C*) shows severe portal vein stenosis with retrograde filling of multiple dilated varices. The poststent image shows good opacification of the portal vein (*D*).

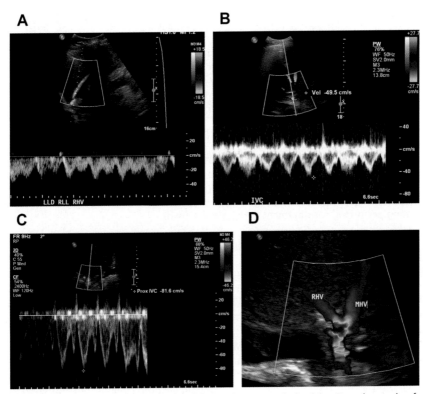

Fig. 9. Normal hepatic venous (*A*) and IVC Doppler (*B*) showing normal phasicity. Doppler study of a man on day 1 after liver transplant shows expected increased velocity (*C*), which should not be considered abnormal in this setting. Also note the normal appearance of the piggyback anastomosis (*D*). MHV, middle hepatic vein; RHV, right hepatic vein.

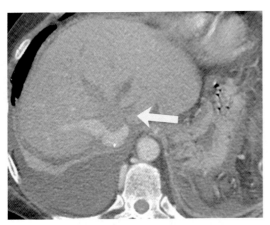

Fig. 10. A 57-year-old man 9 years after liver transplant. Axial venous-phase CT shows filling defects involving the middle and left hepatic veins and extending partially into the IVC (*arrow*), consistent with hepatic venous thrombosis. The patient was treated with anticoagulation, with complete resolution of the thrombus on the follow-up scan (not shown).

Hepatic vein/inferior vena cava stenosis Hepatic vein/IVC stenosis is most common in living donor transplants, and usually presents more than a year after transplant.[40,42] Loss of phasicity and monophasic flow are sensitive but not specific signs for stenosis. Direct signs include turbulent flow and increased PSV (3 to 4 times velocity gradient between the prestenotic and poststenotic segments) at the site of stricture (usually at the anastomosis) (**Fig. 11**).[1–4] A retrospective study of 94 patients found a venous pulsatility index of less than 0.45 to be 95.7% specific for diagnosing stenosis, with the normal mean venous pulsatility being 0.75 in the study.[43] Other findings include prestenotic hepatic venous dilatation, flow reversal, development of venovenous and portovenous collaterals, and reduced caliber at the site of stenosis.[1,2,47,48] CT/MR venography may be used to confirm the findings. Treatment options include balloon angioplasty and stenting.[1,2,4]

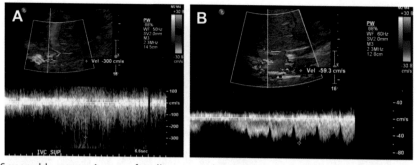

Fig. 11. A 56-year-old woman 1 year after liver transplant with increasing ascites. Doppler shows increased turbulent flow in the IVC at the site of the anastomosis (PSV 300 cm/s compared with 59.3 cm/s in the preanastomotic segment; [A] and [B] respectively), suggestive of IVC stenosis. This finding was confirmed on IVC venography, with stenting performed for treatment (images not shown).

Arterioportal fistula

Hemodynamically significant fistulas are rare, occurring in only 0.2% of patients with transplants.[49] Overall, they are found in 0% to 5.4% of transplant patients undergoing angiography, and are thus a common finding.[49]

Most fistulas are generally small and are seen on Doppler as a focal area of aliasing and turbulent flow, with a low RI (<0.5). Reversal or arterialization of flow may be seen in the draining vein.[41,42,49] Although US is not very sensitive, detecting only half the fistulae, it detects significant lesions.[41,42,49] Hemodynamically significant fistulae show the Doppler findings described earlier in the main portal vein of the graft or its first-order branch.[41,42,49] CT/MR imaging shows early enhancement of the portal venous branches on arterial phase ahead of the main portal vein and the superior mesenteric and splenic veins.[3] Peripheral transient attenuation defects may also be seen (**Fig. 12**). Hemodynamically significant fistulae may show dilated hepatic artery or draining veins and are more commonly central than peripheral.[3,41,42,49] Digital subtraction angiography is the most sensitive and specific modality, with hemodynamically significant fistulae showing arterial phase opacification of the main portal vein of the graft or its first-order branch.[41,42,49] Most fistulas can be safely followed up without treatment unless there is hemodynamic compromise, in which case endovascular embolization is the treatment of choice.[41,42,49]

Biliary complications

Biliary complications are the second most common cause of posttransplant hepatic dysfunction after graft rejection, occurring in 5% to 25% of patients.[2,50] Their incidence is gradually decreasing because of improved surgical techniques and medical management. They occur within the first 3 months after transplant, with some exceptions.[1,2,50]

The normal posttransplant anastomotic site may show mild narrowing caused by differences in caliber of the donor and recipient ducts. Residual cystic ducts may be present in the donor or recipient systems, or both, and should not be confused with a leak.[51] As previously mentioned, a T tube is often left in place after the operation, providing direct access for a cholangiogram.

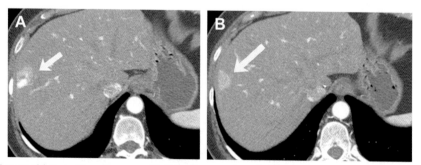

Fig. 12. A 58-year-old asymptomatic man with hepatic transplant following recent liver biopsy. Axial CT shows a focal area of hyperenhancement on the arterial phase (*arrow* in A) associated with a wedge-shaped subcapsular perfusional abnormality on the venous phase (*arrow* in B), consistent with an arterioportal fistula.

Biliary Complications

Biliary leak

Biliary leaks are a common early complication, occurring in 5% to 10% of cases.[50,52] They usually manifest within the first month after transplant, or after the removal of the T tube. The most common sites of leak include the anastomotic site, cystic duct stump, T-tube entry site into the duct, and along the resection margin in a living donor transplant.[2,16,46,53] Visualizing a leak at an atypical site should lead to evaluation for hepatic arterial involvement because ischemia can cause biliary leak. The leak can cause a perihepatic biloma or can lead to diffuse biliary peritonitis. Although sterile, superimposed infection may occur.[2,16,46,53]

If a T tube is in place, a cholangiogram can show extravasation at the site of leak. MR imaging with a hepatocyte-specific contrast agent that is excreted into the biliary tree may be used to detect the biliary leak. A hepato iminodiacetic acid (HIDA) scan is a specific and sensitive test for evaluating biliary leak (**Fig. 13**).[1–4,46] Alternatively, clinicians often directly perform percutaneous drainage of the collection followed by endoscopic retrograde cholangiopancreatography (ERCP) with stenting. Although small leaks may close spontaneously, surgical revision is often eventually needed for larger leaks.[1–4,46]

Biliary stricture

Biliary strictures are the most common complication, with an incidence of 12% for deceased donor and 19% for living donor transplants. They commonly present within a year after transplant, although they can manifest many years after transplant as well.[50,52] They can be anastomotic or nonanastomotic, and present with signs of liver dysfunction and obstructive jaundice.

Anastomotic strictures Anastomotic strictures are more common, with the mean interval at presentation being 5 to 8 months.[50,52] MR cholangiopancreatography (MRCP) and US show biliary dilatation proximal to the anastomosis with normal-sized distal CBD. These conditions can be treated with ERCP (**Fig. 14**A) and balloon dilatation/stenting, or rarely surgery (choledochojejunostomy). Correlation with clinical and laboratory parameters is important because patients with high-grade obstruction may not have dilated ducts and vice versa.[1–4,23]

Nonanastomotic strictures Nonanastomotic strictures may be caused by ischemia (the most common cause), infection, or recurrent PSC. They usually present earlier than anastomotic strictures, with the mean time to stricture being 3 to 6 months (although strictures with immunologic causes usually present beyond 1 year).[50] Although anastomotic strictures are solitary, nonanastomotic strictures can be multifocal. Ischemia usually affects single or multiple hepatic ducts at or proximal to the hilum. Ischemic strictures do not affect the distal (recipient) CBD because it has good collateral supply.[1–4,23] Accordingly, focal or diffuse biliary dilatation may be seen on imaging. Hepatic artery evaluation by Doppler reveals stenosis or thrombosis in such cases. Hepatic arterial abnormality usually precedes stricture formation by 1 to 3 weeks.[1–4,23] Severe ischemia may cause biliary necrosis with sloughing of the biliary epithelium (**Fig. 14**B). US shows echogenic debris within the dilated bile ducts in these cases.[1,23] Treatment with repeated balloon dilatation and stenting is

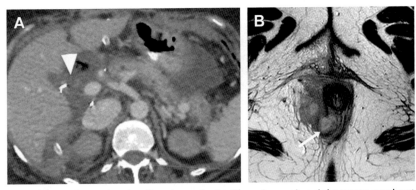

Fig. 13. A 47-year-old man 3 months after liver transplant with an increasing right upper quadrant collection on US (images not shown). Axial venous-phase CT (*A*) shows a collection with its epicenter at the site of the biliary anastomosis, as shown by the suture (*arrowhead*). The CBD could not be completely traced, and the possibility of biliary leak was raised. HIDA scan performed subsequently (*B*) shows complete leakage of the radiotracer into the peritoneal cavity (*arrow*).

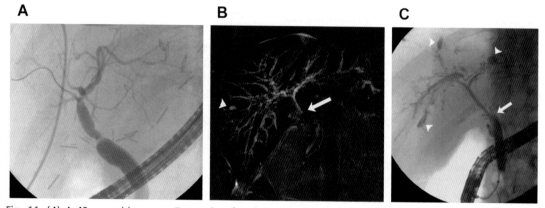

Fig. 14. (*A*) A 49-year-old woman 7 months after liver transplant with progressive jaundice. US (not shown) showed mildly dilated bile ducts. ERCP image shows a severe anastomotic stricture with proximal biliary dilatation. The patient was treated with biliary stenting with good outcome. (*B, C*) A 51-year-old man 5 months after liver transplant presenting with altered liver function tests. Coronal MRCP maximum intensity projection image and ERCP image show multifocal biliary stenosis (including one at the anastomotic site [*arrows*]) with biloma formation (*arrowheads*) suggestive of biliary necrosis and breakdown. MR imaging also showed associated HAS (image not shown). The patient was treated with retransplant, with good outcome.

usually attempted, but patients often require surgical revision or retransplant.[1,23]

Recurrent PSC can also appear similar to ischemic strictures with multifocal biliary strictures. Prior history and lack of hepatic arterial involvement favors PSC.[1,23,53]

Other biliary complications

Dilatation of both the recipient and donor ducts may be seen in sphincter of Oddi dysfunction, secondary to devascularization or denervation of the sphincter during the operation. Sphincterotomy is usually successful.[1,2] Kinking of a redundant CBD also uncommonly causes obstruction.[3]

Cyclosporine-induced biliary stones and sludge are uncommonly seen. Cyclosporine alters biliary composition, increasing the frequency of cholesterol stones and sludge.[1,23,53]

Rarely, patients present with progressive biliary dilatation caused by compression of the CBD by a mucocele of the cystic duct, seen as a rounded collection on imaging. This condition develops because of both proximal and distal ligation of the duct.[1,3]

Other Complications

Postoperative collections

Postoperative fluid collections are a common observation, and may represent a hematoma, seroma, biloma, or abscess.[1–4] Hematomas usually occur at the sites of anastomosis and in the perihepatic and subhepatic spaces. Because the normal peritoneal reflections are removed during the operation, fluid often collects in the right subhepatic space in the bare area of the liver.[1–4]

US is often not able to differentiate between the causes. Bilomas and seromas are often simple anechoic collections, whereas abscesses and hematomas show debris within.[1–4] CT/MR imaging can identify a hematoma as a hyperattenuating/T1 hyperintense collection. ERCP and drainage may be needed for bilomas, whereas abscesses often need aspiration for diagnosis and treatment. Hematomas usually resolve on their own within a few weeks, and can be carefully observed.[1–4]

Postoperative right adrenal hematoma or thickening may be seen because of hemorrhage caused by backpressure changes and venous ischemia during an operation.[23]

Hepatic ischemia/infarction

These occur because of hepatic arterial abnormality in most (85%) cases, or less commonly portal venous involvement.[3] They appear on US as peripheral geographic or round avascular lesions with central hypoechoic areas caused by liquefaction. Intraparenchymal gas is occasionally seen, and hepatic arterial abnormality is usually present on Doppler. On CT, hepatic infarction appears as nonenhancing low-attenuation areas that can be rounded or oval, peripheral, wedge-shaped, or irregularly shaped, paralleling bile ducts (caused by biliary necrosis) (see **Fig. 3**B).[49] The differential diagnosis includes an abscess, which shows peripheral thick enhancement and central necrosis with occasional foci of gas. Infarcts often have superimposed infection, and aspiration is needed for definitive diagnosis. Treatment is in the form of percutaneous drainage or surgical excision of the necrotic tissue.[1,3]

Rejection

The diagnosis of the most common cause of graft failure, rejection, is based on histopathology. The role of imaging in these cases is to rule out other causes of hepatic dysfunction. Acute rejection usually occurs within the first 90 days after transplant.[54] Chronic (ductopenic) rejection manifests as the vanishing bile duct syndrome, with loss of bile ducts and cholestasis on pathology.[55] Graft rejection has a nonspecific appearance on imaging, with heterogeneous hepatic echotexture often being the only abnormality seen on US.[1,2,56]

Apart from rejection, the other causes for diffuse parenchymal abnormality include ischemia, hepatitis (usually recurrent infectious or autoimmune hepatitis), and cholangitis (usually infectious or recurrent PSC).[1,2]

Infections

The immunosuppressed state makes transplant patients vulnerable to local and systemic infections in both acute and chronic settings. Almost half of all transplant patients have at least 1 infectious complication, and more than half of transplant deaths are caused by infection.[6] Imaging

and intervention play major roles in their diagnosis and management, as described earlier.

Neoplasms

Recurrent primary/metastatic hepatic neoplasms can develop in transplant patients. In addition, the chronic immunosuppressed state leads to the development of posttransplant lymphoproliferative disorder (PTLD) and Kaposi sarcoma early on, and nonmelanocytic skin cancers and anogenital cancers later.[1,2,6] A recent single-institute study of 534 patients found a higher de novo cancer incidence in liver transplant patients compared with the general population, with 5-year and 10-year incidences being 11.7% and 24.8% respectively.[57] PTLD is discussed in detail because radiology plays an important part in its diagnosis and management.

The incidence of PTLD has significantly decreased over the last decade because of improved immunosuppression. Narkewicz and colleagues[58] recently showed that the incidence of PTLD in the pediatric liver transplant population (which is higher than in the adult population) decreased to 1.7% in the period 2002 to 2007 compared with 4.2% in 1995 to 2001. PTLD develops in a median interval of 7 to 10 months, although it can develop anytime from a couple of

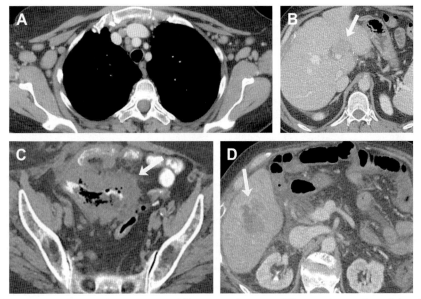

Fig. 15. Different sites of PTLD developing in different patients at different time points. (A) Axial contrast-enhanced CT shows enlarged bilateral axillary, subpectoral, and mediastinal adenopathy seen 7 years after liver transplant in a 52-year-old man. The patient also had infradiaphragmatic lymphadenopathy; biopsy revealed PTLD. (B) Axial venous-phase CT shows hepatic hilar soft tissue (arrow) seen 6 months after hepatic transplant in a 57-year-old man, proved to be PTLD on biopsy. (C) Axial noncontrast CT shows diffuse bowel wall thickening (arrow) seen 2 years after liver transplant in a 56-year-old man; proved to be PTLD on biopsy. (D) Axial venous-phase CT shows an ill-defined heterogeneously enhancing segment V hepatic lesion (arrow) seen 5 years after hepatic transplant in a 62-year-old woman; proved to be PTLD on biopsy.

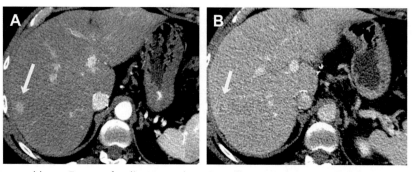

Fig. 16. A 63-year-old man 5 years after liver transplant. Surveillance CT shows a well-defined arterial enhancing lesion in segment VIII (*arrow* in *A*) with subtle washout on the delayed phase image (*arrow* in *B*), suspicious for recurrent HCC. This finding was confirmed on biopsy and treated with radiofrequency ablation.

months to years after transplant.[59,60] Ebstein-Barr virus is the chief causal agent, with EBV-associated PTLD occurring in the first 2 years after transplant and non–EBV-associated PTLD occurring later.[58,60,61]

Abdominal involvement is more common than extra-abdominal involvement. Lymphadenopathy involving single or multiple nodal groups (with or without splenomegaly) is the most common manifestation, followed by a periportal mass (**Fig. 15**A, B). Extranodal involvement can involve any organ, but the common ones are bowel, liver, kidneys, and adrenals (**Fig. 15**C, D). Radiologic appearance of involvement is similar to other lymphomas.[1,58–61]

In transplant patients with hepatocellular carcinoma (HCC), recurrent HCC can also occur, most commonly involving lungs and liver allografts (**Fig. 16**). Other sites include lymph nodes, adrenals, and bones.[1,2,62] The median time to HCC recurrence is greater than a year in most studies, although one study noted that one-third of its patients had recurrence within 1 year of transplant.[51–53]

Recurrent disease

Recurrence (with variable severity) of the disease that required transplant in the first place is a common complication. Recurrent hepatitis C virus (HCV) occurs in as many as 90% to 95% of patients after transplant, with 20% to 30% progressing to cirrhosis.[63,64] A recent pathology study concluded that the development of hepatic steatosis at 1 year is an independent predictor of subsequent development of fibrosis on multivariate analysis.[65] Recent advances in treatment of HCV with the introduction of highly active antivirals such as sofosbuvir and ledipasvir hold promise for reducing this rate.[64] Hepatitis B virus (HBV) recurrence is less common because of treatment with HBV immunoglobulin and antivirals.[66] Autoimmune disease such as autoimmune hepatitis, primary biliary cirrhosis, and PSC may also recur in 10% to 41% of

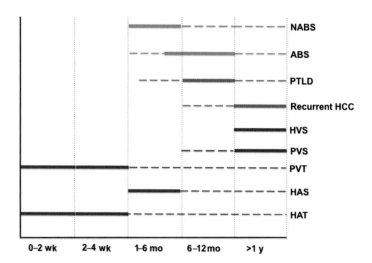

Fig. 17. Timeline for complications of liver transplant. X-axis: Time after transplant; Y-axis: Complications. Bold line: Common timeline for complication to occur; Dashed line: Less common timeline for complication to occur. Note that complications represent a continuum and can occur at any time. ABS, anastomotic biliary stricture; HVS, hepatic vein stenosis; NABS, nonanastomotic biliary stricture; PVS, portal vein stenosis; PVT, portal vein thrombosis.

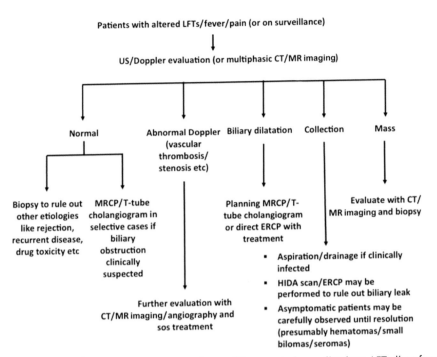

Fig. 18. Algorithm for evaluating liver transplant patients with suspected complications. LFTs, liver function tests.

patients, and is usually treated by increased immunosuppression.[67]

OVERALL APPROACH

Clinically, complications are often approached based on whether they are acute/short-term or long-term based on the time of presentation after an operation. Nevertheless, most complications form a continuum and can present at varying time points.[6] A working clinical differential diagnosis is then made based on the patient's symptoms and laboratory profile. The timeline of development of major complications is given in **Fig. 17**. A simplified algorithm for evaluation of patients with suspected complications is provided in **Fig. 18** based on our experience. US with Doppler is the preferred first modality for evaluation in most cases. Depending on the clinical status of the patient and the US findings, further evaluation with CT/MR imaging/angiography or biopsy may be performed or close clinical and imaging surveillance may be continued.

REFERENCES

1. Bhargava P, Vaidya S, Dick AA, et al. Imaging of orthotopic liver transplantation: review. AJR Am J Roentgenol 2011;196(3 Suppl):WS15–25 [quiz: S35–8].

2. Caiado AH, Blasbalg R, Marcelino AS, et al. Complications of liver transplantation: multimodality imaging approach. Radiographics 2007;27(5):1401–17.

3. Quiroga S, Sebastia MC, Margarit C, et al. Complications of orthotopic liver transplantation: spectrum of findings with helical CT. Radiographics 2001; 21(5):1085–102.

4. Singh AK, Nachiappan AC, Verma HA, et al. Postoperative imaging in liver transplantation: what radiologists should know. Radiographics 2010;30(2): 339–51.

5. Organ Procurement and Transplantation Network. US Department of Health & Human Services Web site. Available at: http://optn.transplant.hrsa.gov. Accessed November 2, 2014.

6. Moreno R, Berenguer M. Post-liver transplantation medical complications. Ann Hepatol 2006;5(2):77–85.

7. Fonseca AL, Cha CH. Hepatocellular carcinoma: a comprehensive overview of surgical therapy. J Surg Oncol 2014;110(6):712–9.

8. Llado L, Figueras J. Techniques of orthotopic liver transplantation. HPB (Oxford) 2004;6(2):69–75.

9. Tzakis A, Todo S, Starzl TE. Orthotopic liver transplantation with preservation of the inferior vena cava. Ann Surg 1989;210(5):649–52.

10. Jovine E, Mazziotti A, Grazi GL, et al. Piggy-back versus conventional technique in liver transplantation: report of a randomized trial. Transpl Int 1997; 10(2):109–12.

11. Sanyal R, Lall CG, Lamba R, et al. Orthotopic liver transplantation: reversible Doppler US findings in the immediate postoperative period. Radiographics 2012;32(1):199–211.

12. Ugurel MS, Battal B, Bozlar U, et al. Anatomical variations of hepatic arterial system, coeliac trunk and

renal arteries: an analysis with multidetector CT angiography. Br J Radiol 2010;83(992):661–7.

13. Covey AM, Brody LA, Maluccio MA, et al. Variant hepatic arterial anatomy revisited: digital subtraction angiography performed in 600 patients. Radiology 2002;224(2):542–7.

14. Ishigami K, Zhang Y, Rayhill S, et al. Does variant hepatic artery anatomy in a liver transplant recipient increase the risk of hepatic artery complications after transplantation? AJR Am J Roentgenol 2004; 183(6):1577–84.

15. Merion RM, Burtch GD, Ham JM, et al. The hepatic artery in liver transplantation. Transplantation 1989; 48(3):438–43.

16. Huang WD, Jiang JK, Lu YQ. Value of T-tube in biliary tract reconstruction during orthotopic liver transplantation: a meta-analysis. J Zhejiang Univ Sci B 2011;12(5):357–64.

17. Quintini C, Hashimoto K, Uso TD, et al. Is there an advantage of living over deceased donation in liver transplantation? Transpl Int 2013;26(1):11–9.

18. Grewal HP, Shokouh-Amiri MH, Vera S, et al. Surgical technique for right lobe adult living donor liver transplantation without venovenous bypass or portocaval shunting and with duct-to-duct biliary reconstruction. Ann Surg 2001;233(4):502–8.

19. Brown RS Jr. Live donors in liver transplantation. Gastroenterology 2008;134(6):1802–13.

20. Nadalin S, Bockhorn M, Malago M, et al. Living donor liver transplantation. HPB (Oxford) 2006; 8(1):10–21.

21. Ito K, Siegelman ES, Stolpen AH, et al. MR imaging of complications after liver transplantation. AJR Am J Roentgenol 2000;175(4):1145–9.

22. Lang P, Schnarkowski P, Grampp S, et al. Liver transplantation: significance of the periportal collar on MRI. J Comput Assist Tomogr 1995;19(4): 580–5.

23. Crossin JD, Muradali D, Wilson SR. US of liver transplants: normal and abnormal. Radiographics 2003; 23(5):1093–114.

24. Chezmar JL, Nelson RC, Bernardino ME. Portal venous gas after hepatic transplantation: sonographic detection and clinical significance. AJR Am J Roentgenol 1989;153(6):1203–5.

25. Clavien PA, Lesurtel M, Bossuyt PM, et al. Recommendations for liver transplantation for hepatocellular carcinoma: an international consensus conference report. Lancet Oncol 2012;13(1):e11–22.

26. Garcia-Criado A, Gilabert R, Salmeron JM, et al. Significance of and contributing factors for a high resistive index on Doppler sonography of the hepatic artery immediately after surgery: prognostic implications for liver transplant recipients. AJR Am J Roentgenol 2003;181(3):831–8.

27. Bekker J, Ploem S, de Jong KP. Early hepatic artery thrombosis after liver transplantation: a systematic review of the incidence, outcome and risk factors. Am J Transplant 2009;9(4):746–57.

28. Gunsar F, Rolando N, Pastacaldi S, et al. Late hepatic artery thrombosis after orthotopic liver transplantation. Liver Transpl 2003;9(6):605–11.

29. Warner P, Fusai G, Glantzounis GK, et al. Risk factors associated with early hepatic artery thrombosis after orthotopic liver transplantation - univariable and multivariable analysis. Transpl Int 2011;24(4): 401–8.

30. Flint EW, Sumkin JH, Zajko AB, et al. Duplex sonography of hepatic artery thrombosis after liver transplantation. AJR Am J Roentgenol 1988;151(3):481–3.

31. Nolten A, Sproat IA. Hepatic artery thrombosis after liver transplantation: temporal accuracy of diagnosis with duplex US and the syndrome of impending thrombosis. Radiology 1996;198(2):553–9.

32. Hom BK, Shrestha R, Palmer SL, et al. Prospective evaluation of vascular complications after liver transplantation: comparison of conventional and microbubble contrast-enhanced US. Radiology 2006; 241(1):267–74.

33. Sidhu PS, Shaw AS, Ellis SM, et al. Microbubble ultrasound contrast in the assessment of hepatic artery patency following liver transplantation: role in reducing frequency of hepatic artery arteriography. Eur Radiol 2004;14(1):21–30.

34. Rostambeigi N, Hunter D, Duval S, et al. Stent placement versus angioplasty for hepatic artery stenosis after liver transplant: a meta-analysis of case series. Eur Radiol 2013;23(5):1323–34.

35. da Silva RF, Raphe R, Felicio HC, et al. Prevalence, treatment, and outcomes of the hepatic artery stenosis after liver transplantation. Transplant Proc 2008; 40(3):805–7.

36. Abbasoglu O, Levy MF, Vodapally MS, et al. Hepatic artery stenosis after liver transplantation–incidence, presentation, treatment, and long term outcome. Transplantation 1997;63(2):250–5.

37. Marshall MM, Muiesan P, Srinivasan P, et al. Hepatic artery pseudoaneurysms following liver transplantation: incidence, presenting features and management. Clin Radiol 2001;56(7):579–87.

38. McNaughton DA, Abu-Yousef MM. Doppler US of the liver made simple. Radiographics 2011;31(1): 161–88.

39. Stell D, Downey D, Marotta P, et al. Prospective evaluation of the role of quantitative Doppler ultrasound surveillance in liver transplantation. Liver Transpl 2004;10(9):1183–8.

40. Tamsel S, Demirpolat G, Killi R, et al. Vascular complications after liver transplantation: evaluation with Doppler US. Abdom Imaging 2007;32(3):339–47.

41. Saad WE. Portal interventions in liver transplant recipients. Semin Intervent Radiol 2012;29(2):99–104.

42. Buell JF, Funaki B, Cronin DC, et al. Long-term venous complications after full-size and segmental

pediatric liver transplantation. Ann Surg 2002; 236(5):658–66.

43. Chong WK, Beland JC, Weeks SM. Sonographic evaluation of venous obstruction in liver transplants. AJR Am J Roentgenol 2007;188(6):W515–21.

44. Glockner JF, Forauer AR. Vascular or ischemic complications after liver transplantation. AJR Am J Roentgenol 1999;173(4):1055–9.

45. Navarro F, Le Moine MC, Fabre JM, et al. Specific vascular complications of orthotopic liver transplantation with preservation of the retrohepatic vena cava: review of 1361 cases. Transplantation 1999; 68(5):646–50.

46. Federle MP, Kapoor V. Complications of liver transplantation: imaging and intervention. Radiol Clin North Am 2003;41(6):1289–305.

47. Garcia-Criado A, Gilabert R, Bargallo X, et al. Radiology in liver transplantation. Semin Ultrasound CT MR 2002;23(1):114–29.

48. Nghiem HV. Imaging of hepatic transplantation. Radiol Clin North Am 1998;36(2):429–43.

49. Holbert BL, Baron RL, Dodd GD 3rd. Hepatic infarction caused by arterial insufficiency: spectrum and evolution of CT findings. AJR Am J Roentgenol 1996;166(4):815–20.

50. Ryu CH, Lee SK. Biliary strictures after liver transplantation. Gut Liver 2011;5(2):133–42.

51. Escartin A, Sapisochin G, Bilbao I, et al. Recurrence of hepatocellular carcinoma after liver transplantation. Transplant Proc 2007;39(7):2308–10.

52. Welker MW, Bechstein WO, Zeuzem S, et al. Recurrent hepatocellular carcinoma after liver transplantation - an emerging clinical challenge. Transpl Int 2013;26(2):109–18.

53. Valdivieso A, Bustamante J, Gastaca M, et al. Management of hepatocellular carcinoma recurrence after liver transplantation. Transplant Proc 2010;42(2): 660–2.

54. Neuberger J, Adams DH. What is the significance of acute liver allograft rejection? J Hepatol 1998;29(1): 143–50.

55. Burton JR Jr, Rosen HR. Diagnosis and management of allograft failure. Clin Liver Dis 2006;10(2): 407–35, x.

56. Berrocal T, Parron M, Alvarez-Luque A, et al. Pediatric liver transplantation: a pictorial essay of early

and late complications. Radiographics 2006;26(4): 1187–209.

57. Chatrath H, Berman K, Vuppalanchi R, et al. De novo malignancy post-liver transplantation: a single center, population controlled study. Clin Transplant 2013;27(4):582–90.

58. Narkewicz MR, Green M, Dunn S, et al. Decreasing incidence of symptomatic Epstein-Barr virus disease and posttransplant lymphoproliferative disorder in pediatric liver transplant recipients: report of the studies of pediatric liver transplantation experience. Liver Transpl 2013;19(7):730–40.

59. Wu L, Rappaport DC, Hanbidge A, et al. Lymphoproliferative disorders after liver transplantation: imaging features. Abdom Imaging 2001;26(2):200–6.

60. Jain A, Nalesnik M, Reyes J, et al. Posttransplant lymphoproliferative disorders in liver transplantation: a 20-year experience. Ann Surg 2002;236(4):429–36 [discussion: 436–7].

61. Borhani AA, Hosseinzadeh K, Almusa O, et al. Imaging of posttransplantation lymphoproliferative disorder after solid organ transplantation. Radiographics 2009;29(4):981–1000 [discussion: 1000–2].

62. Ferris JV, Baron RL, Marsh JW Jr, et al. Recurrent hepatocellular carcinoma after liver transplantation: spectrum of CT findings and recurrence patterns. Radiology 1996;198(1):233–8.

63. Gordon FD, Poterucha JJ, Germer J, et al. Relationship between hepatitis C genotype and severity of recurrent hepatitis C after liver transplantation. Transplantation 1997;63(10):1419–23.

64. Jimenez-Perez M, Gonzalez-Grande R, RandoMunoz FJ. Management of recurrent hepatitis C virus after liver transplantation. World J Gastroenterol 2014;20(44):16409–17.

65. Brandman D, Pingitore A, Lai JC, et al. Hepatic steatosis at 1 year is an additional predictor of subsequent fibrosis severity in liver transplant recipients with recurrent hepatitis C virus. Liver Transpl 2011; 17(12):1380–6.

66. John S, Andersson KL, Kotton CN, et al. Prophylaxis of hepatitis B infection in solid organ transplant recipients. Therap Adv Gastroenterol 2013;6(4):309–19.

67. El-Masry M, Puig CA, Saab S. Recurrence of non-viral liver disease after orthotopic liver transplantation. Liver Int 2011;31(3):291–302.

Renal Pretransplantation Work-up, Donor, Recipient, Surgical Techniques

Carla B. Harmath, MD[a],*, Cecil G. Wood III, MD[a],
Senta M. Berggruen, MD[a], Ekamol Tantisattamo, MD[b]

KEYWORDS

- Kidney • Renal transplant • Computed tomography imaging • MR imaging • Ultrasonography
- Renal donor • Renal transplant recipient

KEY POINTS

- Renal transplant is the single best treatment of end-stage renal disease.
- Multiphase CT is particularly useful because of detailed evaluation of the kidneys, including the vascular anatomy and the collecting system.
- MR imaging can be used with the advantage of no ionizing radiation, but its limitation for stone detection makes it a less preferred method of evaluating potential donors.
- Preoperative knowledge of the renal vascular anatomy is essential to minimize risks for the donor.
- Imaging evaluation of the recipient is also necessary for vascular assessment and detection of incidental findings that could preclude safe transplantation.

INTRODUCTION

End-stage renal disease (ERSD) is increasing in prevalence as the world population ages.[1,2] The most cost-effective treatment of ERSD, which also results in the best quality of life, is renal transplantation. The discrepancy between the need for transplant and cadaveric organ availability has led to the expansion of the donor pool to living donors. Harvesting an organ from an otherwise healthy individual requires careful preoperative assessment in order to minimize risks to the donor. The advent of noninvasive methods for the evaluation of the renal anatomy of potential donors, such as multiphase computed tomography (CT) and magnetic resonance (MR) imaging, along with improvements in laparoscopic surgical techniques, have resulted in safer preoperative evaluation and organ harvesting in living renal donors.

PRETRANSPLANT EVALUATION OF LIVING RENAL DONORS

Before harvesting a kidney for transplant, the potential donor is evaluated to ensure suitable candidacy for the harvesting procedure and that the kidney to be donated is suitable for transplantation. Anatomic evaluation of the transplant kidney as well as its vasculature and collecting system is necessary for optimal surgical planning. A thorough history, physical examination, and blood

Conflicts of interest: The authors have no commercial or financial conflicts of interest to disclose.
[a] Department of Radiology, Northwestern University Feinberg School of Medicine, 676 North Saint Clair, Suite 800, Chicago, IL 60611, USA; [b] Division of Nephrology, Department of Medicine, Comprehensive Transplant Center, Northwestern University Feinberg School of Medicine, 676 North Saint Clair, Suite 1900, Chicago, IL 60611, USA
* Corresponding author.
E-mail address: Charmath@nm.org

radiologic.theclinics.com

tests are obtained and various imaging studies (**Box 1**) are used to evaluate for potential short-term and long-term complications of renal donation.

Cardiovascular complications are the most common short-term complications of living renal donation, and routine chest radiographs in the posteroanterior (PA) and lateral projections are used for routine evaluation. These radiographs are performed to screen for any signs of long-standing hypertension such as left ventricular dilatation/hypertrophy and signs of chronic pulmonary disease. An important long-term complication of donation is the development of chronic kidney disease (CKD) and ESRD. The increased absolute risk of ESRD in donors is small, with an estimated risk of ESRD of 30.8 per 10,000 at 15 years after donation compared with 3.9 per 10,000 in their matched healthy nondonors.[3] However, even with this small risk, estimating glomerular filtration rate (GFR) before kidney donation is necessary to ensure adequate renal function after donation, in both the donor and the recipient. There is no consensus on the lower limit of GFR to determine candidacy for potential living kidney donor. An estimated GFR of greater than or equal to 80 mL/min/1.73 m^2 is an acceptable renal function to provide adequate GFR for both donor and recipient.[4] At our institution we use an estimated GFR of greater than 90 mL/min for any donor less than 50 years of age, and an estimated GFR greater than 80 mL/min for donors more than 50 years of age. Several centers use the 24-hour creatinine clearance (CrCl) to calculate the estimated GFR. However, multiple centers opt for nuclear medicine renal GFR imaging (**Fig. 1**), especially in cases of questionable 24-hour urine CrCl. Usually both kidneys have equal or close to equal GFR. There is a general consensus that the donated kidney relative function should not exceed 55%.[5] If renal scintigraphy shows significant discrepancy in function, the candidate is deemed unsuitable.

Anatomic evaluation before native nephrectomy is crucial. Detailed anatomic evaluation can be performed with CT or MR imaging. Renal ultrasonography (US) is not commonly used for predonation evaluation. The most common indication for US in the predonation evaluation is when the potential donor has a family history of autosomal dominant polycystic kidney disease (ADPKD). US is used as a screening test before a more extensive imaging work-up. If the results are equivocal (ie, when 1 or 2 cysts are detected), gene-based test confirmation should be performed.[6] A screening mammography is required for female living donors more than 50 years of age as a routine cancer screening.[7]

IMAGING PROTOCOLS FOR DONOR EVALUATION

A multiphase cross-sectional examination is preferred for the evaluation of potential donors. Multidetector CT with its optimal spatial resolution is the preferred method in multiple centers. MR imaging has also been used, because it does not expose the donor to ionizing radiation. Although modern MR equipment is capable of the high spatial and temporal resolution necessary to evaluate a potential renal donor, the superiority of CT in detecting calcifications, as well as its lower cost and faster acquisition time, makes it a preferable method. The recently published potential for complications from free circulating gadolinium after contrast-enhanced MR imaging even in the setting of normal renal function has also negatively affected the use of this modality for donor evaluation.[8]

At our institution 3-phase CT is used. Initially a noncontrast thin-section examination of the abdomen is obtained. This thin-section examination is followed by CT angiography (CTA) and excretory phase imaging. Some institutions advocate the use of a topogram for excretory phase imaging in order to decrease the radiation dose. Multiplanar reformations and three-dimensional (3D) reconstructions are used for optimal visualization and are preferred by surgeons because they best simulate their intraoperative plane. The CT technique used at our institution is presented in **Box 2**.

If MR imaging is to be used to evaluate a potential renal donor, it should include MR angiography (MRA) and MR venography phases, T2-weighted images, T1-weighted images obtained before and after the administration of contrast, as well as MR urography. The MR imaging technique for the evaluation of potential renal donors used at our institution is presented in **Box 3**.

Box 1
Imaging evaluation of living renal donors

- Chest radiograph, posteroanterior (PA) and lateral
- Nuclear medicine renal scintigraphy
- Multiphase CT or multiphase MR imaging
- Screening mammography (if female patient >50 years of age)

A

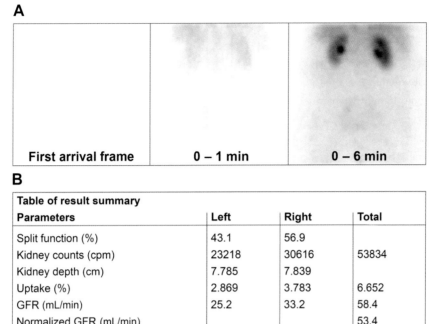

| First arrival frame | 0 – 1 min | 0 – 6 min |

B

Table of result summary

Parameters	Left	Right	Total
Split function (%)	43.1	56.9	
Kidney counts (cpm)	23218	30616	53834
Kidney depth (cm)	7.785	7.839	
Uptake (%)	2.869	3.783	6.652
GFR (mL/min)	25.2	33.2	58.4
Normalized GFR (mL/min)			53.4
GFR low normal (mL/min)			73.0
Mean GFR (mL/min)			96.0
Time of max (min)	5.751	5.001	

C

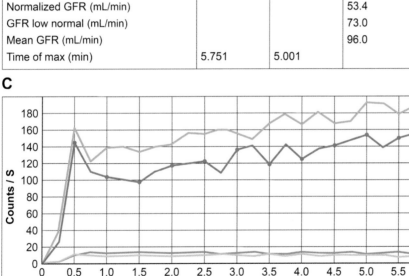

Fig. 1. Nuclear medicine renal scan in a potential donor showing near symmetric GFR. (*A*) Three PA scintigraphic images show symmetric uptake of the radiotracer within the kidneys. (*B*) Table and (*C*) graph corroborate the nearly symmetric uptake of the kidneys.

IMAGING REPORT
Computed Tomography Examination

The precontrast phase allows the optimal detection of stone disease and atherosclerotic calcification. The number, size, and location of the stones can be determined (**Fig. 2**).

Evaluation of the renal parenchyma on the postcontrast images should describe the presence or absence of renal cysts or solid masses and measurement of the kidneys in 3 dimensions. The maximal transverse dimensions are obtained on the axial plane at the level of the renal hilum, whereas the craniocaudal dimension can be obtained from either the coronal or sagittal planes, depending on which best displays the true length, which may vary slightly with the renal orientation (**Fig. 3**).

CTA allows optimal opacification and evaluation of renal arteries. The number of the arteries, their

---

Box 2
Example of comprehensive renal donor CT protocol

Oral contrast type: water

Oral contrast volume: 1 pitcher

Oral prep time: 15 minutes before scan

Scan type: spiral

Breath hold inspiration

Rotation time: 0.5 sec

Protocol step

Series 1

  Preinfusion abdomen

  Thickness/interval: 2 mm/2 mm

Series 2

  CTA abdomen and pelvis

  Intravenous (IV) contrast type: iopamidol 370 mg/mL

  IV contrast dose: 100 mL

  Rate: 4 mL/s

  Delay: bolus tracking (Hounsfield Unit 100)

  Region of interest (ROI) placement: aorta at celiac artery

  Saline volume: 90 mL (test 40 mL/chase 50 mL)

  Track delay/scan delay: 10 sec/5 sec

  Thickness/interval: 1 mm/1 mm

Series 3

  Excretory abdomen and pelvis

  IV contrast delay: 480 seconds

  Thickness/interval: 2 mm/2 mm

Reconstructions

Coronals: 2 × 2 mm

Sagittals: 2 × 2 mm (CT angiography only)

Coronal MIPs: 4 × 2 mm

3D CTA

Box 3
Example of comprehensive renal donor MR imaging protocol

Contrast dose: 0.1 mmol/kg

IV saline: 250 mL, open before positioning patient in the scanner

Nurse to prepare 5 mg of furosemide

Protocol step

Scout abdomen and pelvis

Precontrast images

Scout breath hold

T2 weighted, single shot, fast spin echo

T1 weighted, in phase and opposed phase, gradient echo

Diffusion-weighted imaging

T2 weighted, fat suppressed, fast spin echo

3D, T1 weighted, fat suppressed, spoiled gradient echo

T2-weighted navigator-triggered 3D or rapid acquisition with relaxation enhancement

T1-weighted 3D MRA acquisition × 1

Postcontrast images

T1-weighted 3D MRA acquisition × 3

T1 weighted, fat suppressed, spoiled gradient echo

T1-weighted, 3D MR urography acquisition

---

caliber, and the location of their origin (from aorta or rarely from iliac arteries) should be recorded. The branching pattern should be described (**Fig. 4**). Early branching or prehilar branching is considered when a renal arterial branch arises at 1.5 cm or less from the renal artery origin (**Fig. 5**). When multiple arteries are present, the distance between their origins and the aorta should be recorded (**Fig. 6**). Phrenic and adrenal branches, when present, have to be described

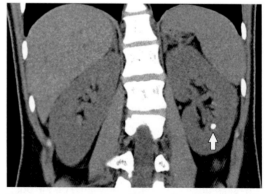

Fig. 2. Precontrast coronal image of a potential donor. Note the 5-mm nonobstructing calculus in the lower pole of the left kidney (*white arrow*).

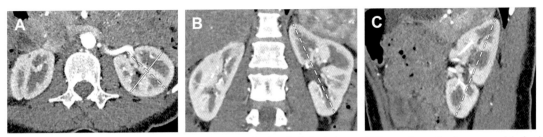

Fig. 3. Renal donor measurements. (*A*) Axial CTA at the level of the left renal hilum where the transverse (*dashed line*) and anterior-posterior (*solid line*) orthogonal dimensions are measured. (*B*) Coronal CTA and (*C*) sagittal CTA images at the maximal renal length. Either one could be used for the craniocaudal or bipolar renal dimension (*dashed lines*).

(**Fig. 7**). Any irregularities, such as are seen in fibromuscular dysplasia (**Fig. 8**), aneurysms (**Fig. 9**), or stenosis, are important findings that should be mentioned. The renal arterial system may be best evaluated on the maximum intensity projection (MIP) images.

The number and course of the renal veins should be evaluated and are easily observed in the arterial phase because of their early opacification (**Fig. 10**). The course of the left renal vein may be anterior or posterior to the aorta, or retroaortic (**Fig. 11**). Also, the convergence pattern of the upper and lower pole veins should be described, because this may affect the surgical clamping technique when it occurs too close to the aorta (**Fig. 12**). A circumaortic left renal vein (with single or multiple branches) should be mentioned (**Fig. 13**). Prominent lumbar veins (**Fig. 14**), adrenal veins, and the insertion point of the gonadal veins (**Fig. 15**) should also be pointed out in the report, because with the laparoscopic approach surgeons need to be forewarned about any variant anatomy in order to minimize potential vascular injuries and bleeding.[9] Accessory veins draining in the gonadal veins at or less than 2 cm from the conversion with the renal vein may be included in the dissection and must be shown. Anomalous right gonadal vein drainage into the right renal vein should be depicted. The presence of retroperitoneal varices may be an exclusion factor and they should be mentioned.

Excretory phase images allow accurate assessment of the renal collecting systems. Some institutions advocate the use of a topogram image for this phase, to decrease the radiation dose to the donor. The number of renal collecting systems in each kidney (**Fig. 16**), their joining point, as well as any aberrant course of the ureters should be noted. Excretory phase imaging is also useful for the detection of urothelial masses. An example of the CT renal donor protocol report used at our institution is shown in **Box 4**. **Box 5** contains a summary of findings to be reported.

MR Imaging

Similar to the CT protocol, multiphase imaging with different sequences is used to evaluate the renal donor with MR imaging, including MRA and MR urography (**Fig. 17**). The detailed anatomy and variance described on the CT approach for

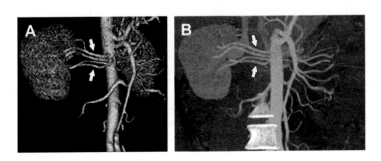

Fig. 4. Multiple renal arteries. (*A*) Coronal 3D and (*B*) maximum intensity projection (MIP) CTA images showing 4 right renal arteries with similar caliber arising in close proximity from the aorta (*arrows*).

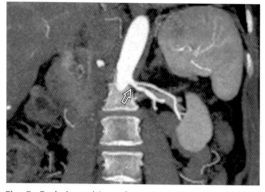

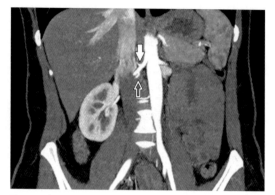

Fig. 5. Early branching of renal arteries. Coronal CTA MIP image showing early branching pattern of the left renal artery. The upper pole branch takes off at 5 mm from the origin (*open arrow*).

Fig. 7. Phrenic artery. Coronal MIP oblique CTA image shows a small right inferior phrenic artery arising from the proximal right renal artery (*solid white arrow*). Note also early branching of the right renal artery (*open arrow*).

the evaluation is also valid when providing the MR imaging report (**Fig. 18**).

Living Donor Selection

Usually a kidney with less vascular complexity is chosen for harvesting; preferably the left because of longer venous pedicle. The largest kidney is usually preferable, because there is a correlation between the renal size and long-term transplant function. If it is not possible to harvest the kidney with lower vascular anatomic complexity, postharvesting and pretransplantation manipulations are necessary. In the kidney with significant vascular anatomic variants, such as multiple renal arteries, multiple renal veins, or duplicated collecting system, these structures must be reconstructed before transplantation, increasing organ ischemic time and placing the donor and recipient at a higher risk of postoperative complications, such as renal artery or venous thrombosis, and urinary leakage. Early branching of the renal arteries makes safe clamp placement difficult. Similarly,

left renal vein conversion close to the aorta may not allow safe clamping.

A single stone measuring less than 5 mm is not an exclusion criterion, as long as the stone is not related to hereditary or systemic disorders potentially leading to the possibility of a high rate of recurrence.[10] If a larger stone burden is present, the kidney is not suitable for transplant. In addition, if both kidneys are affected, harvesting 1 of the organs may be detrimental to the future renal function of the donor. A small (preferably <2 cm) simple-appearing cyst is not an absolute contraindication to transplant, because some peripheral cysts can be decorticated at the time of transplant.[11,12] More complex lesions prevent donation.

In addition to investigating the kidneys, CT provides a good overview of potential extrarenal lesions, especially malignancies that may prevent renal donation in order to prevent transmission of a malignancy from the donor to the recipient. **Box 6** summarizes the factors taken into consideration on selecting a kidney to be harvested.

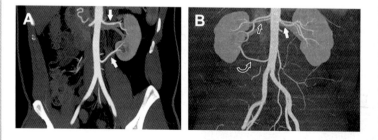

Fig. 6. Multiple renal arteries with variable origins. (*A*) Coronal oblique MIP CTA image showing 2 left renal arteries with distant origins from the aorta (*white arrows*). (*B*) Coronal MIP CTA with bone subtraction showing 2 left renal arteries with close origins from the aorta (*solid white arrow*). On the right, additional to the 2 arteries that arise in close proximity to the aorta (*open arrow*), a third artery supplying the lower pole arises more distally (*curved open arrow*).

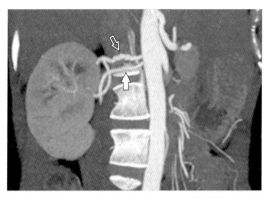

Fig. 8. Fibromuscular dysplasia. Coronal oblique MIP CTA image showing incidental fibromuscular dysplasia in the superiormost right renal artery in this patient with 2 renal arteries of similar caliber. Note the irregularity of the contour of the superiormost artery (*open arrow*) compared with the normal inferior artery (*solid white arrow*).

In the case of a deceased donor, no pretransplant imaging is routinely performed. The cadaveric organ is harvested and suitability for transplant is performed with gross inspection.

PRETRANSPLANT EVALUATION OF KIDNEY TRANSPLANT RECIPIENTS

Similar to living kidney donors, kidney transplant recipients require pretransplant evaluation (**Box 7**). In general, the recipient population has more comorbidities given their stage IV or V CKD or ESRD. Pretransplant imaging evaluation is a universal requirement. The donor kidney is usually placed extraperitoneally in the iliac fossa of the recipient. Preoperative knowledge of the recipient's anatomy, mostly the pelvic vascular anatomy, is important for evaluation of potential vascular targets for the anastomosis. A vascular

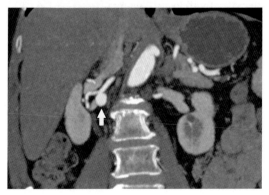

Fig. 9. Aneurysm. Coronal CTA image showing an incidental right renal artery aneurysm (*white arrow*).

inflow abnormality or significant atherosclerotic vascular calcification may affect the surgical technique and impair graft survival. The urinary bladder anatomy is also assessed.

The purpose of recipient imaging is also the detection of conditions that would contraindicate transplantation or that would be affected by the long-term immunosuppression that transplant recipients require. Two main complications of long-term immunosuppression are malignancy and infection. Kidney transplant recipients have a higher overall incidence of posttransplant malignancy (PTM), which is in part attributable to the more frequent surveillance a transplant patient receives compared with the general population.[13,14] With immunosuppression, there is impairment of DNA repair and reduced immune regulation.[15–17] Although most PTM is de novo, donor to recipient transmission can occur. In addition, unidentified malignancy before transplant may be unmasked by immunosuppression.

A chest radiograph is routinely performed to evaluate for lung nodules and infection, and further imaging with CT of the chest may be indicated, depending on the patient's risk factor for bronchogenic carcinoma. CT of the abdomen and pelvis is also performed. The use of intravenous contrast depends on the patient's renal function and dialysis regimen. In patients with ESRD on chronic hemodialysis, the prevalence of acquired renal cystic disease is high, up to 35% to 50%, and is associated with a higher incidence (6%) of renal cancer in the native kidneys, which might necessitate removal of the native kidneys before transplantation[18,19] (**Fig. 19**). If a contrast-enhanced CT examination cannot be performed to further evaluate a suspicious native renal lesion, US and noncontrast MR imaging may be used. However, both of these techniques present challenges. US may be limited because a poor acoustic window and suboptimal visualization of the usually atrophic native kidneys often preclude accurate renal evaluation. With MR imaging, the risk of inducing nephrogenic systemic fibrosis in patients with ESRD precludes the routine use of gadolinium-based contrast agents, which limits the evaluation of renal lesions with MR imaging, but lesions with marked heterogeneous T2 signal should be regarded with high suspicion, especially if associated with restricted diffusion.

Cross-sectional imaging such as CT is the preferred method for the evaluation of potential vascular anastomosis targets and bladder anatomy. Patients with CKD and ESRD have a high prevalence of vascular calcification, particularly medial arterial (Mönckeberg calcification) (**Fig. 20**).[20] Extensive vascular calcification at the

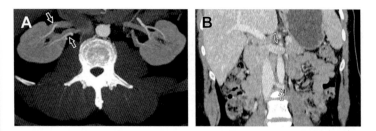

Fig. 10. Duplicate renal veins. (*A*) Axial oblique MIP image showing 2 right renal veins draining into the inferior vena cava (IVC) at the same level (*open arrows*). (*B*) Coronal volume-rendered CTA image showing 2 left renal veins draining into the IVC approximately 5 cm from each other (*open arrows*).

site of anastomosis may make it difficult or impossible for the surgeon to anastomose the donor renal artery to the recipient artery. In addition, extensive atherosclerotic disease in more proximal arteries may prevent adequate blood flow to the transplant kidney. A CT examination is especially indicated in patients with significant risks of peripheral arterial disease (PAD), such as heavy smoking and long-standing diabetes mellitus, as well as with signs of PAD such as diminished pulses in the lower extremities. Although noncontrast CT can show calcific atherosclerosis, contrast-enhanced CTA is best to evaluate for associated noncalcified plaque as a potential source of inflow disease. In addition to evaluating the vascular system, native kidneys, bladder, and any potential infection or malignancy, CT examination is also useful to determine whether the patient has enough intra-abdominal space for a transplant and to plan the operation. This determination is of particular interest in pediatric patients; patients with large nonfunctioning native kidneys, such as those with ADPKD; and in cases of previous failed transplants. An example of the CT protocol used for the evaluation of transplant candidates is provided in **Box 8**. In patients with ADPKD it is also important to screen for intracranial aneurysms (ICAs) before any major surgical interventions, because these patients have a higher incidence of ICAs (up to 10% and 22% in the patients without and with family history of intracranial aneurysm or subarachnoid hemorrhage, respectively) and major elective surgery affects intracranial hemodynamics.[21,22] The imaging of choice is time of flight (TOF) MRA or CTA because contrast-enhanced MRA is contraindicated because of the risk of nephrogenic systemic sclerosis.[23,24]

SURGICAL TECHNIQUE

In the harvesting procedure, a laparoscopic approach is preferred in the case of a living donor renal transplant (LDRT). The preferable kidney, determined preoperatively as described earlier, is harvested. Manipulations of the renal arterial system, venous system, and collecting system are performed. In the case of deceased donor, an open approach is performed. Aortic arterial patches and inferior vena cava patches may be used when working with a deceased donor renal transplant (DDRT). The organ is visually inspected, because these are usually not evaluated pretransplant.

Concomitantly the recipient patient is prepared. The most common location of the transplant is within the iliac fossa, and the usual approach is the lower abdominal Gibson incision[25] (**Fig. 21**). The laterality of the incision depends on the chosen surgical approach. The most common

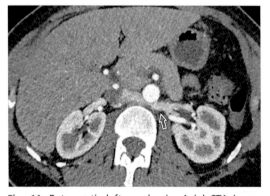

Fig. 11. Retroaortic left renal vein. Axial CTA image showing the left renal vein coursing dorsal to the aorta, also known as retroaortic renal vein (*open arrow*).

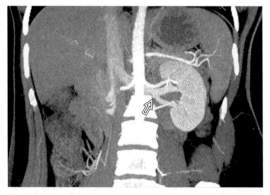

Fig. 12. Renal vein convergence. Coronal oblique MIP CTA image. The left renal veins converge in close proximity to the aorta (*open arrow*).

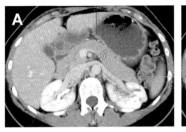

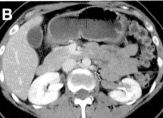

Fig. 13. Circumaortic left renal vein. (A) Superior and (B) inferior axial volume-rendered CTA images showing a circumaortic renal vein, with components anterior and posterior to the aorta (*open arrows*).

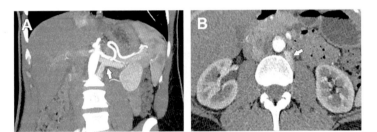

Fig. 14. Lumbar veins. (A) Coronal volume-rendered CTA and (B) axial CTA images show a prominent lumbar vein draining into the left renal vein near the aortic margin (*white arrows*).

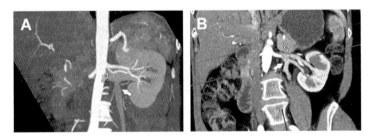

Fig. 15. Gonadal veins. (A) Oblique coronal MIP CTA image shows a prominent left gonadal vein (*solid white arrow*) draining into the left renal vein at less than 2 cm from the aortic margin. Note also the small accessory left renal artery (*open arrow*). (B) Double oblique coronal volume-rendered CTA shows a prominent gonadal vein that joins the inferior left renal vein (*solid white arrow*). The superior and inferior left renal veins merge in close proximity to the aorta (*open arrow*).

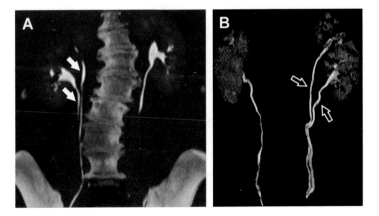

Fig. 16. Partially duplicated collecting systems. (A) Coronal CT excretory volume-rendered image and (B) coronal 3D CT urogram of different patients show partially duplicated collecting systems. The duplicated collecting system on the right in (A) (*solid white arrows*) joins in the mid-abdomen, whereas the duplicated left collecting system in (B) (*open arrows*) joins near the ureterovesical junction.

Box 4
Example template report for CT renal donor protocol

History

Potential renal transplant donor.

Technique

Precontrast helical acquisition of the abdomen and precontrast scout view of the abdomen and pelvis were obtained. Helical CT scans of the abdomen and pelvis were then obtained following the administration of nonionic iodinated IV contrast. Arterial and excretory phase sequences were performed. Multiple 3D reconstructions were created from the arterial data set.

Comparison

Findings

CTA abdomen and renal/CTA pelvis

Precontrast

Postcontrast

Vasculature

Renal arteries

Renal veins

Kidneys

There are bilateral symmetric nephrograms without hydronephrosis. No renal mass is seen. There is symmetric excretion of contrast into the collecting systems.

Right kidney: ___cm (CC) × ___cm (width) × ___cm (AP)

Left kidney: ___cm (CC) × ___cm (width) × ___cm (AP).

Ureters

Pelvic urogenital structures

Lower thorax

The lung bases are clear. There is no pleural effusion. The heart is normal in size.

Liver

Unremarkable.

Biliary tree

There is no biliary ductal dilatation.

Spleen

Unremarkable.

Pancreas

Unremarkable.

Adrenal glands

Unremarkable.

Lymph nodes

Abdomen

There is no abdominal adenopathy.

Pelvis

There is no pelvic adenopathy.

Vasculature

There is no abdominal aortic aneurysm.

Peritoneum/mesentery/omentum

There is no free fluid or free air.

Gastrointestinal tract

There is no bowel obstruction.

Body wall

Impression

Abbreviation: CC, Craniocaudal.

Box 5
Important findings to be included in the report

- Report renal stones and atherosclerotic calcifications
- Report renal size and lesions
- Report complete vascular anatomy (arterial and venous)
- Report collecting system (single/duplicated, obstruction, lesions)

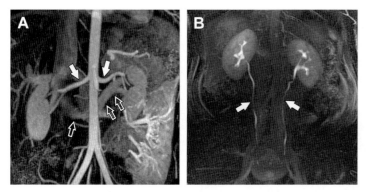

Fig. 17. MRA image and MR urogram of a renal donor. (*A*) Coronal MRA MIP image shows single renal arteries (*solid white arrows*). Note retroaortic left renal vein (*open arrows*). (*B*) Coronal MR urography MIP image shows single collecting systems (*solid white arrows*).

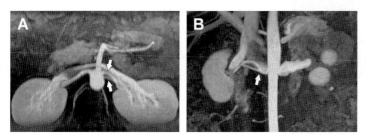

Fig. 18. Variant artery anatomy on MRA. (*A*) Axial volume-rendered MRA with 2 left renal arteries (*white arrows*), and (*B*) coronal volume-rendered MRA with early bifurcation of the right renal artery (*white arrow*).

Box 6
Donor preferred selection

- Larger kidney
- Least vascular and collecting system complexity
- No more than a single stone measuring less than 5 mm
- No more than 1 small simple-appearing cyst

Box 7
Elements to be included in the imaging evaluation of renal transplant recipients

- Chest radiograph, PA and lateral
- CT abdomen and pelvis with or without contrast
- If additional imaging needed: renal ultrasonography and/or MR imaging
- If ADPKD: CTA or time of flight MRA to screen for intracranial aneurysms

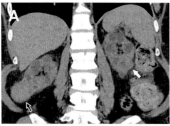
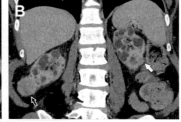

Fig. 19. Pretransplant evaluation in a patient on chronic hemodialysis. (*A*) Precontrast and (*B*) postcontrast CT of the abdomen shows a large enhancing lesion in the lower pole of the right kidney (*open arrows*), and a smaller enhancing lesion in the lower pole of the left kidney (*solid white arrows*), consistent with renal cell carcinomas.

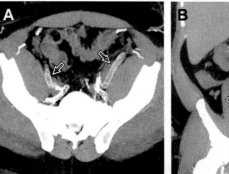
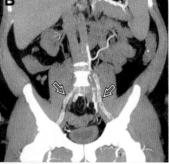
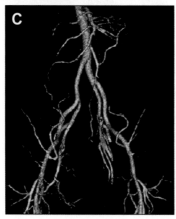

Fig. 20. Atherosclerosis in renal recipient. (*A*) Noncontrast axial volume-rendered and (*B*) coronal MIP images of recipient evaluation show extensive media calcification involving the iliac arterial system (*open arrows*). (*C*) CTA 3D image on the same patient shows no significant inflow stenosis or irregularity of the vessel, characteristic of media calcification.

Box 8
Example of comprehensive renal transplant recipient CT protocol

Oral contrast: none

Scan type: spiral

Rotation time: 0.5 sec

Breath hold inspiration

Protocol step

Series 1

    Preinfusion abdomen and pelvis

    Thickness/interval: 2 mm/2 mm

If patient is on dialysis and able to receive intravenous contrast

Series 2

    CTA abdomen and pelvis

    IV contrast type: iopamidol 370 mg/mL

    IV contrast dose: 100 mL

    Rate: 4 mL/s

    Delay: bolus tracking (Hounsfield Unit 100)

    ROI placement: aorta at celiac artery

    Saline volume: 90 mL (test 40 mL/chase 50 mL)

    Track delay/scan delay: 10 sec/5 sec

    Thickness/interval: 2 mm/2 mm

Reconstructions

Coronals: 2 × 2 mm

Sagittals: 2 × 2 mm (CT angiography only)

Coronal MIPs: 4 × 2 mm

3D CTA

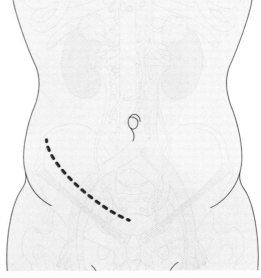

Fig. 21. The usual surgical approach (*dotted line*) for placement of the transplant in the iliac fossa. This approach is also known as the Gibson incision. (*Courtesy of* D.C. Botos, Chicago, IL, 2015.)

approach is to use the right side regardless of the side of the donor kidney because the right iliac vein is easier to access than the left (**Fig. 22**). Another approach is to use the contralateral side of the donor kidney (ie, right kidney in the left side, left kidney in the right side); this technique is used when the internal iliac artery is chosen for the anastomosis, because the vessels are in a convenient position and the renal pelvis is anteriorly oriented, making the ureter accessible if it needs to be repaired. The third option is to use the ipsilateral side to the donor kidney (right kidney to the right side). This option is best when the

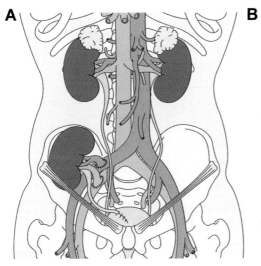 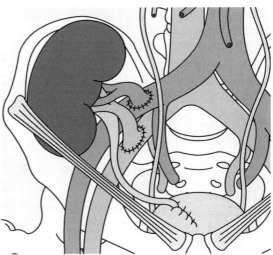

Fig. 22. (*A*, *B*) The renal transplant is placed in the iliac fossa, and the arterial and venous anastomoses are performed to the iliac vasculature. The ureter is anastomosed to the anterior bladder dome. (*Courtesy of* D.C. Botos, Chicago, IL, 2015.)

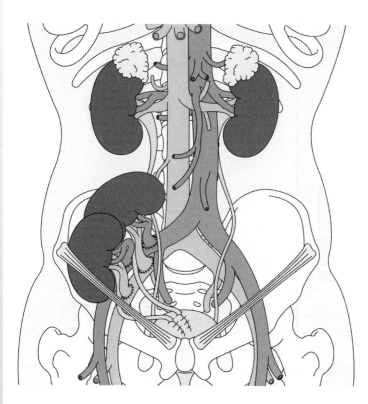

Fig. 23. Ipsilateral placement of a transplant after a failed transplant. The renal vessels are anastomosed to the common iliac vessels. This technique can also be used in a dual transplant in the case of marginal donor kidney function. (*Courtesy of* D.C. Botos, Chicago, IL, 2015.)

external iliac artery is chosen for the anastomosis because the vessels lie without kinking. For re-transplantation, the side opposite to the failed transplant is the usual choice. However, if this is not possible, a transabdominal incision and proximal vessels may be used (**Fig. 23**). In patients in whom a pancreas after kidney transplant is anticipated, the kidney is preferably placed in the left renal fossa in order to facilitate the pancreas transplant.

In simple vascular cases, the renal vein is anastomosed first to minimize ischemia to the leg. Usually it is anastomosed end to side to the external iliac vein. In the case of multiple renal veins, the largest one may be used and the others ligated. If there are 2 renal veins of similar caliber, they may be sewn together with the pair-of-pants technique (**Fig. 24**), or each vein is anastomosed to the external iliac vein. In the case of DDRT, especially when using the right kidney, the donor vena cava may be used as an extension graft, because the right renal vein is usually shorter than the left[26,27] (**Fig. 25**).

The next step is arterial end-to-side anastomosis of the donor renal artery to the external iliac artery. In DDRT, the donor renal artery (or arteries)

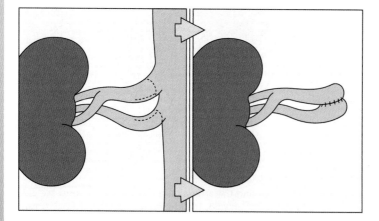

Fig. 24. The pair-of-pants technique used to anastomose a duplicated renal vein before transplant. (*Courtesy of* D.C. Botos, Chicago, IL, 2015.)

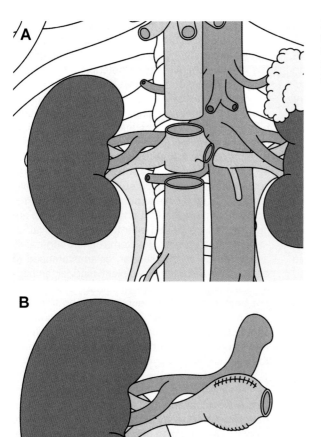

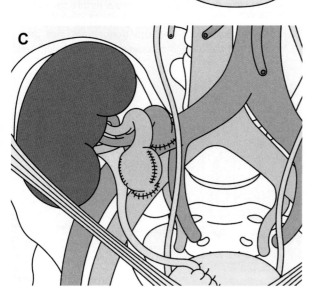

Fig. 25. (*A–C*) Donor vena cava used as an extension to the right renal vein. This procedure can be performed on cadaveric donor transplant. (*Courtesy of* D.C. Botos, Chicago, IL, 2015.)

is usually kept in continuity with a patch of the donor aorta called a Carrel aortic patch (**Fig. 26**) to facilitate the anastomosis, especially in the case of multiple arteries. The aortic (Carrel) patch is not possible in the case of LDRT, and the renal artery is anastomosed directly to the recipient external iliac artery. In rare instances the arterial anastomosis is performed with the internal iliac artery, aorta, or common iliac artery. This technique may be more commonly seen in pediatric or retransplant cases. For multiple arteries, several techniques may be used. An important point is that the lower pole renal artery should never be ligated because this usually supplies the ureter and ligation may lead to ureteral necrosis. Small visible vessels that supply a small part of the cortex may be ligated. In the case of LDRT and multiple arteries, they may be individually anastomosed to the recipient iliac artery or anastomosed to each other before being anastomosed to the recipient iliac artery (**Fig. 27**). Given the high risk of thrombosis in multiple arteries, heparin intravenous bolus before anastomosis and continuous infusion in the period immediately after the operation should be used.

The most complex portion of the procedure, the collecting system, is then addressed. The ureter is most commonly anastomosed to the anterior bladder dome; however, it may also be anastomosed to the ipsilateral ureter (ureterostomy) or the native ureter can be brought up to connect with the renal donor pelvis (ureteropyelostomy). Multiple techniques exist to connect the donor ureter to the urinary bladder. The most common is the Lich-Gregoir technique. The bladder is first distended with saline and the detrusor muscles are dissected. A muscular tunnel is then created by separating the detrusor muscle from the bladder mucosa for a length of approximately 2 to 4 cm. The mucosa is then opened and approximated with the ureter. The detrusor muscle is closed exteriorly, which can function as an antireflux mechanism. A Foley catheter placed preoperatively is retained for at least 3 to 5 days to up to 10 days postoperatively, especially in cases of risk of bladder obstruction, such as neurogenic bladder or benign prostatic hyperplasia, or in cases of possible urinary leak, such as ureteral reconstruction before anastomosis or bladder injury. A ureteral stent is routinely placed to prevent ureteral obstruction/stenosis and is usually removed around 6 week posttransplantation. Prophylactic antibiotics for urinary tract infection are used and discontinued after the stent removal.

Duplicated collecting systems can be separately anastomosed to the bladder, or anastomosed to each other before the recipient bladder anastomosis. Usually the recipient urinary bladder has not been distended by urine for a long time and is contracted; however, it often regains function shortly after transplantation. In cases of nonfunctioning or absent bladder, the ureter can be anastomosed to an ileal or colonic conduit.

In some situations the surgical technique is more complicated. Such is the case with pediatric enbloc transplants and dual transplantation, used for marginal donor kidney function to provide adequate renal allograft function posttransplantation. The recipients of dual transplants are usually older nonobese patients with lower metabolic requirements. One kidney can be placed on each side, or both kidneys on the same side (preferably the right side). Usually the right kidney is placed first, and the donor vena cava extension is anastomosed to the recipient vena cava, followed by the arterial anastomosis to the right common iliac artery. The left kidney is then addressed, and the donor vein and artery anastomosed to the recipient external iliac vein

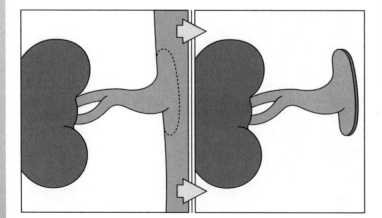

Fig. 26. A portion of the aorta is resected along with the harvested cadaveric kidney. This procedure is called a Carrel aortic patch. (*Courtesy of* D.C. Botos, Chicago, IL, 2015.)

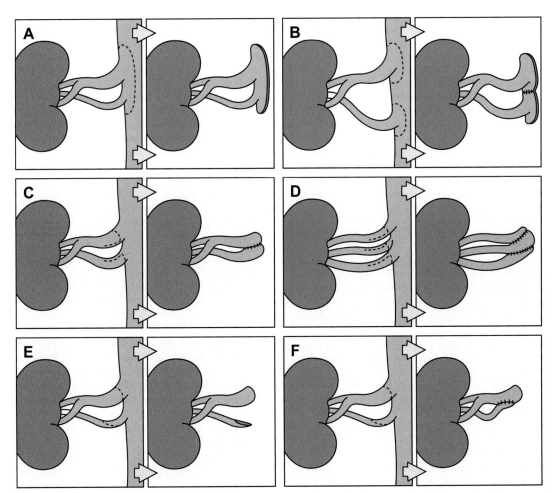

Fig. 27. The types of pretransplant manipulations that can be performed in the case of multiple arteries. (*Courtesy of D.C. Botos, Chicago, IL, 2015.*)

and artery. The ureters are then addressed and can be anastomosed to each other before the bladder anastomosis or they may each be anastomosed separately to the bladder.[28]

SUMMARY

Transplantation remains the single best option for the treatment of CKD and ESRD. Pretransplant evaluation is necessary for both the living donor and the renal transplant recipient to ensure optimal surgical planning and to minimize risks and complications. Knowledge of the imaging and surgical procedures enables best radiology collaboration with the several medical teams involved in the care of transplant patients.

ACKNOWLEDGMENTS

The authors thank David Botos, Visual Communications Specialist, for the figures in this article, and Holly Harper, administrative assistant and fellowship coordinator, for assistance in preparing the tables.

REFERENCES

1. Ferguson TW, Tangri N, Rigatto C, et al. Cost-effective treatment modalities for reducing morbidity associated with chronic kidney disease. Expert Rev Pharmacoecon Outcomes Res 2015;15(2): 243–52.
2. Fishbane S, Hazzan AD, Halinski C, et al. Challenges and opportunities in late-stage chronic kidney disease. Clin Kidney J 2015;8(1):54–60.
3. Muzaale AD, Massie AB, Wang MC, et al. Risk of end-stage renal disease following live kidney donation. JAMA 2014;311(6):579–86.
4. Delmonico F. A Report of the Amsterdam Forum on the Care of the Live Kidney Donor: data and medical guidelines. Transplantation 2005;79(6 Suppl): S53–66.

5. Weinberger S, Bäder M, Scheurig-münkler C, et al. Optimizing evaluation of split renal function in a living kidney donor using scintigraphy and calculation of the geometric mean: a case report. Case Rep Nephrol Urol 2014;4(1):1–4.

6. Huang E, Samaniego-Picota M, McCune T, et al. DNA testing for live kidney donors at risk for autosomal dominant polycystic kidney disease. Transplantation 2009;87(1):133–7.

7. US Preventive Services Task Force. Screening for breast cancer: U.S. preventive services task force recommendation statement. Ann Intern Med 2009; 151(10):716–26. W-236.

8. McDonald RJ, McDonald JS, Kallmes DF, et al. Intracranial gadolinium deposition after contrast-enhanced MR imaging. Radiology 2015;275(3): 772–82.

9. Engels EA, Pfeiffer RM, Fraumeni JF, et al. Spectrum of cancer risk among US solid organ transplant recipients. JAMA 2011;306(17):1891–901.

10. Kim IK, Tan JC, Lapasia J, et al. Incidental kidney stones: a single center experience with kidney donor selection. Clin Transplant 2012;26(4):558–63.

11. Tonyali S, Erdem Y, Yilmaz SR, et al. Urologic disorders in living renal donors and outcomes of their recipients. Transplant Proc 2015;47(5):1306–8.

12. Grotemeyer D, Voiculescu A, Iskandar F, et al. Renal cysts in living donor kidney transplantation: long-term follow-up in 25 patients. Transplant Proc 2009;41(10):4047–51.

13. Sampaio MS, Cho YW, Qazi Y, et al. Posttransplant malignancies in solid organ adult recipients: an analysis of the U.S. National Transplant Database. Transplantation 2012;94(10):990–8.

14. Herman M, Weinstein T, Korzets A, et al. Effect of cyclosporin A on DNA repair and cancer incidence in kidney transplant recipients. J Lab Clin Med 2001; 137(1):14–20.

15. Hojo M, Morimoto T, Maluccio M, et al. Cyclosporine induces cancer progression by a cell-autonomous mechanism. Nature 1999;397(6719):530–4.

16. Guba M, von Breitenbuch P, Steinbauer M, et al. Rapamycin inhibits primary and metastatic tumor growth by antiangiogenesis: involvement of vascular endothelial growth factor. Nat Med 2002; 8(2):128–35.

17. Brennan JF, Stilmant MM, Babayan RK, et al. Acquired renal cystic disease: implications for the urologist. Br J Urol 1991;67(4):342–8.

18. Truong LD, Krishnan B, Cao JT, et al. Renal neoplasm in acquired cystic kidney disease. Am J Kidney Dis 1995;26(1):1–12.

19. Abou-Hassan N, Tantisattamo E, D'Orsi ET, et al. The clinical significance of medial arterial calcification in end-stage renal disease in women. Kidney Int 2015; 87(1):195–9.

20. Xu HW, Yu SQ, Mei CL, et al. Screening for intracranial aneurysm in 355 patients with autosomal-dominant polycystic kidney disease. Stroke 2011; 42(1):204–6.

21. Huston J, Torres VE, Sulivan PP, et al. Value of magnetic resonance angiography for the detection of intracranial aneurysms in autosomal dominant polycystic kidney disease. J Am Soc Nephrol 1993; 3(12):1871–7.

22. Gibbs GF, Huston J, Qian Q, et al. Follow-up of intracranial aneurysms in autosomal-dominant polycystic kidney disease. Kidney Int 2004;65(5):1621–7.

23. Chapman AB, Rubinstein D, Hughes R, et al. Intracranial aneurysms in autosomal dominant polycystic kidney disease. N Engl J Med 1992;327(13):916–20.

24. Park SC, Kim SD, Kim JI, et al. Minimal skin incision in living kidney transplantation. Transplant Proc 2008;40(7):2347–8.

25. Veale JL, Singer JS, Gritsch HA. The transplant operation and its surgical complications. In: Danovitch GM, editor. Handbook of kidney transplantation. 5th edition. Philadelphia: Lippincott Williams & Wilkins; 2010;(8):181–97.

26. Kaufman DB. Kidney transplantation. In: Stuart FP, Abecassis MM, Kaufman DB, editors. Kidney, pancreas and islet cell transplantation. Georgetown (Guyana): Landes Bioscience; 2004. p. 41.

27. Barry JM, Fuchs EF. Right renal vein extension in cadaver kidney transplantation. Arch Surg 1978; 113(3):300.

28. Masson D, Hefty T. A technique for the transplantation of 2 adult cadaver kidney grafts into 1 recipient. J Urol 1998;160(5):1779–80.

Imaging Complications of Renal Transplantation

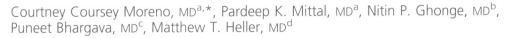

Courtney Coursey Moreno, MD[a],[*], Pardeep K. Mittal, MD[a], Nitin P. Ghonge, MD[b], Puneet Bhargava, MD[c], Matthew T. Heller, MD[d]

KEYWORDS

- Renal transplantation • Complications of renal transplantation • Renal artery stenosis
- Renal vein thrombosis • Collecting system injury • Lymphocele • Urinoma
- Posttransplant lymphoproliferative disorder

KEY POINTS

- Renal transplant complications are categorized as those related to the transplant vasculature, collecting system, perinephric space, renal parenchyma, and miscellaneous complications.
- Ultrasound is often the initial imaging modality used for evaluation of a renal transplant. CT, MR imaging, and nuclear medicine studies are complimentary.
- The most common transplant vascular complications are renal artery stenosis, renal artery thrombosis, renal vein thrombosis, pseudoaneurysm formation, and arteriovenous fistula formation.
- The most common collecting system complications are urine leak and obstruction.
- Renal parenchymal complications include delayed graft function, acute tubular necrosis, rejection (hyperacute, acute, or chronic), and damage caused by nephrotoxic drugs.

INTRODUCTION

Approximately 69,000 kidney transplants are performed annually worldwide.[1] In the United States, approximately 91% of grafts are functional at 1 year, 82% are functional at 3 years, and 72% are functional at 5 years.[2] Because many causes of renal transplant failure are potentially treatable, transplant recipients undergo routine surveillance so that complications are detected in the early and treatable stage. This surveillance consists primarily of ultrasound and monitoring of urine output and serum creatinine values in the immediate postoperative period.[3] Following discharge from the hospital, serum creatinine values are typically checked two to three times per week in the first

several weeks following transplant.[3] For individuals with stable transplant function, surveillance intervals become increasingly spaced out to every 3 to 6 months in long-term follow-up.[3] An elevated serum creatinine value detected during one of these postoperative checks may prompt a renal transplant ultrasound to investigate for potential etiologies.

Renal transplant complications are categorized as involving transplant vasculature, collecting system, perinephric space, parenchyma, and miscellaneous complications. Accurate diagnosis of these complications on imaging is important for appropriate patient management. This article reviews normal renal transplant anatomy, imaging

Financial Disclosure: C.C. Moreno, P.K. Mittal, and N.P. Ghonge have no financial disclosures; P. Bhargava is the Editor-in-Chief of *Current Problems in Diagnostic Radiology*, Elsevier Inc; M.T. Heller is a consultant for Amirsys Inc.
[a] Department of Radiology and Imaging Sciences, Emory University School of Medicine, 1364 Clifton Road, NE, Atlanta, GA 30322, USA; [b] Department of Radiology, Indraprastha Apollo Hospitals, Delhi-Mathura Road, New Delhi 110076, India; [c] Department of Radiology, VA Puget Sound Health Care System, University of Washington Medical Center, 1959 NE Pacific Street, Room BB308, Box 357115, Seattle, WA 98195-7115, USA; [d] Department of Radiology, University of Pittsburgh School of Medicine, 200 Lothrop Street, Suite 174E PUH, Pittsburgh, PA 15213, USA
* Corresponding author.
E-mail address: courtney.moreno@emoryhealthcare.org

Radiol Clin N Am 54 (2016) 235–249
http://dx.doi.org/10.1016/j.rcl.2015.09.007
0033-8389/16/$ – see front matter © 2016 Elsevier Inc. All rights reserved.

techniques, and the appearance of renal transplant complications at imaging. For each complication, typical presenting symptoms and treatment options are also reviewed.

NORMAL ANATOMY

Renal transplants are typically placed in the iliac fossa in an extraperitoneal location. The transplant main renal artery may be anastomosed to either the external iliac artery by an end-to-side anastomosis or the internal iliac artery by an end-to-end anastomosis.[4] The operative technique used for a donor kidney with multiple renal arteries is variable.[5] Small accessory renal arteries may be anastomosed to a larger renal artery with the larger artery anastomosed to the external or internal iliac artery.[5] Alternatively multiple iliac anastomoses may be performed.[5] The transplant main renal vein is most commonly anastomosed to the recipient external iliac vein via an end-to-side anastomosis. The donor ureter is typically anastomosed to the anterior or lateral wall of the recipient urinary bladder.[6] A bladder wall myotomy is performed, and the ureter is directly sutured to the bladder mucosa.[6] For donor kidneys with a duplicated collecting system, both ureters may be implanted separately into the urinary bladder.[7] Alternatively, the ureters may be joined together and implanted as a single ureter.[7]

IMAGING PROTOCOL
Ultrasound

Ultrasound is often the initial imaging modality used for evaluation of a renal transplant. Benefits of ultrasound include its lack of ionizing radiation and ability to assess transplant vasculature without intravenous contrast material. A good acoustic window is usually available because transplanted kidneys are typically placed in the iliac fossa and therefore are not obscured by overlying bowel gas. Gray-scale ultrasound evaluation should include documentation of the greatest length of the transplant, assessment of whether or not hydronephrosis is present, and assessment for a perinephric fluid collection.[8]

A detailed evaluation of transplant vasculature also should be performed with color Doppler and spectral imaging (Table 1). Peak systolic velocity (PSV) should be recorded at the main renal artery anastomosis, distal to the anastomosis, and in the external iliac artery cephalad to the anastomosis so that the renal artery PSV to external iliac artery PSV ratio can be computed.[8] If more than one main renal artery is present, each should be documented separately. Resistive indices should be

Table 1	
Images to be obtained in ultrasound evaluation of transplant vasculature	
Transplant Vessel	**Components of Evaluation**
Main renal artery[a]	Record peak systolic velocity at anastomosis, distal to anastomosis, and any area with color aliasing
Main renal vein	Record peak systolic velocity at anastomosis and distal to anastomosis
External iliac artery	Record peak systolic velocity proximal (cephalad) to the transplant
External iliac vein	Consider recording velocity just distal to the anastomosis
Interlobar and segmental arteries	Record resistive indices in the upper pole, interpolar region, and lower pole

[a] If more than one transplant main renal artery is present, each should be interrogated.

obtained from interlobar or segmental arteries in the upper pole, interpolar region, and lower pole of the transplant kidney.[8] The transplant main renal vein should be evaluated from the kidney to its anastomosis.[8] The external iliac vein should also be evaluated for patency.[8]

Contrast-enhanced ultrasound also is used to evaluate renal transplants. Ultrasound contrast agents are gas-containing microbubbles that remain in the intravascular compartment.[9] These contrast agents therefore are used to evaluate for areas of parenchymal infarction, to assess parenchymal perfusion, and to assess for blood flow within renal masses.[10,11] An advantage of contrast-enhanced ultrasound as compared with contrast-enhanced computed tomography (CT) is that ultrasound microbubble contrast agents are not thought to result in contrast induced nephropathy. A disadvantage of contrast-enhanced ultrasound is that these agents are not currently approved for use by the US Food and Drug Administration. Additional software packages also are required to quantify perfusion with microbubble technology.

Ultrasound elastography is a relatively new ultrasonographic technology that assesses tissue stiffness.[12] The role of ultrasound elastography in the evaluation of renal transplants is yet to be determined because early studies have found poor interobserver agreement in assessment of tissue stiffness and mixed results in terms of whether measurements of tissue stiffness correlate with clinical, laboratory, or histologic findings.[12-14]

Computed Tomography

CT may be complimentary in the evaluation of renal transplant complications. If the patient's renal function allows, intravenous contrast-enhanced CT angiography (CTA) may be performed to noninvasively confirm a diagnosis of renal artery stenosis if, for example, PSVs are elevated at ultrasound. Contrast-enhanced imaging also can be used to characterize indeterminate focal lesions detected at ultrasound as cystic or solid. Additionally, intravenous contrast-enhanced CT with excretory phase imaging (acquired 5–20 minutes after intravenous contrast material administration) can be used to confirm a urine leak or urinoma. Administration of intravenous contrast material should be avoided in individuals with impaired renal function because of the risk of developing contrast-induced nephropathy.[15-17]

Noncontrast CT is helpful to evaluate the full extent of a perinephric fluid collection and its relationship to surrounding structures if portions of the collection are obscured by bowel gas at ultrasound. Also, noncontrast CT is more accurate than ultrasound for the diagnosis of renal and ureteral stones, especially for small stones.[18]

MR Imaging

MR imaging also plays a complimentary role in the evaluation of renal transplant complications. Magnetic resonance angiography (MRA) can be used to noninvasively confirm renal artery stenosis. Contrast-enhanced MR imaging can also characterize focal renal lesions as cystic or solid. Additionally, excretory phase imaging can be performed to diagnose a urine leak or urinoma. Administration of gadolinium-based contrast agents in individuals with impaired renal function has been associated with the development of nephrogenic systemic fibrosis, a potentially fatal fibrosing condition.[17] Contrast agents associated with the greatest number of nephrogenic systemic fibrosis cases are gadodiamide (Omniscan), gadopentetate dimeglumine (Magnevist), and gadoversetamid (OptiMARK) and should not be administered to individuals with impaired renal function.[17] Other gadolinium-based contrast agents are associated with few if any unconfounded cases of nephrogenic systemic fibrosis, and understanding of their potential role in the evaluation of individuals with impaired renal function is evolving.[17]

Nuclear Medicine

Nuclear medicine studies may be used to evaluate transplant perfusion or for collecting system injury following renal transplantation. Technetium-99m (^{99m}Tc) labeled pharmaceuticals are typically used, either ^{99m}Tc-mercaptoacetyl triglycine or ^{99m}Tc-diethylene triamine.[19] The radiopharmaceutical is injected intravenously and sequential images are acquired to evaluate the vascular phase (flow phase), parenchymal phase (functional phase), and washout (excretory phase).[19] Nuclear medicine studies are an option for patients with contraindications to iodinated and gadolinium-based intravenous contrast agents.

RENAL TRANSPLANT COMPLICATIONS

Renal transplant complications can be categorized as complications of the transplant vasculature, collecting system, perinephric space, renal parenchyma, and other miscellaneous complications (**Box 1**).

Vascular Complications

The most common transplant vascular complications are renal artery stenosis, renal artery

---

Box 1
Renal transplant complications

Vascular

Renal artery stenosis

Renal artery thrombosis

Renal vein thrombosis

Pseudoaneurysm

Arteriovenous fistula

Collecting system

Urine leak

Obstruction

Peritransplant collection

Hematoma

Lymphocele

Urinoma

Parenchymal disease

Delayed graft function

Rejection

Drug nephrotoxicity

Miscellaneous

Posttransplant lymphoproliferative disorder

thrombosis, renal vein thrombosis, pseudoaneurysm formation, and arteriovenous fistula (AVF) formation.

Renal artery stenosis

Transplant renal artery stenosis occurs in 0.9% to 8% of patients.[20–23] Clinical findings may include allograft dysfunction, new-onset hypertension, and a bruit over the graft.[23,24] Transplant renal artery stenosis typically presents between 3 months and 2 years following the transplant.[20,25] The stenosis most often occurs at the anastomosis but also can be more diffuse.[25] Stenosis occurs more commonly following an end-to-end anastomosis of the renal transplant artery to the internal iliac artery and less commonly following an end-to-side anastomosis to the external iliac artery.[26] Causes of transplant renal artery stenosis include suture technique, donor or recipient atherosclerotic disease, arterial trauma during graft harvesting, and cytomegalovirus infection.[23,25]

At ultrasound, PSV is the most sensitive and specific finding for the diagnosis of transplant renal artery stenosis (**Fig. 1**).[23,27,28] Velocity thresholds from greater than or equal to 200 to 300 cm/s have been proposed with higher

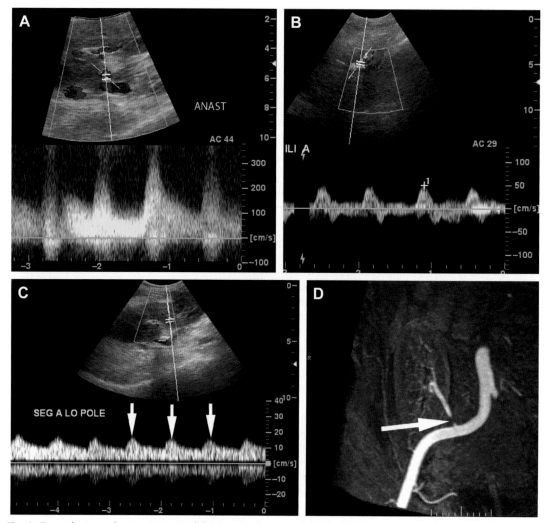

Fig. 1. Transplant renal artery stenosis. (*A*) Spectral ultrasound shows elevated peak systolic velocity at the anastomosis of greater than 300 cm/s. (*B*) The velocity in the ipsilateral iliac artery was approximately 50 cm/s, yielding an anastomotic velocity ratio of six-fold. (*C*) Spectral Doppler interrogation of a segmental renal artery shows delay in the systolic upstroke and rounding of the systolic peak, consistent with a tardus-parvus waveform (*arrows*) caused by the upstream stenosis. The resistive index was 0.43, and the acceleration time was 0.185 seconds. (*D*) Maximum intensity projection image from MRA shows near complete loss of signal at the anastomosis (*arrow*) consistent with high-grade arterial stenosis.

threshold values having a higher specificity and positive predictive value compared with lower thresholds.[23,27,28] Technical parameters must be optimized to avoid spurious velocity values. Angle correction should be less than or equal to 60°, and the angle indicator line should be parallel to the long axis of the vessel. An acceleration time greater than or equal to 0.08 to 0.1 second in the renal or intrarenal arteries is also suggestive of renal artery stenosis.[28] The acceleration time is defined as the time from the beginning of systole to the early systolic peak. A ratio of PSV in the main renal artery to the PSV in the external iliac artery of greater than 1.8 is also suggestive of renal artery stenosis.[28]

In some individuals, vessel tortuosity or a poor acoustic window may limit accurate assessment. CTA or MRA can be complimentary to noninvasively confirm a diagnosis of renal artery stenosis. At CTA or MRA, a hemodynamically significant stenosis is defined as luminal narrowing greater than 50%.[25] Alternatively, if patient presentation and ultrasound findings are convincing, patients with suspected renal artery stenosis may go directly to percutaneous angioplasty with stents placed in individuals with recurrent disease.[29]

Renal artery thrombosis

Transplant renal artery thrombosis occurs in 0.4% to 3.5% of recipients.[25,30,31] Patients typically present with an acute reduction in urine output and an elevation in serum creatinine.[25] Arterial thrombosis most commonly occurs in the immediate postoperative period but may occur at any time following the transplant. Etiologies include technical factors, such as vessel kinking, arterial dissection, acute rejection, hypercoaguable states, and toxicity of immunosuppressive agents.[25,32] At ultrasound, contrast-enhanced CT, and contrast-enhanced MR imaging, renal artery thrombosis appears as absence of flow in the transplant main renal artery and branch vessels (**Fig. 2**).

Unfortunately, the graft is typically lost once arterial thrombosis occurs.[25] Surgical thrombectomy may be attempted. Catheter-directed thrombolysis also may be attempted if the thrombosis occurs outside of the immediate postoperative period but is generally contraindicated within 14 days of the transplant because of the risk of postoperative bleeding.[33]

Renal vein thrombosis

Transplant renal vein thrombosis occurs in 0.55% to 4% of patients.[25,26] Symptoms include pain, fever, swelling in the area of the graft, and/or ipsilateral lower extremity edema.[25] Vein thrombosis most commonly occurs in the early postoperative period because of such factors as prolonged ischemia, extrinsic compression on the vein, vein torsion, or hypercoaguable states.[25,34] Later thrombosis may be caused by acute rejection or immunosuppressive agents.[25,34]

At ultrasound, absence of flow in the transplant main renal vein is diagnostic of renal vein thrombosis (**Fig. 3**). The transplant main renal artery also typically demonstrates an extremely high-resistance waveform with reversal of diastolic flow (see **Fig. 3**). However, reversal of diastolic flow can also be seen in other conditions that result in a high-resistance waveform including hydronephrosis, rejection, and extrinsic compression on the transplant. Contrast-enhanced CT or MR imaging

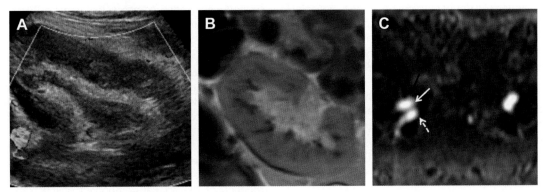

Fig. 2. Transplant renal artery thrombosis. (*A*) Sagittal color Doppler ultrasound image demonstrates no detectable flow within the transplant main renal artery or vein. Because the level of renal artery stenosis or thrombosis could not be determined based on this study, the patient underwent MR imaging. (*B*) Axial T2-weighted MR imaging demonstrates loss of expected corticomedullary differentiation in the transplant. (*C*) Axial T1-weighted MR imaging after administration of intravenous contrast material demonstrates contrast material in the right external iliac artery (*solid white arrow*) and internal iliac artery (*dashed arrow*) and nonopacification of the transplant main renal artery (expected location indicated by *black arrow*).

A

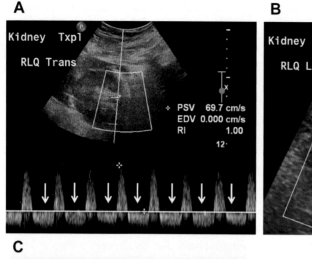

B

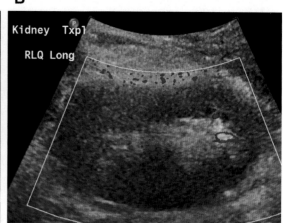

C

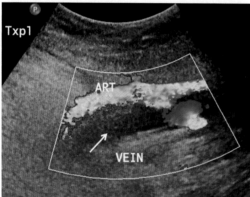

Fig. 3. Renal vein thrombosis. (*A*) Transplant main renal artery demonstrates a high-resistance waveform as indicated by reversal of flow in diastole (*arrows*). Differential diagnosis for this waveform includes renal vein thrombosis, hydronephrosis, extrinsic compression, or renal parenchymal disease. No flow was seen in the transplant main renal vein compatible with renal vein thrombosis. (*B*) Sagittal color Doppler image demonstrates no flow in the transplant main renal vein. (*C*) Thrombus also extends into the right external iliac vein (*arrow*).

usually is not necessary for confirmation because ultrasound and clinical presentation are typically definitive. If contrast-enhanced CT or MR imaging is performed, nonopacification of the transplant main renal vein is seen with thrombus within it.

Historically, immediate transplant removal was performed following a diagnosis of renal vein thrombosis because of concerns regarding potential transplant rupture and even death.[34] Currently, salvage thrombectomy may be performed in the early postoperative period or thrombolytics may be administered for individuals with a late renal vein thrombosis.[34] Unfortunately, the graft is typically lost even despite these interventions.[25]

Pseudoaneurysm
Pseudoaneurysms or AVFs may form as a complication of renal transplant biopsy. At gray-scale ultrasound, pseudoaneurysms appear as a cyst[35] (**Fig. 4**). With application of color Doppler, the "yin-yang sign" is seen in the aneurysm sac

(see **Fig. 4**). With spectral Doppler imaging, "to-and-fro" flow is visible as flow above and below the baseline.[36] Pseudoaneurysms may be treated with graded compression, direct percutaneous thrombin injection, or transcatheter embolization.[37]

Arteriovenous fistula
AVFs also most commonly occur as a complication of a transplant biopsy because of laceration of adjacent arterial and venous structures and resultant creation of a new communication between the two.[35] Most AVFs are not identifiable at gray-scale ultrasound.[35] Spectral waveform analysis is key for the diagnosis of an AVF. Interrogation of the arterial component of the fistula demonstrates a high-velocity, low-impedance arterial waveform.[35] Interrogation of the venous component demonstrates an arterialized waveform.[35] Larger AVFs may result in vibrations of the adjacent tissues, which are detectable at color Doppler imaging, also known as the "soft

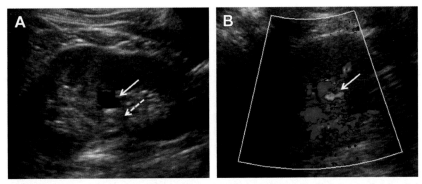

Fig. 4. Pseudoaneurysm. (*A*) Gray-scale ultrasound image demonstrates a well-circumscribed anechoic structure (*solid arrow*) in the renal sinus fat with increased through transmission (*dashed arrow*). Differential diagnosis includes a simple cyst or pseudoaneurysm. (*B*) Color Doppler image demonstrates the yin-yang appearance of a pseudoaneurysm (*arrow*).

tissue bruit."[35] Most AVF are small, asymptomatic, do not require treatment, and many resolve on their own. The optimal management of large symptomatic AVFs is somewhat controversial, and transcatheter embolization may be performed.[37]

Collecting System Complications

An elevated serum creatinine value or decreased urine output may be the first clue to a collecting system abnormality and typically warrants an imaging work-up.[38] The most common complications are urine leak and obstruction.

Urine leak

Urine leak occurs in approximately 1.1% to 6.5% of transplant recipients.[39,40] Leaks are usually diagnosed early in the postoperative period with a median time to diagnosis of 4 to 29 days.[39,40] Urine leaks most commonly involve the lower ureter followed by the urinary bladder and the upper ureter/collecting system.[39] Direct injury may occur during organ harvest or reimplantation or may result from ischemic necrosis caused by vascular compromise.[39]

At imaging, a urine leak appears as ill-defined fluid or a fluid collection. At ultrasound, leaked urine appears hypoechoic or anechoic and may contain internal debris. The differential diagnosis of a perinephric fluid collection at ultrasound also includes a lymphocele or hematoma. At CT, attenuation of urine is essentially that of simple fluid ($\leq$10 HU). CT attenuation values of lymphoceles are also those of simple fluid. By comparison, the attenuation of hematoma is usually greater than 30 to 40 HU. At MR imaging, leaked urine demonstrates predominantly low T1 signal intensity and predominantly high T2 signal intensity. Signal intensity may be heterogeneous because of the presence of debris (**Fig. 5**). Lymphoceles also demonstrate predominantly low T1 signal intensity and predominantly high T2 signal intensity. By comparison, the signal intensity of a hematoma varies based on the age of the blood products. Subacute and chronic blood products or proteinaceous debris typically demonstrate intrinsic T1 bright signal at precontrast MR imaging.

If the patient's renal function allows, contrast-enhanced CT or MR imaging with acquisition of delayed images (5–20 minutes after injection of contrast material) can be used to noninvasively establish a diagnosis of urine leak because excreted contrast material is visible accumulating in the collection (see **Fig. 5**). Alternatively, nuclear medicine studies with ^{99m}Tc can be used to noninvasively diagnose a urine leak in individuals with contraindications to iodine- and gadolinium-based intravenous contrast media.[19,41,42] These radiopharmaceuticals are excreted by the renal transplant into the renal transplant collecting system.

Accurate identification of the site of the leak and leak size is important for optimal patient management. Small defects in the collecting system or ureter may be managed with retrograde stent placement to allow for healing.[39] Larger leaks originating from the ureter may warrant ureteral reimplantation, ureteroureterostomy, and/or nephrostomy tube placement.[39] Small bladder leaks may be treated with catheter drainage to allow for bladder healing.[39] Larger bladder leaks may warrant primary repair.[39] Most urine leaks are treated successfully. In rare cases, patients have died because of sepsis related to a urine leak.[39] An enlarging peritransplant fluid collection or a

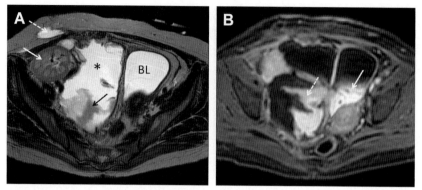

Fig. 5. Urine leak. (*A*) Axial T2-weighted image demonstrates a large area of fluid bright signal intensity (*asterisk*) with dependent debris (*black arrow*) located along the medial aspect of the patient's right lower quadrant renal transplant (*solid white arrow*). Fluid is also present in the subcutaneous tissues (*dashed arrow*). The urinary bladder (BL) is deviated leftward. (*B*) Axial T1-weighted postcontrasted image obtained approximately 20 minutes after administration of intravenous contrast material demonstrates excreted contrast material in the urinary bladder (*solid arrow*) and also in the pelvic collection (*dashed arrow*).

collection that is causing mass effect on the kidney or collecting system is typically drained, often percutaneously and with imaging guidance. Checking the creatinine level in the aspirated fluid can rule in or rule out a diagnosis of urinoma.

Urinary obstruction

Urinary obstruction may be either primary or secondary. Primary obstruction is defined as obstruction related to a primary collecting system stricture. Secondary obstruction is caused by extrinsic compression, most commonly from a fluid collection or crossing vessel. Ureteral strictures occur in 2.6% to 6.5% of patients following transplant.[39,40] Primary ureteral obstruction may present early in the recovery period if related to anatomic or technical factors.[39] By comparison, ureteral obstruction related to ischemia becomes clinically evident at a median of 6 months.[39]

At ultrasound, hydronephrosis appears as a dilated renal collecting system (**Fig. 6**). Acquiring images with color Doppler imaging is important to avoid mistaking hilar vasculature for a dilated collecting system. Both a dilated pelvicalyceal system and renal hilar vasculature appear anechoic at gray-scale ultrasound. Only hilar vessels fill with color at color Doppler imaging. Another potential pitfall is mistaking parapelvic renal cysts for hydronephrosis. When adjusting the plane of imaging, parapelvic renal cysts appear as discrete rounded structures. By comparison, a dilated renal collecting system appears as connected and relatively tubular anechoic structures (see **Fig. 6**). The dilated ureter should be traced all the way to its insertion into the urinary bladder to try to determine the site and cause of obstruction (**Fig. 7**). Identification of a ureteral jet within the bladder indicates that the ureteral obstruction is not complete. A high-resistance

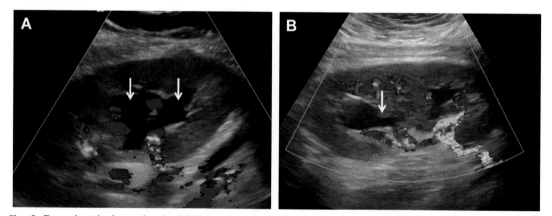

Fig. 6. Transplant hydronephrosis. (*A*) Color Doppler image demonstrates anechoic rounded structures in the renal sinus (*arrows*). (*B*) Color Doppler image in a slightly different plane demonstrates a tubular morphology of these anechoic spaces (*arrow*) indicating hydronephrosis.

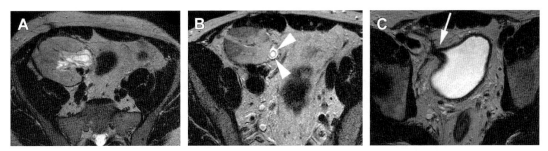

Fig. 7. Ureteral stricture. (A) Axial T2-weighted image demonstrates mild to moderate transplant hydronephrosis with urothelial edema. (B) Axial T2-weighted image demonstrates mild to moderate hydroureter, also with urothelial edema (*arrowheads*). (C) Axial T2-weighted image at the level of the urinary bladder demonstrates tethering of the ureter at the ureterovessicular anastomosis (*arrow*).

waveform with an elevated resistive index and even reversal of diastolic flow can also be seen with obstruction. Resistive index is defined as (PSV - end diastolic velocity)/PSV.

Stenting may be adequate treatment of some patients.[39] In one series of 46 patients with strictures, 33 ultimately required operative repair, most commonly ureteral reimplantation.[39]

Renal Parenchymal Complications

Renal parenchymal complications include delayed graft function, acute tubular necrosis, rejection (hyperacute, acute, or chronic), and damage caused by nephrotoxic drugs. These complications are generally not distinguishable based on imaging, and the role of imaging is to rule out other potentially treatable causes of renal transplant dysfunction including vascular and collecting

system abnormalities. Transplant biopsy may be performed to establish a diagnosis.

Delayed graft function is defined as the need for dialysis within 1 week following transplant.[43] Delayed graft function occurs in 20% to 30% of recipients of cadaveric renal transplants and is thought to be related to cold ischemia time.[44,45] Acute tubular necrosis is a potential cause of delayed graft function.[46] Many patients who experience delayed graft function eventually regain function of the renal transplant. However, recipients who experience delayed graft function have a 41% increased risk of graft loss compared with those who do not experience delayed graft function.[47]

Hyperacute rejection is identified immediately in the operating room at time of initial transplant perfusion and appears as abrupt cessation of transplant perfusion caused at the histologic level

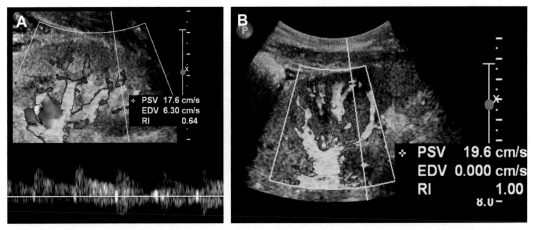

Fig. 8. Acute rejection. (A) Spectral evaluation performed on postoperative Day 1 following renal transplantation demonstrates a normal waveform in an interlobar artery with a resistive index of 0.64 The patient then experienced a marked decline in urine output. (B) Follow-up ultrasound on postoperative Day 3 demonstrates a markedly abnormal high-resistance waveform with no diastolic flow and a resistive index of 1.0. The patient underwent biopsy, which revealed acute cellular rejection.

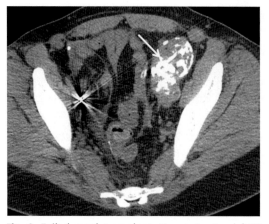

Fig. 9. Failed renal transplant. Noncontrast axial CT image demonstrates a partially calcified mass (*arrow*) in the left iliac fossa reflecting a failed renal transplant that has atrophied and partially calcified.

by small vessel thrombosis and cortical ischemia.[48] Hyperacutely rejected kidneys are not salvageable and are explanted. Acute rejection may present in the immediate postoperative period with deteriorating transplant function and occurs in up to 33% of transplant recipients.[49] Chronic rejection is a cause of the slow deterioration in renal function experienced by many transplant recipients.[50,51] Other medical causes of deteriorating renal function include chronic allograft nephropathy, antibody-mediated microcirculation injury, drug toxicity related to immunosuppressive agents, and recurrent medical renal disease.[50–53]

At ultrasound, elevated resistive indices greater than 0.80 may be seen with rejection and other medical renal diseases (**Fig. 8**).[54,55] Elevated resistive indices are a nonspecific finding that is seen in other conditions including ureteral obstruction, renal vein thrombosis, and extrinsic compression on the transplant.[56] The diagnosis of rejection is established by tissue sampling and is treated by titrating immunosuppressive agents, often with a corticosteroid burst for acute rejection. Other etiologies of medical renal disease also are typically diagnosed by biopsy, and treatment is usually medical management. Ultimately, medical renal disease or rejection may be a cause of transplant loss. Over time, nonfunctional renal transplants slowly atrophy and calcify. A failed renal transplant may appear as a calcified mass at CT (**Fig. 9**).

Peritransplant Collections

The most common peritransplant collections are hematoma, lymphocele, and urinoma.

Hematoma

Peritransplant hematomas are common in the early postoperative period. Small hematomas may be detected incidentally at imaging. Large hematomas may result in patient pain. At ultrasound, blood products appear as a heterogeneous perinephric collection (**Fig. 10**). At CT, a peritransplant hematoma appears as peritransplant fluid with an attenuation value greater than 30 to 40 HU. At MR imaging, the signal intensity of hematomas is typically heterogeneous and varies somewhat based on the age of the blood products. Hematomas may demonstrate areas of low to high T1 and T2 signal intensity.

Small hematomas that are not resulting in deleterious mass effect on the transplanted kidney are typically observed and resolve without

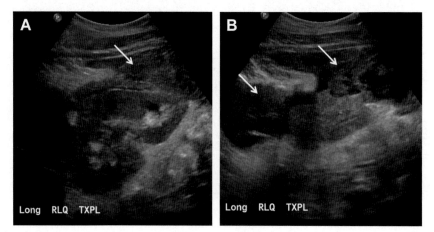

Fig. 10. Perinephric hematoma. (*A*) Gray-scale ultrasound demonstrates heterogeneous material (*arrow*) around the renal transplant compatible with blood products. (*B*) Additional gray-scale image demonstrates additional heterogeneous material (*arrows*) around the renal transplant.

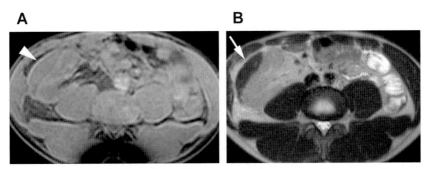

Fig. 11. Subcapsular hematoma. (*A*) T1-weighted image demonstrates a small to moderate subcapsular hematoma demonstrating intermediate T1 signal (*arrowhead*). (*B*) Axial T2-weighted image demonstrates corresponding low T2 signal in the hematoma (*arrow*).

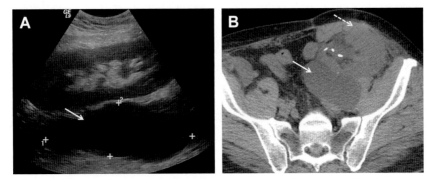

Fig. 12. Lymphocele. (*A*) Gray-scale ultrasound image demonstrates a 13-cm predominantly anechoic cystic structure (*arrow*) along the posterior aspect of the renal transplant. No blood flow was seen in this structure at color Doppler imaging (not shown). (*B*) Axial noncontrast CT image demonstrates a well-circumscribed low-attenuation structure (*solid arrow*) along the posterior aspect of the renal transplant (*dashed arrow*).

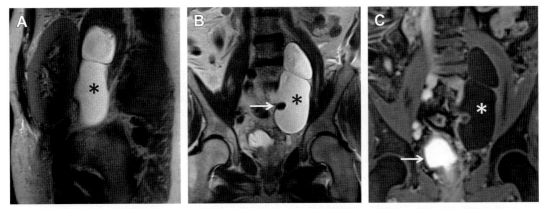

Fig. 13. Lymphocele. (*A*) Sagittal T2-weighted MR imaging demonstrates a tubular area of fluid bright signal (*asterisk*) along the posterior aspect of the renal transplant. (*B*) Coronal T2-weighted image demonstrates encasement of the left common iliac vein (*arrow*) by the lymphocele (*asterisk*). (*C*) Coronal T1-weighted postcontrast image demonstrates excreted contrast material in the urinary bladder (*arrow*). The lymphocele (*asterisk*) demonstrates low T1 signal intensity (*asterisk*) and does not contain excreted contrast material.

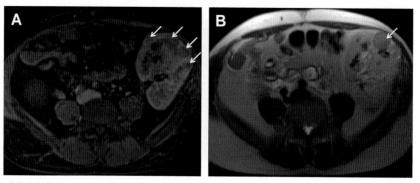

Fig. 14. PTLD. (*A*) Axial T1-weighted postcontrast image of a left lower quadrant renal transplant demonstrates multiple hypoenhancing masses (*arrows*). Tissue sampling revealed PTLD. (*B*) Axial T2-weighted image demonstrates intermediate to low signal in the dominant lesion (*arrow*).

intervention. Percutaneous drainage of a hematoma is generally not advisable because typically clotted blood products do not drain adequately through percutaneous drainage catheters.[57] Additionally, percutaneous drainage may result in infection of a previously sterile hematoma.[57]

Peritransplant hematomas should be distinguished from subcapsular hematomas (**Fig. 11**). Subcapsular hematomas may occur following trauma or transplant biopsy. Subcapsular hematomas appear as an area of blood products that exerts mass effect on the underlying renal parenchyma (see **Fig. 11**). This mass effect may result in hypertension.[58] Subcapsular hematomas typically resolve on their own.[58]

Lymphocele

Lymphoceles form from leakage of lymph from recipient lymphatic channels.[59] Symptomatic lymphoceles develop in 3.3% of patients following renal transplant.[60] Lymphoceles may result in pain in the area of the graft or ipsilateral lower extremity or scrotal edema.[60] Additionally, lymphoceles may result in impaired graft function and/or hydronephrosis.[61]

At ultrasound, lymphoceles appear hypoechoic to anechoic (**Fig. 12**) and may be septated.[62] At CT and MR imaging, lymphoceles appear as well-circumscribed areas of simple fluid attenuation ($\leq$10 HU at CT) (see **Fig. 12**) or fluid signal (low T1 signal intensity and high T2 signal intensity at MR imaging) (**Fig. 13**).

Small, asymptomatic lymphoceles may resolve on their own and may be observed with follow-up imaging. Management options for a symptomatic lymphocele include percutaneous drainage and surgical drainage with fenestration.[60] Percutaneous drainage is associated with a 30% recurrence rate and a 17% rate of infection.[61] Following surgical drainage with fenestration,

lymphoceles recurred in 7% of patients and recurred an average of 7 months following initial surgery in one series.[60]

Urinoma

Urinomas result from a collecting system or bladder injury. The imaging findings of urinoma were discussed previously.

Miscellaneous Complications

Posttransplant lymphoproliferative disorder

Posttransplant lymphoproliferative disorder (PTLD) results primarily from decreased levels of immunosurveillance caused by immunosuppressive agents in patients following transplantation.[63] Most cases are attributed to Epstein-Barr virus.[63] At imaging, PTLD may appear as a solid mass or multiple masses with or without associated lymphadenopathy (**Fig. 14**).[63] When PTLD occurs following renal transplantation, the most common sites of involvement are the gastrointestinal tract, central nervous system, and kidneys.[64]

PTLD can range from a relatively benign lymphoid hyperplasia to aggressive lymphoma. Tissue sampling is required to establish the subtype and guide management.[63] Treatment of PTLD is usually initially reduction in immunosuppressive regimens. Chemotherapeutic agents may be required for some forms of PTLD.

SUMMARY

Many treatable renal transplant complications are diagnosed with imaging. Ultrasound is typically the initial imaging modality used to evaluate vascular patency, the collecting system, and for perinephric fluid collections. CT, MR imaging, and nuclear medicine studies play a complimentary role. Accurate diagnosis of renal transplant complications is important because many complications are potentially treatable if detected early.

REFERENCES

1. World Health Organization. Available at: http://www.who.int/transplantation/gkt/statistics/en/. Accessed May 25, 2015.

2. Organ Procurement and Transplantation Network. 2015. Available at: http://optn.transplant.hrsa.gov/converge/latestData/rptData.asp. Accessed May 25, 2015.

3. Kasiske BL, Vazquez MA, Harmon WE, et al. Recommendations for the outpatient surveillance of renal transplant recipients. J Am Soc Nephrol 2000;11: S1–86.

4. Matheus WE, Reis LO, Ferreira U, et al. Kidney transplant anastomosis: internal or external iliac artery? Urol J 2009;6:260–6.

5. Aydin C, Berber I, Altaca G, et al. The outcome of kidney transplants with multiple renal arteries. BMC Surg 2004;4:4.

6. Mangus RS, Haag BW. Stented versus nonstented extravesical ureteroneocystostomy in renal transplantation: a metaanalysis. Am J Transplant 2004; 4:1889–96.

7. Watson CJE, Harper SJF. Anatomical variation and its management in transplantation. Am J Transplant 2015;15:1459–71.

8. ACR-AIUM-SPR-SRU practice parameter for the performance of an ultrasound examination of solid organ transplants. 2014. Available at: http://www.acr.org/~/media/89C78E344D454E98AF39187781FD864B.pdf. Accessed June 1, 2015.

9. Quaia E. Microbubble ultrasound contrast agents: an update. Eur Radiol 2007;17:1995–2008.

10. Schwenger V, Korosoglou G, Hinkel UP, et al. Real-time contrast-enhanced sonography of renal transplant recipients predicts chronic allograft nephropathy. Am J Transplant 2006;6:609–15.

11. Paudice N, Zanazzi M, Agostini S, et al. Contrast-enhanced ultrasound assessment of complex cystic lesions in renal transplant recipients with acquired cystic kidney disease: preliminary experience. Transplant Proc 2012;44:1928–9.

12. Ozkan F, Yavuz YC, Inci MF, et al. Interobserver variability of ultrasound elastography in transplant kidneys: correlations with clinical-Doppler parameters. Ultrasound Med Biol 2013;39:4–9.

13. Grenier N, Poulain S, Lepreux S, et al. Quantitative elastography of renal transplants using supersonic shear imaging: a pilot study. Eur Radiol 2012;22: 2138–46.

14. Lukenda V, Mikolasevic I, Racki S, et al. Transient elastography: a new noninvasive diagnostic tool for assessment of chronic allograft nephropathy. Int Urol Nephrol 2014;46:1435–40.

15. Gleeson TG, Bulugahapitiya S. Contrast-induced nephropathy. AJR Am J Roentgenol 2004;183: 1673–89.

16. Stacul F, van der Molen AJ, Reimer P, et al. Contrast induced nephropathy: updated ESUR contrast media safety committee guidelines. Eur Radiol 2011; 21:2527–41.

17. ACR Manual on Contrast Media Version 9. ACR committee on drugs and contrast media. Available at: http://www.acr.org/~/media/ACR/Documents/PDF/QualitySafety/Resources/Contrast%20Manual/2013_Contrast_Media.pdf. Accessed May 20, 2015.

18. Ulusan S, Koc Z, Tokmak N. Accuracy of sonography for detecting renal stone: comparison with CT. J Clin Ultrasound 2007;35(5):256–61.

19. Goldfarb CR, Srivastava NC, Grotas AB, et al. Radionuclide imaging in urology. Urol Clin North Am 2006;33:319–28.

20. Hurst FP, Abbott KC, Neff RT, et al. Incidence, predictors and outcomes of transplant renal artery stenosis after kidney transplantation: analysis of USRDS. Am J Nephrol 2009;30:459–67.

21. Polak WG, Jezior D, Garcarek J, et al. Incidence and outcome of transplant renal artery stenosis: single center experience. Transplant Proc 2006;38:31–2.

22. Halimi JM, Al-Najjar A, Buchler M, et al. Transplant renal artery stenosis: potential role of ischemia/reperfusion injury and long-term outcome following angioplasty. J Urol 1999;161:28–32.

23. Patel NH, Jindal RM, Wilkin T, et al. Renal arterial stenosis in renal allografts: retrospective study of predisposing factors and outcomes after percutaneous transluminal angioplasty. Radiology 2001;219:663–7.

24. Fervenza FC, Lafayette RA, Alfrey EJ, et al. Renal artery stenosis in kidney transplants. Am J Kidney Dis 1998;31:142–8.

25. Dimitroulis D, Bokos J, Zavos G, et al. Vascular complications in renal transplantation: a single-center experience in 1367 renal transplantations and review of the literature. Transplant Proc 2009;41: 1609–14.

26. Orlic P, Vukas D, Drescik I, et al. Vascular complications after 725 kidney transplantations during 3 decades. Transplant Proc 2003;35:1381–4.

27. Baxter GM, Ireland H, Moss JG, et al. Colour Doppler ultrasound in renal transplant artery stenosis: which Doppler index? Clin Radiol 1995;50: 618–22.

28. de Morais RH, Muglia VF, Mamere AE, et al. Duplex Doppler sonography of transplant renal artery stenosis. J Clin Ultrasound 2003;31:135–41.

29. Biederman DM, Fischman AM, Titano JJ, et al. Tailoring of endovascular management of transplant renal artery stenosis. Am J Transplant 2015;15: 1039–49.

30. Osman Y, Shokeir A, Ali-El-Dein B, et al. Vascular complications after live donor renal transplantation: study of risk factors and effects on graft and patient survival. J Urol 2003;169:859–62.

31. Rouviere O, Berger P, Beziat C, et al. Acute thrombosis of renal artery: graft salvage by means of intra-arterial fibrinolysis. Transplantation 2002;73:403–9.

32. Groggel CG. Acute thrombosis of the renal transplant artery: a case report and review of the literature. Clin Nephrol 1991;36:42–5.

33. Klepanec A, Balazs T, Bazik R, et al. Pharmacomechanical thrombectomy for treatment of acute transplant renal artery thrombosis. Ann Vasc Surg 2014;28:1314.

34. Sterrett SP, Mercer D, Johanning J, et al. Salvage of renal allograft using venous thrombectomy in the setting of iliofemoral venous thrombosis. Nephrol Dial Transplant 2004;19:1637–9.

35. Dodd GD III, Tublin ME, Shah A, et al. Imaging of vascular complications associated with renal transplants. AJR Am J Roentgenol 1991;157:449–59.

36. Mahmoud MZ, Al-Saadi M, Abuderman A, et al. "To-and-fro" waveform in the diagnosis of arterial pseudoaneurysms. World J Radiol 2015;28(7):89–99.

37. LaBerge JM. Interventional management of renal transplant arteriovenous fistula. Semin Intervent Radiol 2004;21:239–46.

38. Dominguez J, Clase C, Mahalati K, et al. Is routine ureteric stenting needed in kidney transplantation? A randomized trial. Transplantation 2000;70:597–601.

39. Streeter EH, Little DM, Cranston DW, et al. The urological complications of renal transplantation: a series of 1535 patients. BJU Int 2002;90:627–34.

40. Rahnemai-Azar AA, Gilchrist BF, Kayler LK. Independent risk factors for early urologic complications after kidney transplantation. Clin Transplant 2015;29:403–8.

41. Titton RL, Gervais DA, Hahn PF, et al. Urine leaks and urinomas: diagnosis and imaging-guided intervention. Radiographics 2003;23:1133–47.

42. Jiang M, Gandikota N, Ames SA, et al. Identification of urologic complications after kidney transplant. Am J Kidney Dis 2011;58:150–3.

43. Humar A, Ramcharan T, Kandaswamy R, et al. Risk factors for slow graft function after kidney transplants: a multivariate analysis. Clin Transplant 2002;16(6):425–9.

44. Ojo AO, Wolfe RA, Held PJ, et al. Delayed graft function: risk factors and implications for renal allograft survival. Transplantation 1997;63:968–74.

45. Troppmann C, Gillingham KJ, Benedetti E, et al. Delayed graft function, acute rejection, and outcome after cadaver renal transplantation. The multivariate analysis. Transplantation 1995;59:962–8.

46. Olsen S, Burdick JF, Keown PA, et al. Primary acute renal failure ("acute tubular necrosis") in the transplanted kidney: morphology and pathogenesis. Medicine (Baltimore) 1989;68:173–87.

47. Yarlagadda SG, Coca SG, Formica RN Jr, et al. Association between delayed graft function and allograft and patient survival: a systematic review and meta-analysis. Nephrol Dial Transplant 2009;4:1039–47.

48. Williams GM, Hume DM, Hudson PH Jr, et al. "Hyperacute" renal-homograft rejection in man. N Engl J Med 1968;279:611–8.

49. Pallardo Mateu LM, Sancho Calabuig A, Capdevila Plaza L, et al. Acute rejection and late renal transplant failure: risk factors and prognosis. Nephrol Dial Transplant 2004;19(Suppl 3):iii38–42.

50. Einecke G, Sis B, Reeve J, et al. Antibody-mediated microcirculation injury is the major cause of late kidney transplant failure. Am J Transplant 2009;9:2520–31.

51. Halloran PF, Langone AJ, Helderman JH, et al. Assessing long-term nephron loss: is it time to kick the CAN grading system? Am J Transplant 2004;4:1729–30.

52. Sellares J, de Freitas DG, Mengel M, et al. Understanding the causes of kidney transplant failure: the dominant role of antibody-mediated rejection and nonadherence. Am J Transplant 2012;12:388–99.

53. Morales JM, Andres A, Rengel M, et al. Influence of cyclosporine, tacrolimus, and rapamycin on renal function and arterial hypertension after renal transplantation. Nephrol Dial Transplant 2001;16:121–4.

54. Rifkin MD, Needleman L, Pasto ME, et al. Evaluation of renal transplant rejection by duplex Doppler examination: value of the resistive index. AJR Am J Roentgenol 1987;148:759–62.

55. Wollenberg K, Waibel B, Pisarski P, et al. Careful clinical monitoring in comparison to sequential Doppler sonography for the detection of acute rejection in the early phase after renal transplantation. Transpl Int 2000;13:S45–51.

56. Tublin ME, Bude RO, Platt JF. The resistive index in renal Doppler sonography: where do we stand? AJR Am J Roentgenol 2003;180:885–92.

57. Akbar SA, Jafri SZH, Amendola MA, et al. Complications of renal transplantation. Radiographics 2005;25:1335–56.

58. Machida J, Kitani K, Inadome A, et al. Subcapsular hematoma and hypertension following percutaneous needle biopsy of a transplanted kidney. Int J Urol 1996;3:228–30.

59. Howard RJ, Simmons RL, Najarian JS. Prevention of lymphoceles following renal transplantation. Ann Surg 1976;184:166–8.

60. Fuller TF, Kang S-M, Hirose R, et al. Management of lymphoceles after renal transplantation: laparoscopic versus open drainage. J Urol 2003;169:2022–5.

61. Bischof G, Rockenschaub S, Berlakovich G, et al. Management of lymphoceles after kidney transplantation. Transpl Int 1998;11:277–80.

62. Silver TM, Campbell D, Wicks JD, et al. Peritransplant fluid collections. Ultrasound evaluation and clinical significance. Radiology 1981; 138:145–51.

63. Camacho JC, Moreno CC, Harri PA, et al. Posttransplantation lymphoproliferative disease: proposed imaging classification. Radiographics 2014;34: 2025–38.

64. Opelz G, Naujokat C, Daniel V, et al. Disassociation between risk of graft loss and risk of non-Hodgkin lymphoma with induction agents in renal transplant recipients. Transplantation 2006;81:1227–33.

Imaging of Pancreas Transplantation and Its Complications

Ryan B. O'Malley, MD[a], Mariam Moshiri, MD[a,*],
Sherif Osman, MD[a], Christine O. Menias, MD[b],
Douglas S. Katz, MD[c]

KEYWORDS

- Pancreas transplant • Complications • Rejection • Pancreatitis • Vascular thrombosis
- Pancreas kidney transplant

KEY POINTS

- Anatomic detail of pancreatic transplantation is complex and requires consideration of endocrine and exocrine drainage of the pancreatic graft.
- The venous drainage can be via a systemic pathway or portal pathway, whereas the exocrine drainage can be through the bladder or enteric pathways.
- Pancreatic transplantation is associated with several complications, which could be related to vasculature, the pancreatic parenchyma, or related to other surgical factors.

INTRODUCTION

Whole organ pancreas transplantation is an accepted and valid therapeutic option for patients with insulin-dependent diabetes mellitus (type 1 and type 2), or patients who have undergone prior total pancreatectomy. By eliminating the need for daily glucose monitoring and insulin administration, pancreas transplantation can significantly improve quality of life, while also preventing life-threatening complications associated with hypoglycemic unawareness (lack of warning symptoms associated with hypoglycemia). Moreover, transplantation is the only long-term treatment of diabetic patients that can attain insulin-free euglycemia, and prevent, reverse, or delay the onset of end-organ complications such as retinopathy, nephropathy, and coronary artery disease.[1] For patients with diabetes and renal insufficiency, combining pancreas and kidney transplant has also been shown to increase long-term survival.[2]

Approximately 80% of pancreas transplants are performed as simultaneous pancreas-kidney (SPK) transplants; however, they can also be performed successfully as pancreas after kidney (PAK) transplants or as pancreas transplant alone (PTA).[1] SPK transplant is ideal for most patients, particularly those younger than 55 with renal insufficiency, resulting in better graft success due to the ability to use serum creatinine to concurrently monitor both transplants for rejection.[3] PAK transplant offers the ability to perform a living donor renal transplant followed by a deceased donor pancreas transplant, thus reducing time spent on the transplant waiting list for 2 organs. PTA is only appropriate for a minority of patients who have severe hypoglycemic unawareness and preserved renal function. Patients who have SPK transplantation have improved 10-year survival compared with diabetic patients receiving kidney transplantation alone, with 23.4 years versus 12.9 years, respectively.[4]

[a] Department of Radiology, University of Washington Medical Center, Seattle, WA, USA; [b] Department of Radiology, Mayo Clinic, Scottsdale, AZ, USA; [c] Department of Radiology, Winthrop-University Hospital, Mineola, NY, USA
* Corresponding author.
E-mail address: Moshiri@uw.edu

Radiol Clin N Am 54 (2016) 251–266
http://dx.doi.org/10.1016/j.rcl.2015.09.012

During graft procurement, the pancreas is removed along with a variable length of intact duodenal C-loop. Because the gastroduodenal artery is usually divided during liver procurement, pancreas transplant arterial supply primarily consists of the superior mesenteric artery and splenic artery and their branches.[2] To perform the arterial reconstruction, the donor iliac artery bifurcation is most commonly procured simultaneously for vascular reconstruction as a Y graft. The donor common iliac artery (stem of the Y graft) is anastomosed end-to-side to the recipient common iliac artery, while the donor internal and external iliac arteries (limbs of the Y graft) are anastomosed end-to-end to the stumps of the splenic and superior mesenteric arteries of the transplanted pancreas (Fig. 1).

Venous drainage of the pancreas transplant consists of intrapancreatic tributaries that drain into the splenic vein, superior mesenteric vein, and portal vein.[2] The donor portal vein can be anastomosed to the recipient inferior vena cava or iliac vein (systemic drainage), or the superior mesenteric vein (portal drainage). Bypassing the liver in systemic venous drainage can result in systemic hyperinsulinemia, which is thought to adversely affect lipid metabolism and predispose patients to accelerated atherosclerosis, although this has never been shown to be induced by a pancreas transplant or to result in higher cardiovascular mortality.[3,5] By mimicking native pancreatic venous drainage and preserving hepatic first-pass insulin clearance, the portal drainage technique has been purported to be more physiologic but has not been shown to result in better long-term outcomes regarding graft survival, function, rejection rate, or metabolic profile[5,6] (Fig. 2). As such, the technique is dictated by donor and recipient anatomy in conjunction with the individual surgeon's preference[1] (Fig. 3).

Historically, pancreas transplants used the bladder for exocrine drainage via a duodenocystostomy.[7] Bladder drainage offers several advantages, including the ability to assess graft exocrine function by measuring urinary amylase and also access for cystoscopic biopsy. However, this nonphysiologic communication also results in complications due to the inflammatory nature of pancreatic enzymes. These complications include chemical cystitis, hematuria, metabolic acidosis, leak from the duodenal segment, recurrent urinary tract infections, urethritis, and urethral strictures.[8] As a result, nearly 90% of pancreas transplants now use enteric drainage with the donor duodenum anastomosed to a nonexcluded loop of recipient small bowel or a Roux limb.[1] If the pancreas is taken from a live donor, it is divided at the neck, and the donor splenic artery is anastomosed end-to-side to the recipient iliac artery, and the donor splenic vein is anastomosed to the recipient iliac vein (Table 1).

Imaging assessment of a pancreatic transplant requires a thorough understanding of these surgical techniques and the postoperative anatomy, as well as knowledge of the postoperative complications.[9,10] To properly evaluate the graft, radiologists must also recognize that the position of the pancreas transplant varies depending on the surgical technique. Pancreas transplants are most commonly placed intraperitoneally into the right pelvis, whereas the kidney is typically placed extraperitoneally into the left iliac fossa.[2] Grafts using systemic venous drainage are typically placed obliquely with the head inferior to the body and tail, whereas portal venous drainage most commonly requires the head-tail positioning to be reversed and more vertically oriented.[2]

Ultrasonography (US) is the usual first-line imaging modality for evaluation of the transplanted pancreas and its associated vasculature. A complete examination includes grayscale and duplex Doppler imaging. The normal graft on grayscale US should have a homogenous echotexture usually lower than that of the native pancreas and the surrounding fatty tissue[11] (Fig. 4). However, the position of the pancreatic transplant makes

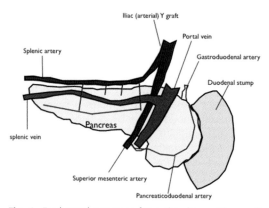

Fig. 1. Explanted pancreas from the donor. The graft is prepared in sterile lactated Ringer at 4-degrees Celsius. Excess tissue, especially fat, is separated from the pancreatic graft. The pancreatic head is supplied by the inferior pancreaticoduodenal artery via the superior mesenteric artery (SMA), and the body and tail are supplied by the splenic artery. The Y graft is connected to SMA and celiac artery proximally to provide a single common arterial conduit to be grafted to the recipient iliac artery. Venous drainage will be established via a portion of the harvested donor portal vein, which connects the superior mesenteric vein (SMV) and splenic vein.

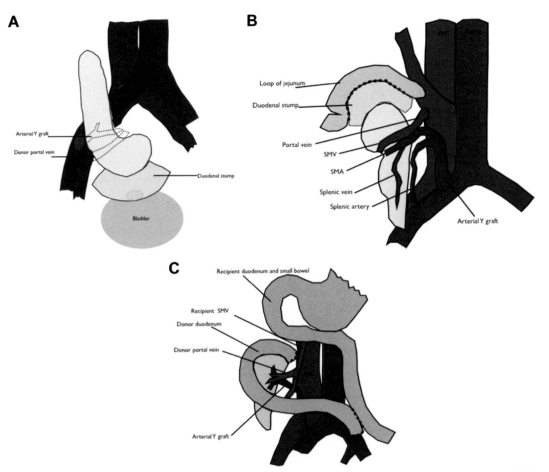

Fig. 2. Various surgical techniques for pancreatic graft implantation. The exocrine and venous drainage of the pancreatic transplant can each be handled in 2 ways. (*A*) Bladder drainage used for PAK transplantation. The second portion of the duodenum is anastomosed in a side-to-side fashion to the bladder dome to facilitate the pancreatic exocrine drainage. The donor portal vein is attached to the recipient external iliac vein. A donor iliac artery Y graft, composed of the donor common iliac artery and the branch points of the internal and external iliac arteries (anastomosed to the explanted SMA and splenic arteries of the pancreas), is anastomosed to the recipient iliac artery. (*B*) Portal-enteric drainage pathway. The second portion of the duodenum is anastomosed to the recipient small bowel via a Roux-en-Y technique. The arterial Y graft (as described earlier) is anastomosed to the recipient iliac artery (common or external) and the SMV is anastomosed to the recipient iliac vein. (*C*) Systemic-enteric drainage pathway. In this variant enteric pathway, the duodenum is anastomosed in a side-to-side fashion to a loop of small bowel (without the Roux-en-Y loop) while the donor portal vein is anastomosed to the recipient portal vein. Using native small bowel allows for endoscopic access and surveillance but carries higher risk for the native small bowel if graft complications develop or if explantation is required. IVC, inferior vena cava; SMA, superior mesenteric artery; SMV, superior mesenteric vein.

sonographic evaluation more limited due to overlying bowel gas, thus computed tomography (CT) or MR imaging may subsequently be required.[12]

CT allows for examination of the graft's parenchyma, vasculature, and enteric anastomosis. The CT examination should be multiphasic, acquired during the arterial and venous phases, to optimally assess the arterial and venous supply and parenchymal enhancement (or lack thereof). CT can also be used to assess for perigraft fluid collections, inflammation, bowel leak, and bowel obstruction. Normal graft tissue should demonstrate homogeneous enhancement with intravenous (IV) contrast (**Fig. 5**).

MR imaging is reserved for select patients in whom complete evaluation with US or CT is not possible or younger patients in whom cumulative radiation risk is a concern. MR angiography (MRA) can help provide an accurate assessment of vascular abnormalities, and MR cholangiopancreatography (MRCP) can help to delineate ductal abnormalities.[13]

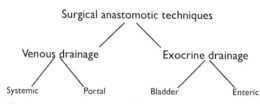

Fig. 3. Various surgical techniques for pancreas transplantation drainage pathways. There are 2 major drainage pathways for the surgeon to handle. The exocrine drainage can be routed to the bladder or to the enteric system, whereas the venous drainage can be routed to the systemic vasculature or a portal venous pathway. Because various options are available to the transplant surgeon, he or she can choose any combination of the options for each category.

The use of both iodinated and gadolinium-based contrast material may be precluded by recovering renal insufficiency in SPK transplants.[5] For these patients, noncontrast MR imaging with or without MRCP is preferred over noncontrast CT. Digital subtraction conventional angiography can be used when necessary for confirmation of vascular abnormalities or when endovascular therapy is needed.[12]

Although pancreatic transplants reportedly have higher rates of postoperative complications compared with other organ transplants, clinical diagnosis is difficult due to lack of reliable laboratory markers for graft function.[14,15] Therefore, the radiologist must be familiar with the spectrum of surgical techniques and the normal postoperative cross-sectional imaging appearances of the whole-pancreas transplant to be able to recognize abnormal postoperative findings.

COMPLICATIONS

Given the complexity of the anatomy and surgical technique related to pancreatic transplantation, postoperative complications can have various causes.

Vascular Complications

Vascular complications are the most common cause of early graft failure. Thrombosis (arterial and venous), the most common technical cause

Table 1
More commonly used surgical techniques for pancreas transplantation

Technique	Advantages	Disadvantage
Systemic-enteric*	• More physiologic • Fewer metabolic imbalances because pancreatic secretions are reabsorbed into the system	• Infections due to anastomotic leak and enteric contamination • Sepsis secondary to fistula or abscess formation • Vascular thrombosis • Complications necessitate more invasive procedures to correct
Portal-enteric*	• More physiologic glucose control • May help lipid profile	• Although purported to be more physiologic, has never been shown to have superior outcomes related to systemic venous drainage • Almost always requires enteric exocrine drainage • Unable to monitor urine amylase • Difficult to biopsy • Requires longer Y graft
Bladder drainage	• Allows direct measurement of graft exocrine function by measuring urine amylase • Complications treated less invasively • Easy access for cystoscopic biopsy	• Nonphysiologic communication between pancreas-duodenum and bladder • Complications warrant conversion to enteric drainage in 15%–30% • Pancreatitis • Bladder leaks • Urethritis • Urinary tract infections • Metabolic acidosis or dehydration from urinary loss of bicarbonate • Hematuria • 35% need enteric conversion

* Systemic-enteric anastomosis is the most commonly used technique, although the portal-enteric anastomotic technique is purported to be more physiologic and superior based on outcomes.

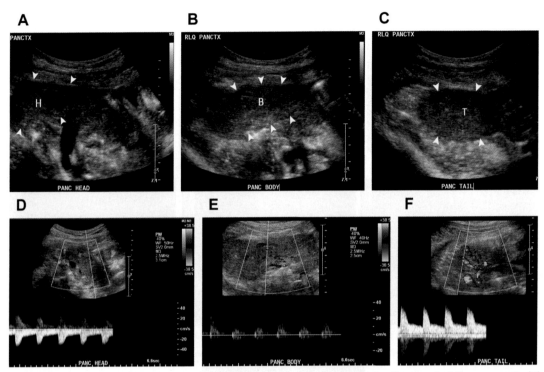

Fig. 4. Normal ultrasound appearance of the pancreatic transplant. Gray scale ultrasound of the pancreatic (*A*) head, (*B*) body, and (*C*) tail show a homogeneously hypoechoic structure relative to adjacent fatty tissue (*arrowheads*). Arterial (*D–F*) and venous (*G–I*) flow should also be assessed via Doppler ultrasound in all 3 segments of the pancreatic transplant, respectively. The splenic vein (*J, K*) and arterial Y graft (*L, M*) also require Doppler evaluation on a routine examination. B, pancreatic body; H, pancreatic head, T, pancreatic tail.

of graft dysfunction, reportedly accounts for 2% to 19% of cases.[16] In addition to thrombosis, other pancreatic transplant vascular complications can occur (**Table 2**). Cross-sectional imaging plays a crucial role because the clinical presentation and laboratory findings are frequently nonspecific and, if unsuspected, vascular dysfunction can rapidly progress to transplant failure.[16,17] Humar and colleagues,[18] in a large multivariate analysis, reported that thrombosis was the most common technical problem leading to graft loss, accounting for 52% of their cases. Percutaneous and surgical interventions may preserve graft viability but require early detection and diagnosis. Assessment for vascular complications requires accurate background knowledge regarding the type of anastomoses that have been performed to ensure comprehensive and accurate imaging assessment.

Thrombosis

Arterial and venous thrombosis affects 5% to 14% of pancreas transplants, usually within the first few weeks posttransplant, and is the most frequent serious surgical complication, predisposing patients to graft infarction, anastomotic dehiscence, bowel strictures, dysmotility, hemorrhagic pancreatitis, and infection.[17,19,20] The cause is typically multifactorial but the smaller microcirculatory blood flow has been implicated as a possible predisposition for thrombosis.[15] Reported causes include phlebitis (related to concomitant pancreatitis), rejection, venous stasis (such as from compression by a fluid collection, twisting of the venous anastomosis, or within vascular stumps), previous venous thrombosis, previous venous surgery, indwelling catheters, and systemic hypercoagulable states. Surgical causes include faulty surgical technique, malalignment or venous redundancy with resultant kinking, and donor–recipient vessel mismatch.[19] Donor risk factors include increased age, obesity, cerebrovascular disease leading to death, and hemodynamic instability requiring large volume resuscitation.[20] Among the types of pancreatic transplants, PAK, PTA, and portal-enteric drainage all have a higher risk of graft thrombosis.[20]

Thrombus can develop within the graft's superior mesenteric vein, splenic vein, or both, and can be completely or partially occlusive. Thrombosis can propagate into the recipient superior mesenteric vein (if portal venous drainage), iliac

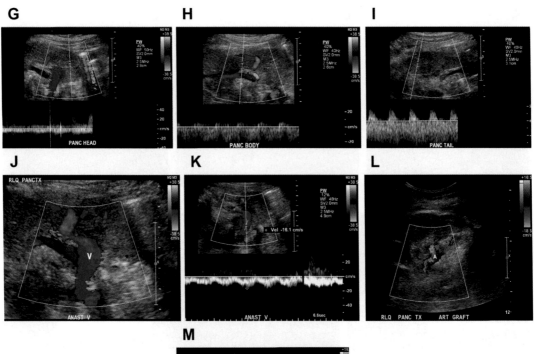

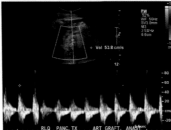

Fig. 4. (*continued*)

vein or inferior vena cava (if systemic venous drainage), or possibly even into the pulmonary arteries. Although most stump thrombi are inconsequential and are not treated, some will propagate into proximal veins and be clinically significant.[21]

The appearance of a thrombosed pancreatic transplant on grayscale ultrasound is nonspecific. Acute venous thrombosis may manifest solely as an edematous enlarged graft with heterogeneous echogenicity, similar to cases of pancreatitis and rejection, or the thrombosed vein may be expanded with an acute thrombus that is central and anechoic. Chronic thrombus is typically echogenic and eccentric.[15,22] Doppler evaluation may demonstrate absent color and spectral signal within the affected veins with high-resistance arterial waveforms demonstrating pandiastolic reversal of flow.[17,22] As isolated findings, high-resistance arterial flow and absent venous flow can both be secondary to other causes (eg, rejection or severe inflammation). However, in the first 12 days posttransplant, this constellation of findings (absent venous flow and diastolic flow reversal in the transplant arteries) has been reported to be highly sensitive and specific for venous thrombosis.[17] Of note, there is commonly mild narrowing of the donor portal vein at its anastomosis to the recipient iliac or superior mesenteric vein, with associated flattening of venous flow waveform, which can be a potential pitfall. Additionally, severe rejection or pancreatitis can result in very slow flow or stasis, which can be very difficult to sonographically distinguish from thrombosis (**Fig. 6**).

On contrast-enhanced CT and MR imaging, thrombus can be seen as a low attenuation or low signal intensity filling defect within the affected veins, possibly with decreased or absent graft enhancement if there is associated necrosis.[12] For patients who cannot receive IV contrast material, noncontrast MR imaging is preferred over noncontrast CT because unenhanced MR imaging may demonstrate increased signal on T1-weighted sequences or loss of normal flow void

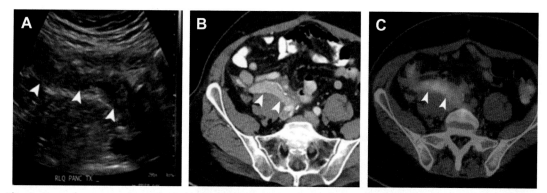

Fig. 5. Normal pancreas transplant. (*A, B*) Axial contrast-enhanced CT with correlative ultrasound image of a pancreas transplant (*arrowheads*) in the right lower quadrant. (*C*) Corresponding normal PET-CT image shows homogeneous [11F]-2-fluoro-2-deoxy-D-glucose (FDG) uptake (*arrowheads*) in the pancreas transplant parenchyma.

within the thrombosed vessel, whereas noncontrast MRA sequences can demonstrate occlusion or absent arterial flow.[15] Although noncontrast CT can be used to suggest the presence of underlying thrombus based on high-attenuation intraluminal material, thrombosis cannot be completely excluded without IV contrast material[15] (**Fig. 7**).

For selected patients with partial portal or isolated splenic venous thrombosis with preserved parenchymal function, anticoagulation can be considered to salvage the graft and to prevent propagation of the thrombus.[20] Endovascular arterial and venous interventions have also been reported for short-segment thrombosis without necrosis.[23] However, to prevent added mortality and to minimize infection-related complications, most recipients with early graft thrombosis require transplant pancreatectomy, sometimes in conjunction with immediate retransplantation.[20] To minimize the risk of graft thrombosis, most centers use routine postoperative anticoagulation, although such prophylaxis has not been proven effective in a prospective randomized fashion to the authors' knowledge.[20] As such, most efforts to prevent venous thrombosis are directed toward careful donor selection and meticulous surgical technique.

Arterial Thrombosis

Arterial thrombosis is the most severe vascular complication that often results in graft dysfunction and failure. Venous and arterial thrombosis combined affect 5% to 10% of pancreas transplants, with arterial thrombosis occurring within the donor superior mesenteric artery, splenic artery, or Y graft.[19] Arterial thrombosis usually occurs within 3 months following transplantation. Increased risk is associated with prolonged cold ischemic time, ABO incompatibility, donor-to-recipient vessel mismatch, small-caliber vessels, low-flow states, faulty surgical technique, and acute

Table 2
Complications associated with pancreatic transplantation

Vascular Complications	Graft-Related Complications	Enteric Complications
Venous thrombosis	Pancreatitis (early or late)	Anastomotic leak or abscess
Arterial thrombosis	Pseudocyst	Postoperative ileus and obstruction
Arterial anastomotic stenosis	Abscess	Typhlitis
AVF	Rejection	PTLD
Arterial dissection	—	—
Y graft kink	—	—
Collections/hematoma	—	—

Abbreviations: AVF, arteriovenous fistula; PTLD, posttransplant lymphoproliferative disorder.

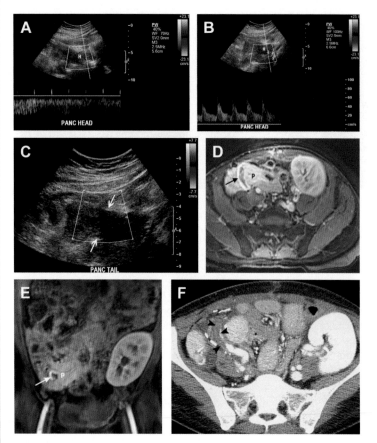

Fig. 6. Pancreatic transplant splenic vein thrombosis. A 50-year-old man presented with abnormal laboratory values. Doppler ultrasound imaging showed (A) venous and (B) arterial flow to the pancreatic head (H). (C) No venous flow to the body and tail of the graft was detected (arrows). Splenic vein thrombosis was suspected. Cather angiography showed partial thrombosis of splenic vein, which was treated with thrombolysis and angioplasty. In a different patient, (D) axial and (E) coronal T1-weighted MR with fat saturation with contrast material administration was obtained after initial ultrasound examination showed lack of flow within the graft splenic vein. MR images show initial arterial flow to the graft with subsequent lack of venous drainage due to thrombus within the splenic vein (seen as a filling defect, arrows) and resultant edematous pancreas (P). (F) Axial CT image with contrast material in a different patient shows a filling defect in the splenic vein (arrowheads). Intraoperative ultrasound (not shown) found blood clot in the vein at the level of the transplanted pancreatic head and body.

rejection.[19] Late thrombosis can occur months to years later and is typically caused by chronic rejection or infection.[9] Thrombosis is more common when portal-enteric drainage is used (compared with systemic-bladder technique), and is more common in PAK and PTA transplants compared with SPK transplants.[15]

Sonographic findings of arterial thrombosis include tardus parvus waveforms of the intrapancreatic arteries; absent arterial signal in the Y graft and the graft itself; and, if there is concomitant necrosis, heterogeneous echogenicity of the graft.[22] On CT and MR imaging, there is abrupt occlusion or cutoff at the site of thrombosis, possibly with a low-attenuation or low-signal intensity filling defect. These findings can be associated with inhomogeneous or absent parenchymal enhancement as it progresses to infarction.[12,16] Notably, these imaging findings may overlap with cases of severe arterial stenosis, diffuse graft edema, and systemic hypotension. Thrombosis within only a single allograft artery (donor superior mesenteric artery or splenic artery) may result in intrapancreatic collateral flow that maintains parenchymal

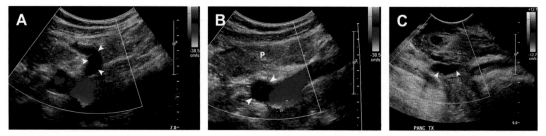

Fig. 7. Portal vein thrombosis. A 39-year-old man 1 month postpancreatic transplant presents. (A–C) Doppler ultrasound of the graft shows lack of venous flow within the transplanted portal vein (arrowheads). P, pancreas.

enhancement and function; this is most readily identified on multiphase CT or MR imaging[2,24] (Fig. 8).

Complications of arterial thrombosis include graft dysfunction and necrosis, pancreatitis, leakage of pancreatic secretions, and sepsis. If untreated, progression of parenchymal necrosis can ultimately lead to emphysematous transformation of the graft, with gas present throughout the parenchyma.[12] For most patients with early thrombosis, repeat laparotomy and transplant pancreatectomy is required.[20]

Arterial Anastomosis or Stenosis

Arterial stenosis in pancreatic transplants is relatively uncommon but if it occurs it is usually in the early postoperative period, most commonly at the site of an anastomosis.[19] Early recognition and diagnosis is critical because stenosis may lead to thrombosis, ischemia, and graft dysfunction.[19] US findings are nonspecific in the early postoperative period (within 72 hours) because stenosis can also be caused by reperfusion edema and altered global hemodynamics. Doppler findings include elevated peak systolic velocity, turbulent flow at the anastomosis, increased resistance, reversed diastolic flow, and tardus parvus waveforms of the intrapancreatic arteries (ie, with spectral broadening, resistive index (RI) <0.5, and a systolic acceleration time >80 ms).[19] Of note, in the immediate postoperative period, velocities up to 400 cm/s at the arterial anastomosis are usually transient, reflecting anastomotic edema or vascular kinking, which improves on follow-up.[25] Hemodynamically significant stenosis is suggested when velocities remain greater than 300 cm/s on follow-up imaging examinations and can be confirmed with CT angiography (CTA), MRA, or catheter angiography.[25] Patients with portal venous-enteric drainage require a longer Y graft, which may kink or twist, resulting in a specific type of stenosis (Y-graft kink).[15,24] Because US often cannot be used to assess contour changes, particularly of long vessels, CTA and MRA are best suited for diagnosis.[14] For a stenosis that is persistent and hemodynamically significant, angioplasty has been reported to be of value.[26]

Pseudoaneurysm

Pseudoaneurysms arise when there is focal disruption or laceration of the arterial wall. They are usually secondary to biopsy, pancreatitis, infection, or surgical trauma.[22,25] Anastomoses are particularly prone to pseudoaneurysm formation due to chemical damage resulting from pancreatic enzyme leakage.[9] Postbiopsy pseudoaneurysms usually occur within the parenchyma at the site of biopsy and can also result in an arteriovenous fistula (AVF).

Sonographically, pseudoaneurysms are seen as anechoic structures or fluid collections immediately adjacent to vessels, with turbulent internal flow (yin-yang appearance) on color Doppler. At the neck, where the pseudoaneurysm communicates with the parent artery, Doppler US demonstrates bidirectional flow with a to-and-fro waveform.[22] If a pseudoaneurysm is suspected on US, then CT or MR imaging is usually performed for confirmation and preprocedural planning. On CT or MR imaging, a pseudoaneurysm will appear as a saccular enhancing outpouching from the injured artery, with enhancement similar to other arteries (Fig. 9).

Endovascular management can include coil embolization or placement of a covered stent. However, a surgical aneurysmectomy is usually

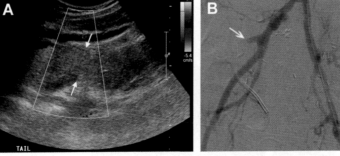

Fig. 8. Pancreatic transplant splenic arterial thrombosis. A 45-year-old man postpancreatic transplant presented with abnormal laboratory values and pain over the region of the transplant. (A) Ultrasound evaluation of the pancreatic transplant showed no detectible arterial perfusion in the transplant (arrows). A complete arterial occlusion was suspected. (B) Catheter angiography confirms complete arterial occlusion (arrow) and nonenhancement of the pancreatic transplant.

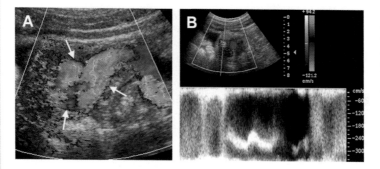

Fig. 9. Arterial pseudoaneurysm. A 42-year-old woman postpancreatic transplant. (A) Doppler ultrasound of the graft shows a pseudoaneurysm (arrows) at the level of the pancreatic head with (B) turbulent flow within the nidus.

required when there is a peritransplant abscess resulting in an infected pseudoaneurysm.[2] Rarely, a pseudoaneurysm can rupture into the donor duodenum, resulting in an arterioduodenal fistula with massive gastrointestinal hemorrhage.[27]

Arteriovenous Fistula

An AVF is usually a postsurgical or postbiopsy complication, occurring when the arterial and venous walls are both lacerated. AVFs can sometimes occur in conjunction with a pseudoaneurysm. On US, there is focal aliasing and turbulent flow within a high-velocity, low-resistance inflow artery, and pulsatile arterialized venous outflow.[19,22] When imaged during the arterial phase, CT and MR imaging may demonstrate early abnormal opacification of the donor draining veins.[22] Dilation of the Y graft may be an additional secondary sign of an underlying fistula. Small AVFs often resolve spontaneously, whereas larger fistulas require endovascular or surgical management[12,28,29] (Fig. 10).

Collection or Hematoma

Peritransplant fluid collections are very common in the first month posttransplantation but usually do not adversely affect outcome.[25] Many cases of early postoperative bleeding and hematoma formation are secondary to perioperative

anticoagulation.[20] Imaging evaluation should be used to assess the size and extent of the collection, as well as any sequelae related to mass effect, particularly vascular compression with resultant stenosis and/or thrombosis.

Sonographically, a hematoma will appear as a peritransplant collection with internal debris, which is difficult to distinguish from abscess, pseudocyst, or lymphocele on the basis of sonography alone. Similar findings may also be seen with a dilated duodenal bulb, which is a potential sonographic pitfall. A hematoma is usually distinguished by the presence of high attenuation with corresponding T1 hyperintensity, on CT and MR imaging, respectively. If the collection is small, precontrast images may be needed to help distinguish a small perigraft hematoma from a pseudoaneurysm. The hematoma is characterized by lack of enhancement on postcontrast images. Secretin MR imaging can be used to distinguish hematoma from pseudocyst, with the latter filling and enlarging 20 to 30 minutes following secretin injection.[2] Nonetheless, for collections that persist, enlarge, or result in significant compression, percutaneous aspiration may be required for definitive diagnosis and treatment.[15] Larger collections may also require surgical management, either due to vascular compression or to prevent subsequent infection (Fig. 11).

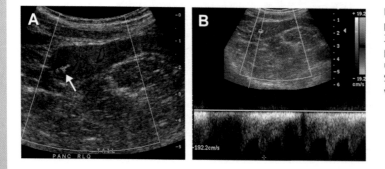

Fig. 10. AVF. A 24-year-old man postpancreatic transplant; biopsy done 3 weeks earlier for assessment of persistent graft rejection. (A) Doppler ultrasound finds and AVF (arrow). (B) Spectral Doppler shows arterialized venous flow within the nidus.

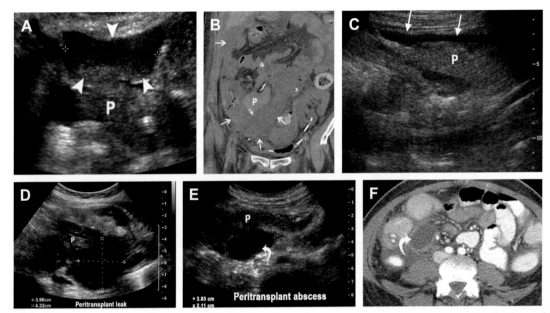

Fig. 11. Peritransplant collections. A 30-year-old woman postpancreatic transplant presented with elevated serum glucose level. (*A*) Gray-scale ultrasound of the pancreatic transplant postgraft biopsy shows complex fluid collection surrounding the graft (*arrowheads*). A large hematoma was suspected due to a drop in the patient's hematocrit level after biopsy. (*B*) A non-contrast CT examination was performed for confirmation. Coronal reformatted images show a large peritransplant hematoma (*arrows*). (*C*) Ultrasound image of the same patient a week later shows interval decrease in the size of hematoma, which is now a peritransplant seroma (*arrows*). (*D*) Different patient postpancreatic transplant biopsy presenting with nausea and vomiting. Ultrasound reveals a peritransplant collection (*calipers*), which was later proven to be a transplant leak. (*E*, *F*) Different patient presenting with nausea and fever. Ultrasound revealed a peritransplant collection (*curved arrow* and calipers), which was suspected to be an abscess, which was then confirmed by CT. Note the thick enhancing capsule of the collection on axial contrast-enhanced CT (*curved arrow*). P, pancreas.

Graft-related Complications

Pancreatitis (early or late)

Most pancreatic transplants have some underlying pancreatitis in the immediate postoperative period, which is described as less than 4 weeks after transplant. This is thought to reflect reperfusion injury. It is usually subclinical and self-limited.[12,22,30] Severe pancreatitis occurs in approximately 10% of grafts, with necrotizing pancreatitis occurring in 2% to 4%.[25] Identifying the more severe cases of posttransplant pancreatitis can be quite difficult because traditional serum markers of native pancreatitis (amylase and lipase) correlate poorly with the severity of graft pancreatitis. Moreover, up to 35% of recipients will have hyperamylasemia in the early postoperative period.[20] Risk factors for early posttransplant pancreatitis include donor quality, use of histidine-tryptophan-ketoglutarate (HTK) solution, prolonged preservation time, graft handling, reperfusion injury, pancreatic duct outflow obstruction, and bladder drainage (reflux pancreatitis).[2,20] Specific risk factors for late pancreatitis are less known.

Imaging evaluation and findings are similar to native pancreatitis, including the possibility of a normal appearance in early or mild cases.

Sonographically, the graft may be enlarged and edematous, although this appearance is nonspecific and can overlap with findings of rejection and early thrombosis.[2] Resistive indices of intrapancreatic arteries may be elevated, although their utility is questionable because values often overlap between normal and abnormal grafts.[24] Moreover, resistive indices for pancreatic transplants are typically higher compared with their renal transplant counterparts, probably reflecting subclinical pancreatitis.[25] Dual-phase pancreatic CT or multiphase MR imaging are primarily used to assess absent enhancement in cases of parenchymal necrosis, as well as associated complications, particularly thrombosis, abscess, hemorrhage, pseudoaneurysm, and pseudocyst formation (**Fig. 12**).

Standard management is typically conservative, including bowel rest and parenteral nutrition; however, severe cases may require debridement.[20]

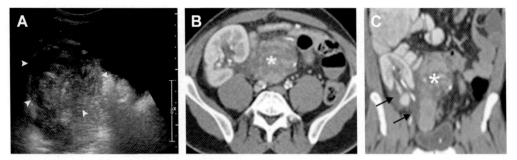

Fig. 12. Graft pancreatitis. A 38-year-old woman presents with significantly elevated amylase and lipase levels. (*A*) Ul-trasound revealed a swollen pancreatic graft with heterogeneous echogenicity (*arrowheads*). (*B*) Axial and (*C*) coronal contrast-enhanced CT images of a different patient after kidney-pancreas (*asterisk*) transplant with graft pancreatitis. Note the heterogeneous enhancement of the pancreatic parenchyma and small amount of free fluid around the pancreatic tissue (*arrows*).

Cases of necrotizing pancreatitis almost always require necrosectomy or graft pancreatectomy.[12] Patients with bladder drainage may ultimately require conversion to enteric drainage.

Pseudocyst

A pseudocyst can occur when pancreatitis or ischemia results in pancreatic duct disruption and fluid collection formation.[2] The cross-sectional imaging appearance of the collection is typically nonspecific but aspiration of the fluid will yield markedly elevated concentration of amylase.[22] Similar to the native pancreas, trans-plant pseudocysts can be complicated by second-ary infection and require percutaneous drainage.

Abscess

Abscesses most commonly occur within the first 30 days posttransplant and represent a serious threat to graft viability and patient survival. The work-up should define the size and extent of the abscess and carefully assess for an underlying anastomotic leak, which is present in up to 30% of patients with abscesses.[20] Other risk factors include older donor age, retransplantation, pretransplant peritoneal dialysis, extended preser-vation time, graft pancreatitis, and immunosup-pression with sirolimus.[20] For patients with enteric drainage, abscess, and anastomotic leak, a repeat laparotomy is almost always required. Most (up to 80%) of the remainder of patients can be successfully managed with conservative therapy (eg, with a percutaneous drainage cath-eter or with a Foley catheter).[20] A potential pitfall exists when the donor duodenum is distended and thick-walled but is not opacified with oral contrast material, thus simulating an abscess (see **Fig. 11**).[15,25]

Rejection

Although rates of acute rejection have been decreasing in recent years, rejection remains the most common cause of graft loss overall.[15] Acute rejection has been reported in up to 40% of pancreatic transplants, usually occurring 1 week to 3 months after transplantation. Acute rejection is thought to be secondary to small vessel autoim-mune arteritis resulting in small vessel occlusion followed by large vessel occlusion.[15,22,30] Chronic rejection remains the major cause of long-term failure (after 6 months), occurs in 4% to 10% of pa-tients, and can result from recurrent episodes of acute rejection with subsequent fibrosis, atrophy, and eventual loss of graft function.[15,30]

Imaging findings in both acute and chronic rejection are relatively nonspecific and unreliable, making prospective diagnosis difficult.[22] The most common sonographic finding in acute pancreatic transplant rejection is graft enlarge-ment, with a reported sensitivity of 58% and a specificity of 100%.[30] However, graft enlargement and heterogeneity are also seen in patients with pancreatitis that affected their transplants. Thus, the primary role of US is to exclude underlying major vessel thrombosis as the cause of graft dysfunction. CT may demonstrate an enlarged pancreas with heterogeneous enhancement, peri-graft fluid, and duodenal edema, which are similarly nonspecific findings.[15] MR imaging is more sensitive for the identification of acute rejec-tion and can be useful in particular when IV contrast cannot be administered. In cases of acute rejection, the graft usually demonstrates diffuse increased signal intensity on T2-weighted sequences. However, MR imaging lacks speci-ficity in this situation due to the overlap of findings with otherwise normal grafts, as well as with graft pancreatitis and with graft rejection.[15,30] Contrast-enhanced MR imaging will demonstrate a significantly decreased mean percentage of parenchymal enhancement in case of rejection, but this is also seen with pancreatic transplant necrosis. Findings in cases of chronic rejection usually reflect an underlying atrophic fibrotic graft, with increased parenchymal echogenicity and decreased signal intensity on both T1-weighted and T2-weighted MR images[15,30] (**Fig. 13**). In the setting of hyperglycemia, a small atrophic allograft is virtually diagnostic of chronic pancreatic transplant rejection.[26] However, percutaneous biopsy is still the primary means for diagnosing and grading both acute and chronic rejection.[15]

ENTERIC COMPLICATIONS
Anastomotic Leak or Abscess

Anastomotic leaks occur in up to 10% of pancreatic transplants but account for fewer than 0.5% of all graft losses. The impact and clinical course after a leak depends on the type of anastomosis.[20,30] Leaking bowel contents from an enteric-drained graft may result in chemical peritonitis, fluid collection, and sepsis. As a result, there is a much higher risk for graft loss and the need for immediate repeat surgery.[20] Either CT with oral contrast material or fluoroscopy can be used to identify extravasated contrast material at the site of a leak.[25] Leak from a bladder-drained graft is usually less severe and can be identified using retrograde instillation of intravesical contrast, either with a CT cystogram or by conventional cystography. Early leaks usually occur at the duodenocystostomy and can be managed

conservatively with bladder decompression.[15] Late (>4 weeks postoperative) leaks usually occur at the oversewn duodenal stump and may require anastomotic revision of the enteric drainage[15,30] (see **Fig. 11**).

Postoperative Obstruction

Obstruction can develop at the duodenojejunal anastomosis via a mesenteric defect (internal hernia) or from adhesions.[2] Adhesion-related bowel obstruction will show typical cross-sectional imaging findings of dilated bowel upstream from a discrete transition point with relatively decompressed distal bowel, with the adhesion itself rarely directly seen. If a mesenteric defect is created during intraperitoneal placement or when forming the duodenojejunal anastomosis, an internal hernia can occur with a resultant closed-loop obstruction, which will appear as a radial arrangement of bowel small loops with 2 adjacent transition points corresponding to the site of the defect.[25] Although closed-loop small bowel obstruction has a higher risk of strangulation, signs of bowel ischemia (eg, decreased mural enhancement) may be present with any type of small bowel obstruction.

Posttransplant Lymphoproliferative Disorder

Posttransplant lymphoproliferative disorder (PTLD) is a rare long-term complication, reported in 2.4% to 6.1% of patients, with a higher incidence in patients who are Epstein-Barr virus–negative and who have undergone pancreatic transplantation alone.[31] PTLD can present with findings related to the transplanted pancreas itself, including diffuse graft enlargement or focal lesions in or around the graft. Other findings include enlarged regional or distant lymph nodes or distant extranodal findings. The latter includes organomegaly; focal lesions in the liver, spleen, kidney, or bowel; gallbladder wall thickening; and bowel wall thickening.[25,30] Of these, the lymph nodes and liver are most frequently involved (39%–40% of cases), whereas the pancreas transplant is less commonly involved (10%).[15] Compared with patients with PTLD following liver or kidney transplants, pancreas transplant recipients with PTLD more commonly present with widespread disease, with more extranodal sites of involvement, as well as significantly worse overall survival.[32] Establishing the correct diagnosis of PTLD relies heavily on these findings combined with the clinical scenario because imaging appearance of the graft itself is nonspecific and usually cannot be differentiated from pancreatitis or rejection.[12]

Fig. 13. Pancreatic graft rejection. A 37-year-old man with questionable abnormal function of the pancreatic graft. Ultrasound shows a mildly enlarged graft (*arrowheads*). Biopsy was positive for lymphocyte infiltration.

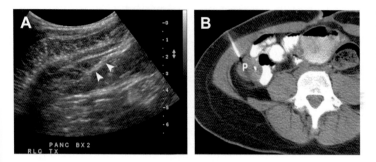

Fig. 14. Pancreas transplant biopsy techniques. (*A*) Ultrasound is the first modality of choice used to guide the biopsy needle (*arrowheads*) into the pancreatic parenchyma. (*B*) If the pancreas (P) was not accessible by ultrasound, then CT is used for guidance of the biopsy needle.

IMAGE-GUIDED PROCEDURES
Biopsy

Despite perceived technical challenges, pancreatic transplant biopsy is effective, resulting in adequate specimens in 96% of patients, with a low procedure-related complication rate of 1.9% to 2.6%, which is similar to rates reported for renal transplant biopsies.[33,34] Because establishing or excluding the clinical diagnosis of rejection is difficult, and because cross-sectional-imaging findings are frequently nonspecific, as noted above, US-guided or CT-guided percutaneous biopsy is the standard procedure for diagnosing and grading rejection, particularly for the 10% of SPK transplant patients in whom rejection only affects the pancreatic graft.[15,26] Allograft biopsy also allows for diagnosis of other entities, including drug-related islet cell toxicity, cytomegalovirus pancreatitis, and PTLD.[34]

If feasible, US-guided percutaneous biopsy is the preferred technique due to its real-time guidance, absence of ionizing radiation, and relatively low cost. Intraabdominal hemorrhage is the most common reported complication. Other clinically important complications include pancreatitis, hematuria (for bladder-drained allografts), inadvertent biopsy of another organ, and pancreatic-cutaneous fistula.[33,34] A relatively avascular segment of the graft is targeted for biopsy, preferably directed parallel to the long axis of the graft, taking care to avoid overlying bowel and vasculature. It is critical for the radiologist performing the procedure to be aware of the type of anastomosis which has been performed, because the location and orientation of the allograft may differ from patient to patient. When the pancreatic allograft cannot be adequately visualized sonographically, a CT-guided approach is an acceptable second choice for biopsy[26] (**Fig. 14**).

Historically, for bladder-drained pancreas transplants, cystoscopic transduodenal biopsy has been an option. However, it is now less preferred because it requires an operating room, general anesthesia, and overnight hospitalization.[33] Open surgical biopsy is currently rarely required.

Fluid Collection Drainage

Most peritransplant fluid collections are hematomas or seromas, which generally resolve with conservative management and do not adversely affect graft outcomes. However, because transplant recipients receive long-term immunosuppression, timely identification and drainage of an abscess, or hematoma or seroma with superimposed infection is critical. For those collections that develop into abscesses, percutaneous aspiration and drainage can be diagnostic as well as therapeutic. Percutaneous drainage can be performed using US or CT guidance, as with management of many abscesses elsewhere in the body.[26]

SUMMARY

Pancreatic transplantation is surgically challenging, even with current techniques, and is usually accompanied by simultaneous renal transplantation. Similar to other solid organ transplants, sonography is usually the first-line imaging modality when evaluating for potential complications, as well as for routine postoperative assessment. However, the position of the pancreatic transplant makes sonographic evaluation more limited due to overlying bowel gas. For this and other reasons, CT or MR imaging may also be required. The use of both iodinated and gadolinium-based contrast material may be precluded by recovering renal insufficiency in these patients. Unenhanced MR imaging with or without MRCP is preferred over unenhanced CT in this subset of patients. Knowledge of the surgical techniques, location of the anastomoses, and possible related complications will assist the radiologist in performing an accurate assessment of pancreas transplants using cross-sectional imaging.

REFERENCES

1. Rogers J, Farney AC, Orlando G, et al. Pancreas transplantation with portal venous drainage with an emphasis on technical aspects. Clin Transplant 2014;28:16–26.

2. Tolat PP, Foley WD, Johnson C, et al. Pancreas transplant imaging: how I do it. Radiology 2015; 275:14–27.

3. White SA, Shaw JA, Sutherland DE. Pancreas transplantation. Lancet 2009;373:1808–17.

4. Ojo AO, Meier-Kriesche HU, Hanson JA, et al. The impact of simultaneous pancreas-kidney transplantation on long-term patient survival. Transplantation 2001;71:82–90.

5. Bazerbachi F, Selzner M, Marquez MA, et al. Portal venous versus systemic venous drainage of pancreas grafts: impact on long-term result. Am J Transplant 2012;12:226–32.

6. Oliver JB, Beidas AK, Bongu A, et al. A comparison of long-term outcomes of portal versus systemic venous drainage in pancreatic transplantation: systematic review and meta-analysis. Clin Transplant 2015;29(10):882–92.

7. Hampson FA, Freeman SJ, Ertner J, et al. Pancreatic transplantation: surgical technique, normal radiological appearances and complications. Insights Imaging 2010;1:339–47.

8. Sollinger HW, Messing EM, Eckhoff DE, et al. Urological complications in 210 consecutive simultaneous pancreas-kidney transplants with bladder drainage. Ann Surg 1993;218:561–8.

9. Heller MT, Hattoum A. Kidney-pancreas transplantation: assessment of key imaging findings in the acute setting. Emerg Radiol 2012;19:527–33.

10. Ming CS, Chen ZH. Progress in pancreas transplantation and combined pancreas-kidney transplantation. Hepatobiliary Pancreat Dis Int 2007;6: 17–23.

11. Nikolaidis P, Amin RS, Hwang CM, et al. Role of sonography in pancreatic transplantation. Radiographics 2003;23:939–49.

12. Freund MC, Steurer W, Gassner EM, et al. Spectrum of imaging findings after pancreas transplantation with enteric exocrine drainage: Part 2, posttransplantation complications. AJR Am J Roentgenol 2004;182:919–25.

13. Franca M, Certo M, Martins L, et al. Imaging of pancreas transplantation and its complications. Insights Imaging 2010;1:329–38.

14. Liu Y, Akisik F, Tirkes T, et al. Value of magnetic resonance imaging in evaluating the pancreatic allograft transplant complications. Abdom Imaging 2015; 40(7):2384–90.

15. Vandermeer FQ, Manning MA, Frazier AA, et al. Imaging of whole-organ pancreas transplants. Radiographics 2012;32:411–35.

16. Hagspiel KD, Nandalur K, Pruett TL, et al. Evaluation of vascular complications of pancreas transplantation with high-spatial-resolution contrast-enhanced MR angiography. Radiology 2007;242:590–9.

17. Foshager MC, Hedlund LJ, Troppmann C, et al. Venous thrombosis of pancreatic transplants: diagnosis by duplex sonography. AJR Am J Roentgenol 1997;169:1269–73.

18. Humar A, Ramcharan T, Kandaswamy R, et al. Technical failures after pancreas transplants: why grafts fail and the risk factors–a multivariate analysis. Transplantation 2004;78:1188–92.

19. Low G, Crockett AM, Leung K, et al. Imaging of vascular complications and their consequences following transplantation in the abdomen. Radiographics 2013;33:633–52.

20. Troppmann C. Complications after pancreas transplantation. Curr Opin Organ Transplant 2010;15: 112–8.

21. Dobos N, Roberts DA, Insko EK, et al. Contrast-enhanced MR angiography for evaluation of vascular complications of the pancreatic transplant. Radiographics 2005;25:687–95.

22. Dillman JR, Elsayes KM, Bude RO, et al. Imaging of pancreas transplants: postoperative findings with clinical correlation. J Comput Assist Tomogr 2009; 33:609–17.

23. Stockland AH, Willingham DL, Paz-Fumagalli R, et al. Pancreas transplant venous thrombosis: role of endovascular interventions for graft salvage. Cardiovasc Intervent Radiol 2009;32:279–83.

24. Norton PT, DeAngelis GA, Ogur T, et al. Noninvasive vascular imaging in abdominal solid organ transplantation. AJR Am J Roentgenol 2013;201:W544–53.

25. Sandrasegaran K, Lall C, Berry WA, et al. Enteric drainage pancreatic transplantation. Abdom Imaging 2006;31:588–95.

26. Daly B, O'Kelly K, Klassen D. Interventional procedures in whole organ and islet cell pancreas transplantation. Semin Intervent Radiol 2004;21:335–43.

27. Dalla Valle R, Capocasale E, Mazzoni MP, et al. Embolization of a ruptured pseudoaneurysm with massive hemorrhage following pancreas transplantation: a case report. Transplant Proc 2005;37: 2275–7.

28. Barth MM, Khwaja K, Faintuch S, et al. Transarterial and transvenous embolotherapy of arteriovenous fistulas in the transplanted pancreas. J Vasc Interv Radiol 2008;19:1231–5.

29. Buttarelli L, Capocasale E, Marcato C, et al. Embolization of pancreatic allograft arteriovenous fistula with the Amplatzer Vascular Plug 4: case report and literature analysis. Transplant Proc 2011;43: 4044–7.

30. Liong SY, Dixon RE, Chalmers N, et al. Complications following pancreatic transplantations: imaging features. Abdom Imaging 2011;36:206–14.

31. Kandaswamy R, Skeans MA, Gustafson SK, et al. OPTN/SRTR 2013 annual data report: pancreas. Am J Transplant 2015;15(Suppl 2):1–20.

32. Paraskevas S, Coad JE, Gruessner A, et al. Post-transplant lymphoproliferative disorder in pancreas transplantation: a single-center experience. Transplantation 2005;80:613–22.

33. Atwell TD, Gorman B, Larson TS, et al. Pancreas transplants: experience with 232 percutaneous US-guided biopsy procedures in 88 patients. Radiology 2004;231:845–9.

34. Klassen DK, Weir MR, Cangro CB, et al. Pancreas allograft biopsy: safety of percutaneous biopsy-results of a large experience. Transplantation 2002;73:553–5.

Interventional and Surgical Techniques in Solid Organ Transplantation

Christopher R. Ingraham, MD[a],*, Martin Montenovo, MD[b]

KEYWORDS

- Liver transplantation • Kidney transplantation • Pancreas transplantation • Surgical techniques
- Complications and interventions

KEY POINTS

- The most commonly used methods and techniques for solid organ transplantation are reviewed in this article. Attention is given to the surgical technique and rationale for each anastomosis, with a discussion of commonly encountered post transplant complications.
- Vascular complications after solid organ transplantation include stenosis, thrombosis, or occlusion and can involve the arterial and/or venous structures.
- Interventional therapy used to treat both vascular and nonvascular (eg, biliary duct or ureteral) complications include thrombolysis, angioplasty, and stent or catheter placement.

SURGICAL TECHNIQUES IN SOLID ORGAN TRANSPLANTATION

Liver Transplantation

Since the pioneering times, innumerable improvements have been made that have transformed the modern liver transplant procedure from an experimental undertaking to a therapeutic and lifesaving procedure. Included in these improvements are the evolution of anesthesia techniques, the introduction of electrocautery and hemostatic agents, the contribution of venovenous bypass to provide more hemodynamic stability and a more suitable atmosphere for the education of liver transplant trainees, and the use of modern mechanical retractors that permit an unrestricted exposure of the surgical field.

Transplant techniques

Liver transplantation is now typically performed using one of two different techniques and is based on the anastomosis of the inferior vena cava (IVC)[1]:

- The classic technique using vena cava interposition
- The piggyback technique, which leaves the native cava behind

There are several potential advantages of the piggyback technique[1]:

- Partial and transient clamping of the IVC maintains continuity of the IVC during the anhepatic phase, minimizing hemodynamic disturbances
- Decrease in warm ischemia time because of the need for only one caval anastomosis
- Decreased retroperitoneal dissection, potentially decreasing blood loss
- Preservation of the native IVC allows adjustment of vessel size disparity between the donor and recipient when the donor liver is small

Venovenous bypass

Venovenous bypass can be performed during liver transplantation (typically with the classic

Conflicts of interest: All authors declare that they have no financial conflicts of interest with this article or its content. This study was not supported by grant funding.

[a] Department of Interventional Radiology, University of Washington, 1959 Northeast Pacific Street, Box 357115, Seattle, WA 98195-7115, USA; [b] Division of Transplant Surgery, Department of Surgery, University of Washington, 1959 NE Pacific Street, Box 356410, Seattle, WA 98195, USA
* Corresponding author.
E-mail address: cringra@uw.edu

technique), and is the extracorporeal circulation of blood from the venous system, typically from the portal and femoral veins, with a return of blood from the circuit to the central veins, usually via an axillary or internal jugular vein.[2]

Potential advantages for venovenous bypass[3,4]:

- Preservation of cardiac, pulmonary, renal, and cerebral blood flow (especially important in patients with fulminant hepatic failure)
- Maintenance of hemodynamic stability during the anhepatic phase
- Reduction of intraoperative blood loss

Potential disadvantages for the use of venovenous bypass include[3–6]:

- Pulmonary or air embolus
- Longer operative and warm ischemia times
- Increased bleeding caused by hemolysis and fibrinolysis in the bypass circuit
- Higher procedural cost
- Lack of clear evidence showing improved clinical outcomes

Controversy still exists over the use of venovenous bypass. Most centers believe that its routine use is no longer necessary for either surgical technique.[2]

Surgical technique for orthotopic liver transplantation Successful organ engraftment begins with a controlled recipient hepatectomy. This hepatectomy can be a challenging task in individuals with prior upper abdominal surgery or in patients with severe portal hypertension and extensive collateral formation. The abdomen is opened via a bilateral subcostal incision with midline extension, termed a Mercedes incision. A mechanical retractor is placed with the blades under both costal margins to pull the rib cage laterally and anteriorly.

Surgical steps for recipient hepatectomy

1. The falciform ligament is divided down to the suprahepatic vena cava and the round ligament is tied, given frequent recanalization of the umbilical vein in patients with portal hypertension.
2. The left triangular ligament is then opened with cautery followed by opening of the gastrohepatic ligament. The ligated round ligament is now lifted superiorly to allow visualization of the porta hepatis.
3. Dissection is then carried down to the hepatic artery, which is then divided above its bifurcation.
4. The common bile duct is then divided. Once the bile duct is divided, the dissection is completed

around the portal vein and the right triangular ligament is dissected into the right hepatic vein. The portal vein is then transected above its bifurcation using mechanical staplers.

5. The anterior aspect of the infrahepatic IVC is then exposed to allow easy circumferential mobilization for placement of a vascular clamp. The retrohepatic caval tissue can be dissected with the surgeon's finger.

At this point in the operation, the patient is prepared for venovenous bypass (if used) by cannulation of the femoral vein using a 15-F cannula. The return cannula is inserted into the left axillary vein or internal jugular vein using an 18-F or 12-F cannula, respectively. In addition, a 28-F cannula is introduced in the portal vein. Bypass can then be commenced. After initiation of bypass, vascular clamps are placed on the suprahepatic and infrahepatic IVC and the IVC is divided proximally and distally. The native liver is then removed. The donor liver is now brought onto the surgical field. When performing the classic technique, the suprahepatic IVC is first anastomosed, followed by the infrahepatic IVC (**Fig. 1**).

When performing the piggyback technique, venovenous bypass is almost never needed and a partial clamping of the suprahepatic IVC is performed (**Fig. 2**). The right, middle, and left hepatic veins are then divided as far into the liver as possible, so that the 3 hepatic veins can be connected into a common cloaca. The donor suprahepatic vena cava is anastomosed to the recipient common cloaca in an end-to-side fashion. The donor infrahepatic IVC is closed with a stapler during bench preparation, creating an IVC stump (**Fig. 3**).

Surgical steps for donor graft placement after inferior vena cava anastomosis

1. After the IVC anastomosis has been made, the portal anastomosis is created.[7]
   a. The time period to complete the caval and portal vein anastomoses before reperfusion (the warm ischemia time) ideally should not exceed 45 minutes.
   b. If venovenous bypass was used, then the portal bypass cannula is now removed and only the systemic venovenous bypass is continued. After reperfusion of the liver, the systemic bypass can be discontinued.
   c. When the portal vein is unsuitable for anastomosis because of significant thrombosis, a conduit using donor iliac vein is created to anastomose with the recipient superior mesenteric vein and the donor portal vein.

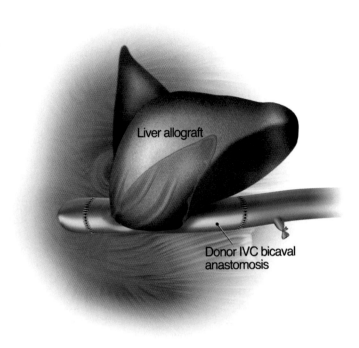

Fig. 1. Bicaval anastomosis of the liver allograft using the classic caval anastomosis technique. The suprahepatic IVC is first anastomosed followed by the infrahepatic IVC (suture lines).

Liver allograft

Donor IVC bicaval anastomosis

The conduit is created posterior to the stomach in front of the pancreas through a tunnel in the transverse mesocolon.

2. The hepatic artery anastomosis is the final vascular step in the procedure.
   a. Most commonly, the anastomosis is performed at the level of the recipient's gastroduodenal artery.
   b. In cases with low arterial flow (<150 mL/min) or with a known history of hepatic artery dissection or stenosis of the celiac trunk, then an aortic conduit using donor iliac artery must be created from the supraceliac or infrarenal aorta.

3. The biliary anastomosis can performed using one of two main techniques:
   a. A duct-to-duct anastomosis has become the most widely used technique.
   b. A Roux-en-Y hepaticojejunostomy may be used in the following circumstances:
      i. Insufficient length of the bile duct in the donor and/or recipient
      ii. A small pediatric recipient
      iii. A severe mismatch in size between the donor and recipient's common bile ducts
      iv. Disease of the extrahepatic bile ducts, biliary atresia, bile duct injury, or cholangiocarcinoma

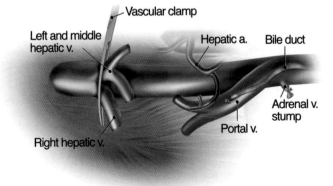

Vascular clamp

Left and middle hepatic v.

Hepatic a.   Bile duct

Adrenal v. stump

Portal v.

Right hepatic v.

Fig. 2. Exposure of the recipient IVC and hepatic veins when piggyback technique is used. The diseased liver has been removed. Note the native IVC is intact and a vascular clamp can be placed across the IVC at the level of the hepatic veins. a, artery; v, vein.

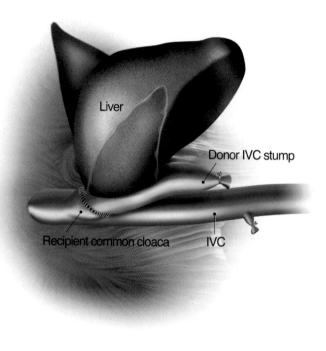

Liver

Donor IVC stump

Recipient common cloaca   IVC

Fig. 3. Piggyback technique of the liver allograft. The donor suprahepatic vena cava is anastomosed to the recipient common cloaca in an end-to-side fashion. The donor infrahepatic IVC is closed with a stapler or tied with a suture.

Renal Transplantation

Surgical technique for renal transplantation

Renal transplantation is a major surgical procedure that combines both vascular and urologic elements. The recipient, who is uremic and usually being maintained on hemodialysis or peritoneal dialysis, often is a high-risk patient with comorbid disease (eg, diabetes, cardiovascular disease, obesity). Patients on dialysis frequently have coagulopathy and platelet dysfunction, making bleeding during the procedure a known risk.[8] Meticulous technique is imperative given that the transplant operation may be the patient's only opportunity for a successful kidney transplant.

The operation begins with a curvilinear (hockey-stick) incision made in the right or left lower quadrant of the abdomen. The inferior epigastric vessels are ligated and divided, unless the graft has multiple arteries. If the graft has multiple arteries, the inferior epigastric artery should be preserved for anastomosis to a lower polar renal artery. In male patients, the spermatic cord is isolated and retracted medially. In female patients, the round ligament is ligated and divided. After the transversalis fascia is opened, the peritoneal reflection is retracted superiorly and medially to expose the psoas muscle and the iliac vessels. Dissection of the external, common, and internal iliac arteries is then performed, followed by dissection of the external iliac vein.

After the donor kidney has been prepared, the recipient vessels are ready for clamping. A venotomy and arteriotomy are performed and the lumen is flushed with heparinized saline. If the renal graft has a lower polar artery, it is imperative that this vessel be revascularized because it nearly universally gives rise to the ureteric blood supply. If more than one renal vein is present, smaller veins can be ligated. Both the artery and vein are anastomosed in an end-to-side fashion (**Fig. 4**).

Ureteroneocystostomy is the usual form of urinary tract reconstruction. Potential advantages include that it can be performed regardless of the quality or presence of the recipient ureter, it is several centimeters away from the vascular anastomoses, and the native ureter remains available for the treatment of ureteric complications. Ideally a 2-cm to 3-cm submucosal tunnel with detrusor muscle backing of the ureter is constructed so that, when the bladder contracts, there is a valve mechanism to prevent reflux of urine up the ureter. The prophylactic use of ureteric stents for all kidney transplants was shown in a randomized prospective trial to reduce the incidence of urologic complications but their widespread use has not gained universal acceptance.[9]

Pediatric en-block donor

When a pediatric patient's kidney is used as a donor kidney and the patient is very small (usually

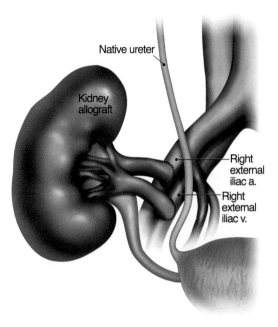

Fig. 4. Renal allograft located in the right lower quadrant. Note the renal artery anastomosed to the right external iliac artery and the renal vein anastomosed to the right external iliac vein.

<10 kg), both kidneys are transplanted en block into the adult recipient.[10,11] For an en-block transplantation, both kidneys are removed with a segment of aorta and vena cava. The cranial ends of the aorta and vena cava are then oversewn. The caudal ends of the aorta and vena cava are then anastomosed end to side with the iliac vessels. Ureters are implanted into the bladder separately or are joined together to form a common funnel.

Pancreas Transplantation

The success of pancreas transplantation is critically dependent both on sound judgment in donor selection and on technical perfection in all phases of organ recovery, preparation, and implantation. It is in many ways, the most fastidious transplantable organ, in that it there is almost zero tolerance for even minor complications involving all phases of organ transplantation.

A lower midline incision is preferable in the case of a combined pancreas/kidney transplant, and/or for access to the recipient's superior mesenteric vein, in the case of portal venous drainage of the transplanted pancreas. If the iliac vein is to be used for the venous anastomosis, the distal external iliac vein is mobilized. If the superior mesenteric vein is to be used for the venous anastomosis, it is exposed below the root of the mesentery. A venous extension graft is frequently needed if this approach is chosen. The arterial exposure is at the level of the common iliac artery. During the benching of the pancreas, the splenic and superior mesenteric arteries are reconstructed with an iliac arterial Y graft from the donor.

When drained into the portal system, the pancreas is transplanted head up (**Fig. 5**). The donor portal vein, with an iliac vein extension, is anastomosed to the superior mesenteric vein. When systemic venous drainage is used, the pancreas is transplanted upside down (**Fig. 6**). The portal vein of the graft is anastomosed end to side to the distal external iliac vein. The artery is then anastomosed to the proximal external iliac artery. After completion of the vascular anastomosis, the vascular clamps are removed for reperfusion of the graft.

Drainage of the exocrine pancreas can be done into the bladder or the small bowel. Bladder drainage involves suturing the side of the duodenum to the dome of the bladder. Enteric drainage has become more popular in the last decade. The anastomoses can be constructed

Fig. 5. Posterior view of the pancreas allograft after benching. Note that the splenic and superior mesenteric arteries are reconstructed with an iliac arterial Y graft from the donor. SMA, Superior mesenteric artery.

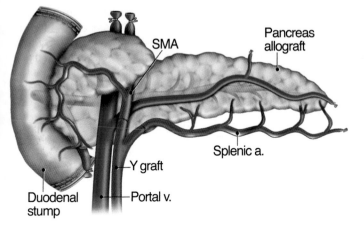

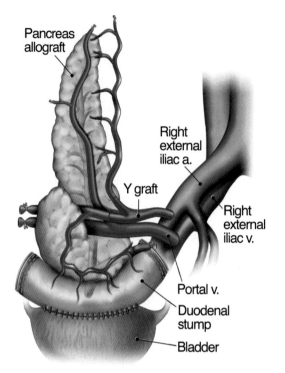

Pancreas allograft

Right external iliac a.

Y graft

Right external iliac v.

Portal v.

Duodenal stump

Bladder

Fig. 6. Pancreas allograft with bladder drainage located in the right lower quadrant. Note the upside down position of the pancreas. The arterial Y graft is anastomosed to the external iliac artery. The portal vein of the allograft is anastomosed to the external iliac vein. The duodenum of the graft is anastomosed to the bladder dome of the recipient.

from the distal end or the side of the donor duodenum into the side of the recipient jejunum.

INTERVENTIONAL RADIOLOGY TECHNIQUES IN POST TRANSPLANT PATIENTS
Liver Transplantation

Vascular complications after liver transplantation
Overview and incidence
- Up to 15% of liver transplant recipients can develop vascular complications[12]
- Bleeding, stenosis, or thrombosis can occur at any of the sites of vascular anastomosis: hepatic artery, portal vein, or hepatic vein/IVC
- Hepatic artery thrombosis (HAT) and portal vein thrombosis are the most common vascular complications, occurring (in total) in approximately 7% of liver transplant patients

Imaging diagnosis of a vascular complication
- The diagnosis of a vascular complication in a transplant patient is typically made by Doppler sonography[13,14]

- Computed tomography or magnetic resonance angiography may also be used to assist in diagnosis or further elucidate ultrasonography findings
- If imaging findings are equivocal, catheter angiography may provide further characterization and allow for possible treatments
- Hemodynamically significant stenoses can be verified during angiography by obtaining intraprocedural pressure gradients

Hepatic arterial thrombosis
HAT has been reported to occur in approximately 3% to 5% of cases, occurring most frequently in the pediatric population, and typically within the first 3 months after transplantation.[12,14,15] HAT can result from kinking of the anastomosis, surgical error or injury to the artery during creation of the anastomosis, dissection of the artery, or from rejection. The clinical consequences of HAT can be grave given that the biliary tree is more dependent, if not completely dependent, on hepatic arterial flow compared with a native liver.[12,14] Ischemia to the bile ducts can cause biliary strictures, bilomas, or ischemic cholangiopathy.[14]

Treatment of HAT can consist of surgical exploration with thrombectomy or anastomotic revision, catheter-based thrombolysis, retransplantation, biliary drainage, or systemic anticoagulation. In one recent large series of patients with HAT, 65% of patients required surgical exploration, thrombectomy, and/or anastomotic revision; 17% required retransplantation; and 3% underwent catheter-directed thrombolysis.[12] Of all patients who experience HAT, 75% require retransplantation, and HAT is the leading cause of graft loss, occurring in 53% of patients with graft loss after transplantation.[12,15]

Hepatic artery stenosis
Hepatic artery stenosis (HAS) occurs less frequently than HAT, but when untreated HAS can progress to HAT.[16,17] Causes of HAS include vascular injury or technical error at the time of transplantation (eg, intimal dissection, clamp injury), kinking of the vessel, extrinsic compression, differences in caliber of the donor and native hepatic arteries, and rejection.[17,18]

Findings on sonographic Doppler suggestive of hepatic artery stenosis
- Resistive index of less than 0.5[19,20]
- Peak hepatic artery velocity greater than 200 to 300 cm/s
- Systolic acceleration time greater than 0.08 seconds
- A parvus et tardus waveform

Treatment of HAS includes angioplasty and/or stent placement, or surgical revision. Endovascular management is the preferred treatment strategy, with surgical revision reserved for cases of endovascular technical failure or complication.[21] Balloon angioplasty for HAS is considered first-line therapy and technical success rates are reported to be approximately 80% at experienced centers[17,21] (**Fig. 7**). Restenosis rates are reported to be approximately 33%.[17,22] In cases in which balloon angioplasty is not successful at treating the stenosis, stent placement can be considered, with restenosis rates approaching 30% to 40%[21,23] (**Fig. 8**).

Portal vein stenosis, thrombosis, and occlusion

Portal vein stenosis or thrombosis has been reported to occur in approximately 3% to 8% of cases of transplantation, most commonly in pediatric patients.[12,24] Diagnosis of portal vein complications can be delineated on Doppler ultrasonography or cross-sectional imaging. However, catheter angiography remains the gold standard given the opportunity for real-time imaging evaluation and the ability to evaluate for a pressure gradient.[25]

Technical considerations and treatment options for portal complications

- Access into the portal system can be achieved either via a transjugular intrahepatic portosystemic shunt approach, or via a percutaneous transhepatic approach[24–26]
- Pressure gradients can be obtained across the region of the stenosis to verify imaging findings or validate clinical suspicion
  - A gradient greater than or equal to 5 mm Hg is generally considered significant
- If significant thrombus is present within the portal vein, mechanical and/or chemical

thrombolysis should be performed 12 to 48 hours before considering balloon angioplasty to treat the underlying stenosis
- If no underlying thrombus is present and only a stenosis is observed, balloon angioplasty is performed
  - Angioplasty is considered successful if the pressure gradient is reduced to less than 5 mm Hg
- If angioplasty is unsuccessful at treating the stenosis (ie, there is a recoil stenosis or >30% residual stenosis is present, or a pressure gradient remains), stenting should be performed

Technical success rates after angioplasty are variable and are reported to be in the range of 36% to 71% at 2 to 3 years.[25,26] Many patients require repeat interventions after balloon angioplasty and ultimately undergo stent placement. Success after stent placement for portal vein stenosis approaches 100% at 3 to 5 years post-treatment.[25,27] However, longer follow-up studies are needed to verify long-term patency. Success rates and patency rates after portal vein thrombolysis are not well established in the literature. However, case reports have described patency greater than 2 years posttreatment.[24,28]

Hepatic venous outflow stenosis and occlusion

Stenosis or occlusion of the hepatic venous outflow can involve either the hepatic vein or IVC, particularly after cases using the piggyback technique.[29] Venous outflow complications affect 1% to 6% of patients after liver transplantation. Early complications can be secondary to technical issues at the surgical anastomosis or venous kinking, and late complications can occur secondary to intimal hyperplasia or perianastomotic fibrosis.[30]

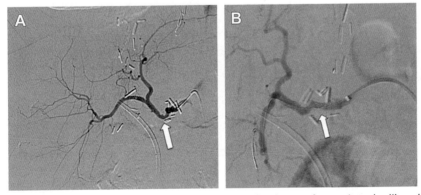

Fig. 7. (A) Transplant hepatic artery angiogram showing a small focal area of stenosis and caliber change (*white arrow*). (B) Transplant hepatic artery angiogram showing resolution of stenosis (*white arrow*) after balloon angioplasty using a 4-mm monorail balloon.

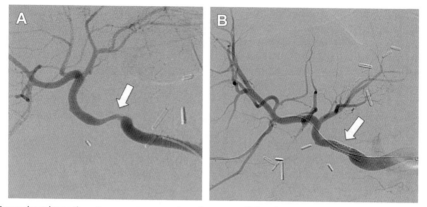

Fig. 8. (*A*) Transplant hepatic artery angiogram showing a small focal area of stenosis and caliber change at the anastomosis (*white arrow*). (*B*) Transplant hepatic artery angiogram showing resolution of stenosis after balloon angioplasty using a 5 mm × 19 mm uncovered balloon-mounted stent (*white arrow*).

Similar to portal venous complications, diagnostic imaging for cases of hepatic venous outflow complications may consist of Doppler sonography or cross-sectional imaging.[31] However, catheter venography remains a gold standard, allowing the opportunity for both diagnostic evaluation and pressure gradient evaluation.

Technical considerations and treatment options for venous outflow complications

- In any hepatic venous outflow stenosis or occlusion, diagnostic and interventional techniques are typically performed via the internal jugular vein, although a percutaneous transhepatic approach may be necessary[30–32]
- Pressure gradients can be obtained across the region of the stenosis to verify imaging findings or validate clinical suspicion
  ○ A gradient greater than 3 to 10 mm Hg is generally considered significant
- If significant thrombus is present within the hepatic vein, mechanical and/or chemical thrombolysis should be performed 12 to 48 hours before considering balloon angioplasty to treat the underlying stenosis
- If no underlying thrombus is present and only a stenosis is observed, balloon angioplasty is performed
  ○ Angioplasty is considered successful if the pressure gradient is reduced to less than 3 to 5 mm Hg
- If angioplasty is unsuccessful at treating the stenosis (ie, during the procedure or within the first 3 months after treatment), stenting should be performed
- For the unique scenario of stenoses involving both the hepatic vein and IVC,

kissing angioplasty or stent placement may be required

Indications for lysis, angioplasty, and stenting in IVC occlusions or stenoses are similar to those for hepatic venous stenosis or occlusion.[30,31] Treatment is considered successful if the pressure gradient is reduced to less than 3 to 5 mm Hg.[30,31]

Technical success rates approach 100% in treatment of venous outflow complications.[30,31,33] The 1-year patency rate for hepatic venous angioplasty is 60% and the assisted patency rate approaches 100%.[34] Given the lack of durable results with angioplasty alone, some interventionalists recommend primary stent placement in the treatment of hepatic venous stenosis.[31] For IVC angioplasty and stent placement, 1-year patency rates are 40% and greater than 91%, respectively.[30–32] Many interventionalists recommend primary stent placement for IVC complications as well.

Biliary complications
Overview and incidence

- Biliary complications occur in 5% to 30% of patients after liver transplant[12,14,35–37]
  ○ Graft loss can occur in 3% to 12% of these patients
- Types of complications include biliary stricture; bile leak; biloma formation; sphincter of Oddi dysfunction; and stone, sludge, and cast formation in the biliary tree
- Complications can result from:
  ○ Surgical error or technique, such as kinking or narrowing at the level of the anastomosis
  ○ The anastomosis or bile ducts may develop a compromise to the arterial blood supply, resulting in bile duct ischemia, biliary duct

stricture, biloma formation, or ischemic cholangiopathy

- The biliary tree in a transplanted liver is heavily, if not completely, reliant on the hepatic arterial blood supply

Clinical presentation and imaging evaluation in biliary complications

- Patients may be asymptomatic or may present with jaundice, increased liver function tests, abdominal pain, and/or cholangitis[36,38]
- Doppler ultrasonography and/or computed tomography angiography of the abdomen should be obtained to exclude an arterial complication
- Magnetic resonance cholangiopancreatography (MRCP) is the imaging modality of choice for biliary complications
  - MRCP can assist with diagnosis of anastomotic, hilar, and intrahepatic complications

Biliary stricture The most commonly encountered biliary complication after transplantation is biliary stricture. In a recent meta-analysis of more than 14,000 patients, the incidence of biliary stricture was estimated to occur in 13% of patients after liver transplantation.[39] Biliary strictures occur in greater than 75% of affected patients at the level of the biliary anastomosis.[35,40] The remainder are nonanastomotic strictures, which typically occur secondary to graft injury and are much more difficult to treat.[35,40] An increased incidence of biliary strictures is observed in patients receiving living donor liver transplant (LDLT) versus orthotopic liver transplant, given the inherent difficulties encountered with smaller grafts and bile ducts

in LDLT patients.[39] Endoscopic retrograde cholangiopancreatography (ERCP)–guided drainage is the most common first-choice treatment strategy (58%), followed by percutaneous transhepatic biliary drainage (PTBD) (15%) and surgical revision (4%). The remainder undergoes a combination of these therapies. There is a 98% rate of salvage using these strategies, with only 1% of patients requiring retransplantation, and 1% of patients experiencing graft loss.[39]

ERCP-guided therapy allows for diagnostic and therapeutic treatment and is frequently the first-choice method for treating biliary strictures, particularly those in patients with a duct-to-duct anastomosis. Balloon angioplasty and plastic stent placement is standard therapy. However, multiple treatment sessions (often 2–3 months apart) are often required for successful therapy. Treatment success ranges from 85% to 90% for patients treated in this fashion.[35,40,41]

In patients in whom ERCP-guided therapy has failed or is challenging (ie, biliary-enteric anastomosis), percutaneous transhepatic biliary (PTB) intervention is warranted. Transhepatic catheter placement and balloon angioplasty are performed as treatment from this approach. Once a transhepatic catheter is placed across the stricture, access to the bile ducts and the stricture is maintained. Repeated serial balloon angioplasty with or without catheter upsizing is performed for treatment of the stricture[42–44] (**Fig. 9**). Treatment may require multiple rounds of angioplasty and prolonged catheter placement to adequately treat the stricture. Using this method, 51% to 57% of strictures are successfully treated, and secondary patency has been reported up to 88% at 5 years.[42,43] Of those patients who fail ERCP or

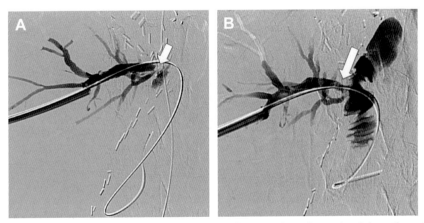

Fig. 9. (A) Cholangiogram in an LDLT patient showing a tight stenosis at the patient's hepaticoenteric anastomosis (*white arrow*). (B) Post-angioplasty cholangiogram with a 6 mm × 4 cm high-pressure balloon showing resolution of the stenosis (*white arrow*).

PTB interventions, surgical revision is often necessary.

Biliary leak and bilomas Biliary leakage post-transplantation is reported to occur in up to 8% of cases.[39] Leaks can occur at the site of anastomosis, at the cystic duct stump, or along the edges of the graft in the case of LDLT.[36] Treatment strategies are similar to those for biliary stricture, with surgical drainage or percutaneous drainage of contained leaks offered as possible additional treatment options. In a large recent meta-analysis of post-transplant biliary complications, PTBD was performed for treatment in only 10% of cases of bile leak.[39] ERCP or PTBD methods are frequently successful at diverting bile so that bilomas associated with biliary leaks can be decompressed and thus can heal.[40] Bilomas that do not communicate with the biliary tree can often be treated by antibiotics with or without percutaneous drainage.[35,39]

Complications After Kidney Transplantation

Vascular complications
Overview and incidence
- Up to 25% of renal transplant recipients develop vascular complications[14,45–47]
- Renal arterial stenosis is the most common vascular complication, occurring in 4% to 10% of all transplant patients
- Less commonly encountered vascular complications include arterial thrombosis or renal vein thrombosis
  - Usually secondary to operative injury of the involved vessel

Imaging diagnosis of a vascular complication
- The diagnosis of a vascular complication in a transplant patient is typically made by Doppler sonography[13,14]

- Computed tomography or magnetic resonance angiography may also be used to assist in diagnosis or further elucidate ultrasonography findings
- If imaging findings are equivocal, catheter angiography may provide further characterization and allow for possible treatments
- Hemodynamically significant stenoses can be verified during angiography by obtaining intraprocedural pressure gradients

The most common location for a renal arterial stenosis is at the site of the anastomosis, and less commonly in the recipient or graft artery. However, inflow lesions, such as underlying iliac lesions caused by atherosclerosis or clamp injury occurring during the transplant operation, can also occur (**Fig. 10**).

Treatments for vascular complications after renal transplantation include angioplasty, stent placement, and/or thrombolysis. Balloon angioplasty for arterial stenosis is usually the first-line treatment, followed by stent placement for cases of angioplasty failure (**Fig. 11**). Technical success rates approach 100% and long-term salvage of the graft approaches 90% of cases.[13,46,48–51] For cases of arterial or venous thrombotic occlusion, surgical thrombectomy is typically performed. However, several cases of successful endovascular lysis for both arterial and venous thrombosis have been described.[52–55] Operative treatment of stenoses or occlusions is typically reserved for cases that do not respond to endovascular therapy or for cases of acute thrombosis.[14]

Urinary complications
Urinary complications after kidney transplant are estimated to occur in approximately 6% of

Fig. 10. (A) Transplant renal angiogram performed from the right common iliac artery showing a focal stenosis (*white arrow*) in the right external iliac artery caused secondary to vascular clamp injury. (B) Right common iliac angiogram following placement of a balloon-mounted 10 mm × 25 mm uncovered stent showing resolution of the stenosis (*white arrow*).

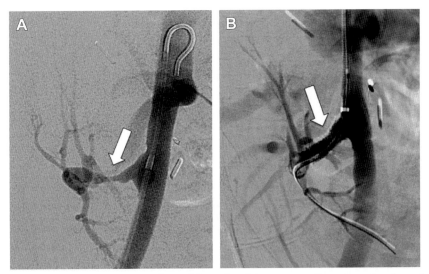

Fig. 11. (*A*) Transplant renal angiogram performed from the right common iliac artery showing a focal stenosis (*white arrow*) in the main renal artery. (*B*) Transplant renal angiogram performed from the right common iliac artery following placement of a balloon-mounted 6 mm × 18 mm uncovered stent showing resolution of the stenosis (*white arrow*).

transplant recipients, as shown in a large recent retrospective study of nearly 1700 patients.[56] In this series, 2.8% of patients developed a ureteral stricture, 1.7% of patients developed a urinary leak and a stricture, and 1.6% of patients developed a urine leak after transplant. Of the patients who experienced a complication, 70% were successfully managed by percutaneous intervention, and the remainder were treated operatively. Median time to develop a stricture occurred at 19 days, and all cases of urine leaks, with or without associated strictures, occurred within 100 days of transplantation.

Stricture of the transplanted ureter most commonly occurs at the distal ureter or at the ureterovesical anastomosis.[57] External compression of the ureter and/or transplanted kidney can be assessed by ultrasonography or cross-sectional imaging. For a ureteral stricture, initial treatment usually consists of percutaneous nephrostomy with the ultimate goal of nephroureteral stent or double-J stent placement. Internal stents are preferred to external catheters because of the risk of infection in this immunocompromised population.[57] These catheters extend from the renal pelvis to the urinary bladder and are placed in patients with normal bladder function. Double-J stents can be placed via an antegrade approach (via the nephrostomy access) or via a retrograde, cystoscopic approach.

In cases of isolated ureteral stricture, nephroureteral stent with or without ureteral angioplasty is successful in 68% of cases; in cases of urine leak with ureteral stricture, nephroureteral

stent with or without ureteral angioplasty is successful in 75% of cases; and in patients with an isolated urine leak, nephroureteral or double-J stent placement is successful in 67% of cases[56,58,59] (**Fig. 12**). In patients who fail percutaneous approaches to management, surgical intervention is often necessary.[57]

Biopsy complications

Transplant recipients frequently require percutaneous biopsy to assess graft function. Given that large core samples are commonly required for tissue analysis, significant arterial bleeding, traumatic pseudoaneurysms, or arteriovenous fistulae may result.[14] Most of these injuries are subclinical and inconsequential. Clinically significant complications (eg, decreasing hematocrit or increasing serum creatinine level) can be confirmed by imaging, such as duplex ultrasonography, or angiography if ultrasonography is equivocal. Transcatheter embolization of the biopsy-related vascular injury can be performed safely and effectively with a low probability of affecting long-term graft function.[60,61]

Complications After Pancreas Transplantation

Given the infrequency of pancreatic transplantation at many institutions, complications after pancreatic transplantation may be rarely encountered. However, radiologists and interventionalists should be familiar with the most common complications, which are usually vascular.[62,63]

Vascular complications after pancreatic transplant include arterial stenosis or thrombosis,

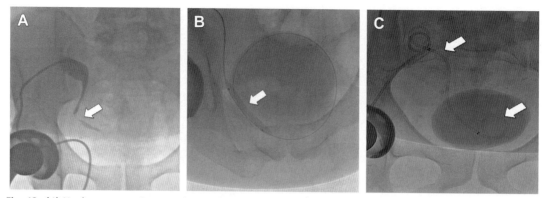

Fig. 12. (*A*) Nephrostogram in a renal transplant showing a partially obstructing stricture/stenosis involving the distal ureter (*white arrow*). (*B*) Ureteroplasty of the same patient's distal ureter performed with a 6 mm × 4 cm high-pressure balloon (*white arrow*). (*C*) Double-J 8-F ureteric stent placement in the same patient after ureteroplasty (*white arrows*). An 8-F nephrostomy tube is also present in the pelvis of the transplant kidney.

pseudoaneurysm or arteriovenous fistula formation, and venous thrombosis. Given the scarcity of literature on these topics, most recommendations are anecdotal based on case reports, and thus no general consensus exists.

In cases of pancreatic arterial stenosis, either anticoagulation or interventional therapy (eg, balloon angioplasty or stent placement) may be beneficial depending on the particular patient.[63] Pancreatic arterial thrombosis does not appear to respond well to pharmacomechanical lysis, likely secondary to the small size of pancreatic vessels that may be involved.[63] However, arteriovenous fistulae and pseudoaneurysms involving the graft vessels do appear to respond well to endovascular therapy depending on the ease with which the involved vessels can be approached endovascularly.[63,64] Depending on the case, venous thrombosis may respond to either anticoagulation, surgical thrombectomy, or endovascular lysis with favorable results.[65,66]

REFERENCES

1. Tzakis A, Todo S, Starzl TE. Orthotopic liver transplantation with preservation of the inferior vena cava. Ann Surg 1989;210(5):649–52.
2. Reddy K, Mallett S, Peachey T. Venovenous bypass in orthotopic liver transplantation: time for a rethink? Liver Transpl 2005;11(7):741–9.
3. Grande L, Rimola A, Cugat E, et al. Effect of venovenous bypass on perioperative renal function in liver transplantation: results of a randomized, controlled trial. Hepatology 1996;23(6):1418–28.
4. Shaw BW Jr, Martin DJ, Marquez JM, et al. Venous bypass in clinical liver transplantation. Ann Surg 1984;200(4):524–34.
5. Fan ST, Yong BH, Lo CM, et al. Right lobe living donor liver transplantation with or without venovenous bypass. Br J Surg 2003;90(1):48–56.
6. Kuo PC, Alfrey EJ, Garcia G, et al. Orthotopic liver transplantation with selective use of venovenous bypass. Am J Surg 1995;170(6):671–5.
7. Wilson CH, Rix DA, Manas DM. Routine intraoperative ureteric stenting for kidney transplant recipients. Cochrane Database Syst Rev 2013;(6):CD004925.
8. Hedges SJ, Dehoney SB, Hooper JS, et al. Evidence-based treatment recommendations for uremic bleeding. Nat Clin Pract Nephrol 2007;3(3):138–53.
9. Tavakoli A, Surange RS, Pearson RC, et al. Impact of stents on urological complications and health care expenditure in renal transplant recipients: results of a prospective, randomized clinical trial. J Urol 2007;177(6):2260–4 [discussion: 2264].
10. Amante AJ, Kahan BD. En bloc transplantation of kidneys from pediatric donors. J Urol 1996;155(3):852–6 [discussion: 856–7].
11. Dreikorn K, Rohl L, Horsch R. The use of double renal transplants from paediatric cadaver donors. Br J Urol 1977;49(5):361–4.
12. Duffy JP, Hong JC, Farmer DG, et al. Vascular complications of orthotopic liver transplantation: experience in more than 4,200 patients. J Am Coll Surg 2009;208(5):896–903 [discussion: 903–5].
13. Pappas P, Zavos G, Kaza S, et al. Angioplasty and stenting of arterial stenosis affecting renal transplant function. Transplant Proc 2008;40(5):1391–6.
14. Valji K. The practice of vascular and interventional radiology. 3rd edition. Philadelphia: Saunders Elsevier; 2012.
15. Pareja E, Cortes M, Navarro R, et al. Vascular complications after orthotopic liver transplantation: hepatic artery thrombosis. Transplant Proc 2010;42(8):2970–2.

16. Abbasoglu O, Levy MF, Vodapally MS, et al. Hepatic artery stenosis after liver transplantation–incidence, presentation, treatment, and long term outcome. Transplantation 1997;63(2):250–5.

17. Saad WE, Davies MG, Sahler L, et al. Hepatic artery stenosis in liver transplant recipients: primary treatment with percutaneous transluminal angioplasty. J Vasc Interv Radiol 2005;16(6):795–805.

18. Vivarelli M, Cucchetti A, La Barba G, et al. Ischemic arterial complications after liver transplantation in the adult: multivariate analysis of risk factors. Arch Surg 2004;139(10):1069–74.

19. Dodd GD 3rd, Memel DS, Zajko AB, et al. Hepatic artery stenosis and thrombosis in transplant recipients: Doppler diagnosis with resistive index and systolic acceleration time. Radiology 1994;192(3):657–61.

20. Vit A, De Candia A, Como G, et al. Doppler evaluation of arterial complications of adult orthotopic liver transplantation. J Clin Ultrasound 2003;31(7):339–45.

21. Saad WE. Management of hepatic artery steno-occlusive complications after liver transplantation. Tech Vasc Interv Radiol 2007;10(3):207–20.

22. Kodama Y, Sakuhara Y, Abo D, et al. Percutaneous transluminal angioplasty for hepatic artery stenosis after living donor liver transplantation. Liver Transpl 2006;12(3):465–9.

23. Ueno T, Jones G, Martin A, et al. Clinical outcomes from hepatic artery stenting in liver transplantation. Liver Transpl 2006;12(3):422–7.

24. Woo DH, Laberge JM, Gordon RL, et al. Management of portal venous complications after liver transplantation. Tech Vasc Interv Radiol 2007; 10(3):233–9.

25. Saad WE. Portal interventions in liver transplant recipients. Semin Intervent Radiol 2012;29(2):99–104.

26. Funaki B, Rosenblum JD, Leef JA, et al. Percutaneous treatment of portal venous stenosis in children and adolescents with segmental hepatic transplants: long-term results. Radiology 2000;215(1): 147–51.

27. Ko GY, Sung KB, Yoon HK, et al. Early posttransplantation portal vein stenosis following living donor liver transplantation: percutaneous transhepatic primary stent placement. Liver Transpl 2007;13(4): 530–6.

28. Ueda M, Egawa H, Ogawa K, et al. Portal vein complications in the long-term course after pediatric living donor liver transplantation. Transplant Proc 2005;37(2):1138–40.

29. Navarro F, Le Moine MC, Fabre JM, et al. Specific vascular complications of orthotopic liver transplantation with preservation of the retrohepatic vena cava: review of 1361 cases. Transplantation 1999; 68(5):646–50.

30. Darcy MD. Management of venous outflow complications after liver transplantation. Tech Vasc Interv Radiol 2007;10(3):240–5.

31. Wang SL, Sze DY, Busque S, et al. Treatment of hepatic venous outflow obstruction after piggy-back liver transplantation. Radiology 2005;236(1): 352–9.

32. Weeks SM, Gerber DA, Jaques PF, et al. Primary Gianturco stent placement for inferior vena cava abnormalities following liver transplantation. J Vasc Interv Radiol 2000;11(2 Pt 1):177–87.

33. Ko GY, Sung KB, Yoon HK, et al. Endovascular treatment of hepatic venous outflow obstruction after living-donor liver transplantation. J Vasc Interv Radiol 2002;13(6):591–9.

34. Kubo T, Shibata T, Itoh K, et al. Outcome of percutaneous transhepatic venoplasty for hepatic venous outflow obstruction after living donor liver transplantation. Radiology 2006;239(1):285–90.

35. Atwal T, Pastrana M, Sandhu B. Post-liver transplant biliary complications. J Clin Exp Hepatol 2012;2(1): 81–5.

36. Macias-Gomez C, Dumonceau JM. Endoscopic management of biliary complications after liver transplantation: an evidence-based review. World J Gastrointest Endosc 2015;7(6):606–16.

37. Wojcicki M, Milkiewicz P, Silva M. Biliary tract complications after liver transplantation: a review. Dig Surg 2008;25(4):245–57.

38. Novellas S, Caramella T, Fournol M, et al. MR cholangiopancreatography features of the biliary tree after liver transplantation. AJR Am J Roentgenol 2008; 191(1):221–7.

39. Akamatsu N, Sugawara Y, Hashimoto D. Biliary reconstruction, its complications and management of biliary complications after adult liver transplantation: a systematic review of the incidence, risk factors and outcome. Transpl Int 2011;24(4): 379–92.

40. Kothary N, Patel AA, Shlansky-Goldberg RD. Interventional radiology: management of biliary complications of liver transplantation. Semin Intervent Radiol 2004;21(4):297–308.

41. Rerknimitr R, Sherman S, Fogel EL, et al. Biliary tract complications after orthotopic liver transplantation with choledochocholedochostomy anastomosis: endoscopic findings and results of therapy. Gastrointest Endosc 2002;55(2):224–31.

42. Sung RS, Campbell DA Jr, Rudich SM, et al. Long-term follow-up of percutaneous transhepatic balloon cholangioplasty in the management of biliary strictures after liver transplantation. Transplantation 2004;77(1):110–5.

43. Roumilhac D, Poyet G, Sergent G, et al. Long-term results of percutaneous management for anastomotic biliary stricture after orthotopic liver transplantation. Liver Transpl 2003;9(4):394–400.

44. Venbrux AC, Osterman FA Jr. Percutaneous management of benign biliary strictures. Tech Vasc Interv Radiol 2001;4(3):141–6.

45. Bruno S, Remuzzi G, Ruggenenti P. Transplant renal artery stenosis. J Am Soc Nephrol 2004;15(1):134–41.

46. Henning BF, Kuchlbauer S, Boger CA, et al. Percutaneous transluminal angioplasty as first-line treatment of transplant renal artery stenosis. Clin Nephrol 2009;71(5):543–9.

47. Singh AK, Sahani DV. Imaging of the renal donor and transplant recipient. Radiol Clin North Am 2008;46(1):79–93, vi.

48. Libicher M, Radeleff B, Grenacher L, et al. Interventional therapy of vascular complications following renal transplantation. Clin Transplant 2006; 20(Suppl 17):55–9.

49. Beecroft JR, Rajan DK, Clark TW, et al. Transplant renal artery stenosis: outcome after percutaneous intervention. J Vasc Interv Radiol 2004;15(12): 1407–13.

50. Hagen G, Wadstrom J, Magnusson M, et al. Outcome after percutaneous transluminal angioplasty of arterial stenosis in renal transplant patients. Acta Radiol 2009;50(3):270–5.

51. Valpreda S, Messina M, Rabbia C. Stenting of transplant renal artery stenosis: outcome in a single center study. J Cardiovasc Surg (Torino) 2008;49(5): 565–70.

52. Modrall JG, Teitelbaum GP, Diaz-Luna H, et al. Local thrombolysis in a renal allograft threatened by renal vein thrombosis. Transplantation 1993;56(4):1011–3.

53. Melamed ML, Kim HS, Jaar BG, et al. Combined percutaneous mechanical and chemical thrombectomy for renal vein thrombosis in kidney transplant recipients. Am J Transplant 2005;5(3):621–6.

54. Rouviere O, Berger P, Beziat C, et al. Acute thrombosis of renal transplant artery: graft salvage by means of intra-arterial fibrinolysis. Transplantation 2002;73(3):403–9.

55. Klepanec A, Balazs T, Bazik R, et al. Pharmacomechanical thrombectomy for treatment of acute transplant renal artery thrombosis. Ann Vasc Surg 2014; 28(5):1314.e11–4.

56. Englesbe MJ, Dubay DA, Gillespie BW, et al. Risk factors for urinary complications after renal transplantation. Am J Transplant 2007;7(6):1536–41.

57. Kobayashi K, Censullo ML, Rossman LL, et al. Interventional radiologic management of renal transplant dysfunction: indications, limitations, and technical considerations. Radiographics 2007; 27(4):1109–30.

58. Benoit G, Alexandre L, Moukarzel M, et al. Percutaneous antegrade dilation of ureteral strictures in kidney transplants. J Urol 1993;150(1):37–9.

59. Fontaine AB, Nijjar A, Rangaraj R. Update on the use of percutaneous nephrostomy/balloon dilation for the treatment of renal transplant leak/obstruction. J Vasc Interv Radiol 1997;8(4):649–53.

60. Perini S, Gordon RL, LaBerge JM, et al. Transcatheter embolization of biopsy-related vascular injury in the transplant kidney: immediate and long-term outcome. J Vasc Interv Radiol 1998;9(6):1011–9.

61. Loffroy R, Guiu B, Lambert A, et al. Management of post-biopsy renal allograft arteriovenous fistulas with selective arterial embolization: immediate and long-term outcomes. Clin Radiol 2008;63(6): 657–65.

62. Gruessner AC, Gruessner RW. Pancreas transplant outcomes for United States and non United States cases as reported to the United Network for Organ Sharing and the International Pancreas Transplant Registry as of December 2011. Clin Transpl 2012;23–40.

63. Saad WE, Darwish WE, Turba UC, et al. Endovascular management of vascular complications in pancreatic transplants. Vasc Endovascular Surg 2012;46(3):262–8.

64. Barth MM, Khwaja K, Faintuch S, et al. Transarterial and transvenous embolotherapy of arteriovenous fistulas in the transplanted pancreas. J Vasc Interv Radiol 2008;19(8):1231–5.

65. Delis S, Dervenis C, Bramis J, et al. Vascular complications of pancreas transplantation. Pancreas 2004; 28(4):413–20.

66. Stockland AH, Willingham DL, Paz-Fumagalli R, et al. Pancreas transplant venous thrombosis: role of endovascular interventions for graft salvage. Cardiovasc Intervent Radiol 2009;32(2):279–83.

Pediatric Abdominal Organ Transplantation
Current Indications, Techniques, and Imaging Findings

A. Luana Stanescu, MD[a], Anastasia L. Hryhorczuk, MD[b],
Patricia T. Chang, MD[c], Edward Y. Lee, MD, MPH[d],
Grace S. Phillips, MD[a],*

KEYWORDS

- Pediatric renal transplantation • Liver transplantation • Multivisceral transplantation
- Doppler ultrasound • Hepatic artery thrombosis • Renal artery stenosis • Intestinal failure

KEY POINTS

- Vascular complications in pediatric renal transplants, including renal artery thrombosis, renal vein thrombosis, and renal artery stenosis, remain the main cause for graft loss.
- Compared with adults, a higher rate of complications is seen with pediatric liver transplantation.
- Accurate and timely radiological diagnosis of transplant complications facilitates appropriate treatment and minimizes morbidity and mortality.
- Doppler ultrasound is the mainstay of imaging after transplantation.
- Computed tomography (CT) and CT angiography, MR imaging and magnetic resonance (MR) angiography, MR cholangiopancreatography, conventional angiography, and nuclear medicine imaging may be used for problem-solving in pediatric transplant patients.

RENAL TRANSPLANTATION
Introduction

End-stage renal disease (ESRD) affects pediatric patients of all ages, with an incidence of 14.1 cases/million in 2012.[1] The most common causes for pediatric ESRD in young children are renal dysplasia and congenital urinary tract obstruction/reflux nephropathy, whereas acquired glomerular disease, such as focal glomerular sclerosis, is more commonly seen in older pediatric patients. Treatment is usually sequential, initiated with hemodialysis and followed by peritoneal dialysis

and renal transplant.[1,2] In recent years, renal transplant has become the optimal therapeutic option for pediatric patients with end-stage kidney disease, providing the most effective long-term renal replacement therapy, with the advantages of significantly improved survival as compared with long-term dialysis as well as a better growth potential and overall quality of life.[3–5] The main contraindications for renal transplantation include active or chronic sepsis, active malignancy, and ESRD from autoimmune disease with elevated levels of circulating antiglomerular basement membrane

The authors have no disclosures.
[a] Department of Radiology, Seattle Children's Hospital, University of Washington School of Medicine, 4800 Sand Point Way NE, Seattle 98105, WA, USA; [b] Department of Radiology, Floating Hospital for Children, Tufts Medical Center, 800 Washington Street, Boston, MA 02111, USA; [c] Department of Radiology, Boston Children's Hospital, Harvard Medical School, 300 Longwood Avenue, Boston, MA 02115, USA; [d] Division of Thoracic Imaging, Department of Radiology, Boston Children's Hospital, Harvard Medical School, 300 Longwood Avenue, Boston, MA 02115, USA
* Corresponding author.
E-mail address: grace.phillips@seattlechildrens.org

Radiol Clin N Am 54 (2016) 281–302
http://dx.doi.org/10.1016/j.rcl.2015.09.011

antibodies like Goodpasture disease and systemic lupus erythematosus.[6,7]

Normal Anatomy and Imaging Techniques

Ultrasound is the anatomic imaging modality of choice in renal transplant, providing a comprehensive assessment including gray-scale and color Doppler evaluation of the renal graft and spectral Doppler interrogation of the transplant vasculature. At the authors' institution, an initial baseline ultrasound examination is performed immediately after surgery (**Box 1**). Short-term follow-up sonographic evaluations are obtained as needed depending on clinical evolution and initial imaging findings, whereas long-term follow-up includes yearly ultrasound examinations.[8,9] Ultrasound also provides guidance for renal graft biopsies. Contrast-enhanced ultrasound using gas-filled microbubbles can assess graft microvascular perfusion and was found to have prognostic value for long-term kidney function in adults,[10,11] therefore, potentially representing a future imaging modality in pediatric renal transplantation patients as well.

Renal scintigraphy using Technetium mertiatide (99m Tc [MAG 3]) is currently the preferred functional imaging method of evaluating the transplanted kidney given its capability to assess the graft perfusion, parenchymal uptake, and excretion. For many years, renal scintigraphy was performed routinely for all pediatric patients immediately after transplant, but is now used as a problem-solving tool for suspected complications after surgery.

Cross-sectional imaging with computed tomography (CT) or magnetic resonance (MR) has limited indications in pediatric renal transplants and is primarily used for evaluating vascular complications after transplantation. CT is now infrequently used in children with renal grafts given concerns for radiation and the nephrotoxic potential of CT contrast. MR has the advantage of a nonradiating anatomic technique with excellent angiographic capabilities and essentially nonnephrotoxic contrast agents; however, the utilization is compromised by the need for sedation in young children, its high cost, and its limited availability. MR renography is emerging as a powerful functional imaging tool, potentially able to differentiate noninvasively acute rejection from acute tubular necrosis, currently diagnosed by renal biopsy.[12,13] Although this technique may have an important role in the future, to the authors' knowledge, no data are yet available for pediatric renal transplant recipients.

Preoperative Assessment

Abdominal Doppler ultrasound is routinely performed during pretransplant assessment to evaluate the vascular anatomy, including the aorta, inferior vena cava (IVC), and common iliac vessels[14] (**Box 2**). Contrast-enhanced CT angiogram is indicated in pediatric patients on peritoneal dialysis, in whom the aorta and IVC are incompletely visualized and assessed by ultrasound as well as in those with prior invasive vascular procedures/long-standing central lines with vascular occlusion detected by ultrasound. A chest radiograph is obtained the day before surgery to screen for active infection.[6,7]

More comprehensive pretransplant imaging studies are reserved for pediatric patients with specific urinary abnormalities, such as neurogenic

---

Box 1
Imaging techniques

Doppler ultrasound

- Gray-scale imaging of the renal transplant
- Color and spectral Doppler evaluation of renal inflow and outflow including all anastomoses and sampling of parenchymal arteries

Renal scintigraphy with 99m Tc (MAG 3)

- Evaluates graft perfusion, parenchymal uptake, and excretion

MR and CT

- MRA may be used in vascular complications such as renal artery stenosis if indicated, with time-of-flight technique or contrast-enhanced time-resolved MR angiogram
- CTA is infrequently used; in select cases it can be performed with thin collimation and bolus tracking on the abdominal aorta tailored to individual pediatric patients
- Maximum-intensity-projection images can be obtained with both modalities

---

Box 2
Preoperative imaging in renal transplantation

Routine

- Abdominal Doppler ultrasound of the aorta, IVC, and common iliac vessels
- Chest radiograph

Advanced imaging

- CTA
- Voiding cystourethrogram
- Urodynamic studies

bladder, prune belly syndrome or posterior ure-thral valves, recurrent urinary tract infections, or voiding abnormalities. In these patients, voiding cystourethrography and urodynamic studies may be indicated to detect any underlying abnormality that could potentially affect the renal graft and should be surgically corrected before transplantation.[6,7]

Postoperative Assessment

Although surgical techniques may vary, renal trans-plants in children are always heterotopic allografts, obtained from living donors in approximately 50% of the cases,[15] usually the patient's parents.[16] Adult-sized kidney transplants from living donors are associated with better graft outcome even in small children, despite the vascular size discrep-ancy and the high blood flow/perfusion require-ment relative to the child cardiac output.

In older children with body weight of 30 kg or more, the surgical technique is identical to adults, with the renal graft placed in an extraperitoneal location in the right iliac fossa, and end-to-side vascular anastomosis to the ipsilateral common iliac artery and vein.[2,9] In pediatric patients with body weight less than 10 kg, the extraperitoneal space may not accommodate the size of the renal graft, which can be placed intraperitoneally and anastomosed to the aorta and IVC to allow a better perfusion.[2] Despite technical difficulties related to vascular access for anastomosis, a recent study showed similar outcomes when comparing intra-peritoneal and extraperitoneal transplantation in small children.[17] Surgical technique for children with body weight between 10 and 30 kg depends on body habitus and surgeon preference. Uretero-neocystostomy remains the preferred surgical method for ureteral anastomosis, independent of age or body habitus.[16,18] Ureteral stenting tech-nique after transplant is variable.[9,18]

The gray-scale sonographic features of the renal graft are slightly different as compared with native kidneys, with improved details given the superfi-cial position, closer to the transducer. The renal cortex may be more echogenic, with an accentu-ated corticomedullary differentiation, while the renal sinus fat may also demonstrate increased echogenicity. Mild prominence of the ureter and renal pelvis can be present due to absent peri-stalsis related to denervation.[19] Small perinephric hematomas or seromas represent an expected finding after surgery (**Fig. 1**).

Global parenchymal perfusion evaluated quali-tatively with color or power Doppler should be homogenous, with cortical interlobular vessels visualized to the capsule. Spectral Doppler arterial waveforms in a normal renal transplant demon-strate a low resistance waveform with continuous antegrade flow throughout the cardiac cycle and sharp systolic upstroke. The normal range of peak systolic velocities in the extrarenal artery is between 50 and 200 cm/s, with transient turbu-lence and high velocity often present immediately after surgery because of perianastomotic edema (see **Fig. 1**). Renal artery velocities should always be correlated with peak velocities in the aorta/iliac vessels (renal/aortic ratio). Diffusely increased peak systolic velocities in the graft artery are typi-cally seen in the setting of increased systemic

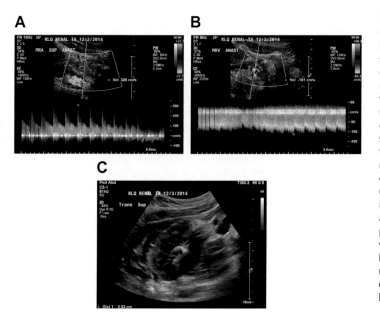

A **B** **C**

Fig. 1. Expected immediate postop-erative findings in a renal transplant. (*A*) Spectral waveform analysis of the superior-most of 2 renal arteries on day 1 after surgery demonstrates normal waveforms and elevated velocity of 306 cm/s near the anasto-mosis. (*B*) Spectral waveform analysis of the main renal vein demonstrates slightly phasic, normal-directional flow with high velocity at the anasto-mosis of 186 cm/s. Follow-up Doppler examination on day 2 after surgery (not shown) demonstrated normal-ized velocities in the renal artery and vein, consistent with decreased perianastomotic edema. (*C*) Trans-verse gray-scale image shows a small, heterogeneous crescentic perineph-ric fluid collection on postoperative day 2, consistent with evolving hematoma.

velocities, often related in the immediate postoperative period to overhydration. Spectral Doppler interrogation of the interlobar renal arteries allows assessment of the intrarenal vascular resistance through the resistive index (RI), calculated as (peak systolic velocity − end diastolic velocity)/peak systolic velocity. Normal values range between 0.4 and 0.8 and may increase up to 1.0 in the immediate postoperative period because of graft edema, causing decreased diastolic flow.

Renal vein waveform is usually monophasic and in the opposite direction of the renal artery. Similar to the renal artery, high velocities and turbulent waveform may be present immediately after surgery because of perianastomotic edema (see **Fig. 1**).

Normal posttransplant renal scintigraphy with 99m Tc mertiatide shows prompt perfusion and uniform cortical uptake, with time to peak less than 5 minutes and time to half activity of up to 11 minutes. Normal excretion in the renal pelvis and spontaneous drainage in the ureter and bladder should be present.

Complications

Hematoma and seroma

Perinephric fluid collections, including hematomas, seromas, urinomas, abscesses, and lymphoceles, represent a common occurrence, seen in up to 50% of renal transplant patients.[19,20] Subcapsular or perinephric hematomas are typically detected by ultrasound immediately after surgery as a crescentic homogenous hypoechoic fluid collection (see **Fig. 1**). Small hematomas usually resolve spontaneously or may evolve into chronic seromas, depicted as homogenous anechoic fluid collections. Larger perinephric hematomas may cause hydronephrosis through mass effect on the ureter, whereas significant subcapsular hematomas can result in parenchymal compression and hypoperfusion, leading to the so-called Page kidney and pseudorejection.[9] Percutaneous ultrasound-guided drainage is indicated in these cases. Perinephric hematomas may also occur after renal biopsies and trauma.

Abscess

Perinephric abscesses are rare, presenting with fever and graft pain in the first month after surgery in affected pediatric patients. Underlying cause may include superinfection of a prior sterile perinephric collection or direct extension from surgical wound or extensive renal graft pyelonephritis.[9] Although the presence of gas foci is highly concerning for an infected fluid collection, more often the ultrasound appearance of an abscess is nonspecific, showing a complex perinephric fluid collection with thick septations and echogenic debris, difficult to differentiate from a resolving hematoma. Percutaneous ultrasound-guided fluid aspiration followed by fluid analysis can provide a definitive diagnosis.

Lymphocele

Lymphoceles represent a late complication of renal transplant, seen usually 4 to 8 weeks after surgery, with a variable incidence reported to be up to 15%.[8] The cause is likely related to the surgical disruption of lymphatic channels along the great vessels during dissection near the site of anastomosis or in the renal hilum. Additional factors, such as high-dose steroids, certain immunosuppressives, and high body mass index, were found to be associated with an increased risk of developing lymphatic complications after renal transplant.[21] Most lymphoceles are small in size and incidentally discovered during routine ultrasound examinations. Large lymphoceles can be symptomatic, presenting with graft pain and mass effect on the renal transplant and adjacent common iliac vessels, causing decreased renal function and ipsilateral lower extremity swelling. Lymphoceles appear on ultrasound as a well-defined, predominantly anechoic fluid collection with possible thin echogenic internal septations.[8,21] On renal scintigraphy with 99m Tc mertiatide, lymphoceles are photopenic, which differentiates them from urine leak.

Vascular Complications

Vascular complications in pediatric renal transplants, including renal artery thrombosis, renal vein thrombosis, and renal stenosis, remain the main cause for graft loss, with a reported incidence between 8.5% and 10%.[22,23]

Renal artery thrombosis

Renal artery thrombosis is a rare immediate complication present in up to 1% of renal grafts, seen in correlation with young age of recipients, deceased donors, and prolonged ischemic cold time. Renal artery thrombosis has been infrequently reported in the last decade with the advent of increasing living adult donor transplantation. The cause is usually arterial kink or an intimal flap, while severe rejection and hypercoagulability can be precipitating factors.[8,9]

Global renal infarction is virtually always associated with renal artery thrombosis. Ultrasound evaluation depicts an enlarged, edematous kidney with absent parenchymal Doppler color flow and absent color flow and spectral Doppler waveforms in the renal vessels. A similar sonographic appearance may however be seen in severe rejection.

Further evaluation with renal scintigraphy may clarify the diagnosis, absent perfusion and cortical uptake being diagnostic for renal artery thrombosis. Segmental infarcts seen on ultrasound as wedge-shaped hypoechoic regions with absent perfusion result from thrombosis of an accessory renal artery or in grafts with multiple renal arteries and may be detected immediately after surgery as well as a delayed complication related to rejection, when a focal area of increased renal echogenicity will be present (**Fig. 2**).[9,24]

Renal vein thrombosis

Renal vein thrombosis is also a rare adverse event seen in the first month after surgery, presenting with pain, occurring in up to 7% of pediatric renal transplants.[22,23] Possible causes include venous compression from perinephric fluid collection and technically difficult venous anastomosis with ischemic changes, with predisposing factors including hypercoagulability, hypovolemia, or slow flow from acute rejection.[19,23,24] Ultrasound evaluation will show an enlarged edematous kidney with absent color and spectral Doppler flow in the renal vein, which may contain echogenic clot. Decreased peak systolic velocity and reversed diastolic flow are present on renal artery spectral Doppler waveform. On 99m Tc mertiatide renal scintigraphy, the findings are nonspecific, with delayed perfusion, decreased cortical uptake, and no excretion, similar to acute rejection or pseudorejection.

Renal artery stenosis

Renal artery stenosis is a late complication of renal transplant, reported lately in up to 4% of pediatric patients.[22,23] Affected pediatric patients typically present with new onset hypertension with or without graft dysfunction. Color and spectral Doppler ultrasound findings of renal artery stenosis include focal narrowing and turbulent flow, usually in the region of the anastomosis, with spectral broadening of the arterial waveform, decreased diastolic flow, and peak systolic velocity higher than 200 cm/s. Tardus parvus waveforms with decreased resistive indices may be present distally in the renal parenchyma. Perivascular soft tissue vibrations, seen as low-frequency reflections on each side of the baseline on spectral Doppler, are caused by turbulent flow in the stenotic segment.[25] MR angiography (MRA) or CT angiography (CTA) can be used for confirmation, because ultrasound cannot always differentiate arterial kink from stenosis. Conventional angiography remains the gold standard for diagnostic as well as treatment of hemodynamically significant stenosis.

Urologic Complications

Urologic complications after renal transplantation include obstruction, urinary leak, and vesicoureteral reflux, present in up to 21% of pediatric patients.[18,26]

Urinary tract obstruction

Urinary tract obstruction is seen more frequently in the first month after transplant, although it may have a delayed presentation after months or years. Stricture at the anastomosis in the distal ureter is the most common cause of obstruction, with approximately 90% of the cases presenting with stenosis in the distal third of the ureter.[24] Renal stones, fungus balls, and sloughed papilla account

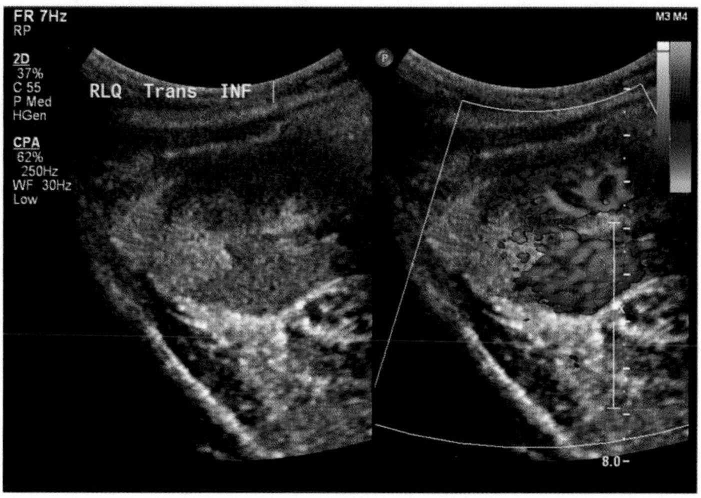

Fig. 2. Segmental infarct. Transverse sonogram obtained 2 years after transplant shows a wedge-shaped area of increased echogenicity in the inferior pole on gray-scale imaging (*left*), with absent flow on color Doppler (*right*), suggestive of infarct.

for the remainder of the cases. Affected pediatric patients are usually asymptomatic given that renal colic cannot occur in the setting of kidney and ureter denervation. Although mild collecting system dilation may represent a normal finding in renal transplants, moderate and particularly progressive hydronephrosis is highly concerning for obstruction. Nuclear medicine renogram can help differentiate a patulous system from obstruction (**Fig. 3**).

Urine leak and urinoma
Urine extravasation is relatively rare, presenting early after surgery with severe pain, swelling,

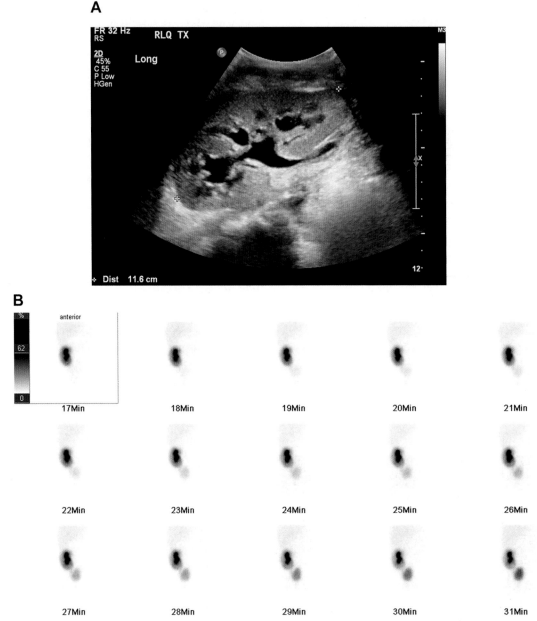

Fig. 3. Ureteral obstruction. (*A*) Longitudinal gray-scale sonogram of the renal transplant 1 day after stent removal demonstrates new mild to moderate pelvicaliectasis and ureterectasis. (*B*) Nuclear medicine renal scintigraphy with 99m Tc mertiatide shows prompt perfusion with delayed cortical transit. There was no significant spontaneous excretion before Lasix, with mild excretion after Lasix. (*C*) Time activity curve reflects these findings, consistent with high-grade obstruction. On retrograde pyelogram (not shown), patient was found to have distal ureteral narrowing at the anastomosis.

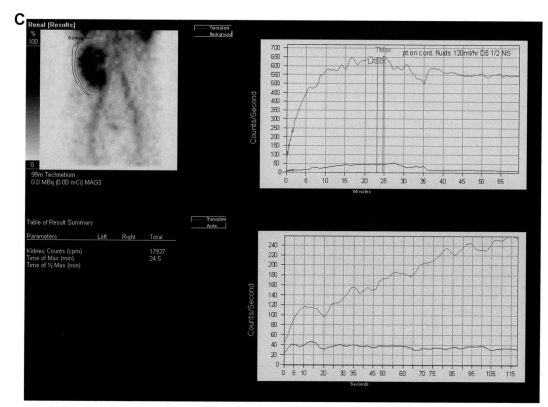

Fig. 3. *(continued)*

and decreased urine output. Vascular insufficiency and subsequent necrosis of the renal collecting system represent the most frequently encountered cause, affecting the distal ureter and the vesicoureteral anastomosis more commonly than the proximal ureter and renal calyces.[21] Ultrasound evaluation demonstrates a nonspecific anechoic fluid collection without septations, which may increase in size rapidly, requiring emergent ultrasound-guided aspiration/decompression.[24] Urinary ascites is present in intraperitoneal transplants. Renal scintigraphy with 99m Tc mertiatide is diagnostic and highly specific, demonstrating progressive radiotracer uptake in the extraluminal fluid.

Vesicoureteral reflux

Vesicoureteral reflux may be seen in up to 10% of pediatric renal patients and is more likely to be present in children with prior urologic abnormality, especially posterior urethral valves.[18] Currently, it is not clear if the presence of vesicoureteral reflux is associated with increased frequency of graft infection or decreased graft survival.[9,18] Similar to native kidneys, voiding cytoureterography and nuclear medicine cystogram are diagnostic (Fig. 4).

Parenchymal Abnormalities

Three main diffuse parenchymal abnormalities of the renal graft in the immediate postoperative period include acute tubular necrosis, rejection, and drug nephrotoxicity. Acute tubular necrosis, also known as preservation injury, is related to ischemic time, more commonly seen in grafts from deceased donors (Fig. 5). Acute rejection, humoral or cellular, is the most common type of rejection and may occur within 1 to 3 weeks after transplantation (Fig. 6).[24] Advances in immunosuppressive therapy over the last 10 to 15 years led to a significant decrease in the incidence of acute rejection episodes.[5] Calcineurin inhibitors remain the mainstay of immunosuppressive therapy in pediatric renal transplant. Unfortunately, their nephrotoxic potential can lead to graft injury. Ultrasound findings in all 3 clinical entities, when present, are usually nonspecific, with loss of the corticomedullary differentiation of the enlarged, edematous renal graft. Moderate urothelial thickening without evidence of pyelonephritis or associated hydronephrosis is thought, however, to be highly suggestive of acute rejection.[27] Doppler ultrasound may show decreased diastolic flow with increased RI in the parenchymal arteries. 99m Tc mertiatide renal scintigraphy may help differentiate

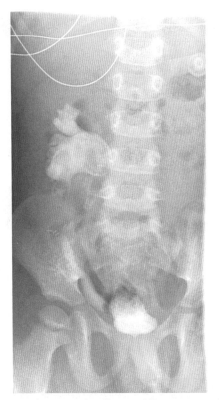

Fig. 4. Vesicoureteral reflux. Voiding cystourethrogram demonstrates reflux during voiding into a dilated collecting system with blunted fornices in a patient presenting with urinary tract infection 2 years after renal transplant.

between acute tubular necrosis and acute rejection. Prompt perfusion and uptake are typically seen in acute tubular necrosis as well as in acute drug toxicity, with decreased or absent perfusion in acute rejection. Excretion is decreased or absent in all clinical entities. Definitive diagnosis is usually made by biopsy and histologic analysis.

Chronic allograft dysfunction, typically occurring 3 months after transplantation, may be seen in chronic rejection as well as in chronic use of calcineurin inhibitors. Ultrasound features of chronic allograft dysfunction include progressive volume loss of the renal graft on serial ultrasounds, with cortical thinning and increased cortical echogenicity.

Postbiopsy Complications

Ultrasound-guided core needle biopsy of the renal graft remains an important diagnostic method for graft surveillance and in allograft dysfunction. Common postbiopsy complications include perinephric hematomas, arteriovenous (AV) fistulas (**Fig. 7**), and pseudoaneurysms. The vast majority

of AV fistulas and pseudoaneurysms do not require treatment and resolve/thrombose spontaneously. Transcatheter embolization is indicated in symptomatic, enlarging AV fistulas causing renal ischemia due to the steal phenomenon as well as in pseudoaneurysms larger than 2 cm.[24]

Summary

Ultrasound remains the primary imaging tool in renal transplant monitoring and detection of complications, while nuclear medicine renal scintigraphy is valuable as a problem-solving tool in selected cases. Cross-sectional imaging using CT and MR has a limited role. Increased awareness of the imaging appearances in renal transplant complications can help in early diagnostic and therapeutic management, potentially extending the graft life.

Pitfalls

- Adult-sized kidney transplants from living donors are associated with better graft outcome even in small children.
- Urinary tract obstruction is painless in patients after renal transplant due to renal and ureteral denervation.
- The greatest reduction in renal graft volume in the first 6 months after transplantation is seen in the youngest transplant recipients, thought to reflect adaptation of the adult size kidney to the lower pediatric vascular supply.

What the Referring Physician Needs to Know

- Are there any focal or diffuse gray-scale or color flow abnormalities of the renal transplant parenchyma?
- Is there new/increasing moderate hydronephrosis to suggest obstruction?
- For extraperitoneal renal transplants, are there any focal perinephric fluid collections to suggest hematoma or abscess? If present, is there mass effect on the renal graft or renal vessels, causing decreased renal perfusion?
- Are there any abnormalities of the Doppler evaluation to suggest vascular complication?

LIVER TRANSPLANTATION
Introduction

Advances in surgical technique and immunosuppressive regimens have allowed pediatric liver transplantation to be an accepted treatment of end-stage liver disease in children. According to the Organ Procurement and Transplantation Network database, in 2014, there were 530 liver transplants in children under the age of 18.[28] In

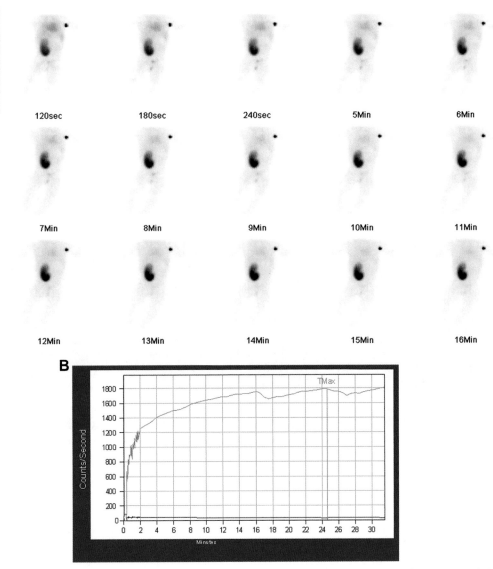

Fig. 5. Acute tubular necrosis day 1 after renal transplant. (*A*) Nuclear medicine renogram with 99m Tc mertiatide shows prompt and homogenous uptake of radiotracer in the right lower quadrant renal transplant, and continued accumulation of tracer without excretion in the collecting system and urinary bladder. (*B*) Time activity curve redemonstrates these findings with delayed time to peak (TMax) uptake (24.6 minutes). The renal Doppler ultrasound examination showed mildly increased resistive indices of 0.8, otherwise unremarkable.

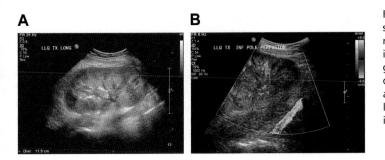

Fig. 6. Acute rejection. (*A*) Grayscale longitudinal sonogram of the renal graft demonstrates diffusely increased echogenicity of the renal graft with loss of corticomedullary differentiation. (*B*) Focal areas of absent perfusion in the upper and lower pole are consistent with focal infarcts.

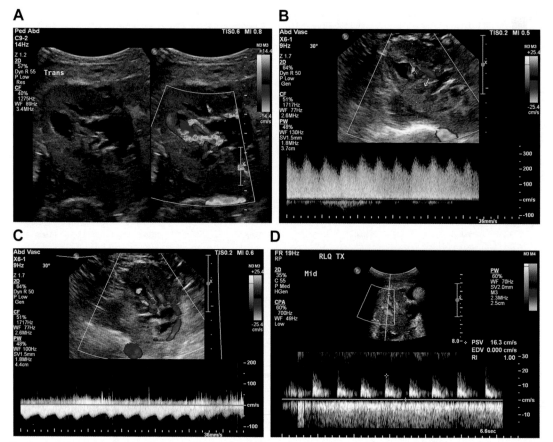

Fig. 7. Arteriovenous fistula after renal biopsy. (*A*) Transverse color Doppler image of the renal transplant shows a focal area of turbulent flow and aliasing in the interpolar region. (*B*) There is increased peak velocity of 300 cm/s in the feeding artery (a midsegmental renal artery branch) with increased diastolic flow. (*C*) The draining vein demonstrates an arterialized waveform. (*D*) Increased RI in the lower pole (RI = 1) consistent with hypoperfusion due to steal phenomenon. Patient underwent successful coil embolization of the AV fistula.

the pediatric population, biliary atresia is the most common underlying cause of end-stage liver disease requiring transplantation. However, a variety of other diseases may be addressed with pediatric liver transplantation, including primary liver malignancies, such as hepatoblastoma, and various metabolic disorders.

Normal Anatomy and Imaging Technique

In children, liver transplantation often makes use of a reduced-sized or segmental transplant, which may consist of a lateral segment, left lobe, right lobe, or extended right lobe,[29] so that the graft is size appropriate for the child. The liver's segmental anatomy and ability to regenerate make this approach feasible. Although there is variability in technique among transplant centers, the vascular anastomoses typically consist of a hepatic artery end-to-end anastomosis, a portal vein end-to-end anastomosis, and a "piggy-

back" side-to-side or end-to-side cavo-caval anastomosis (**Fig. 8**). The biliary anastomosis typically consists of a choledochojejunostomy, particularly in the setting of biliary atresia, or a choledochocholedochostomy.

Sonographic gray-scale, color Doppler, and spectral Doppler evaluation are the mainstay of radiographic assessment of the liver transplant (**Box 3**). Transverse and longitudinal gray-scale imaging should be performed of the entire liver to assess for focal or diffuse parenchymal abnormalities as well as to evaluate the biliary tree.[30] When a segmental graft is used, some mild heterogeneity may be visible on sonographic gray-scale imaging along the cut edge in the immediate postoperative period, and mild periportal edema may be evident (**Fig. 9**). Often, small, transient perioperative fluid collections can also be visualized. Hepatic inflow and outflow should be evaluated with color and spectral Doppler, specifically examining the main, right, and left hepatic arteries, the main and

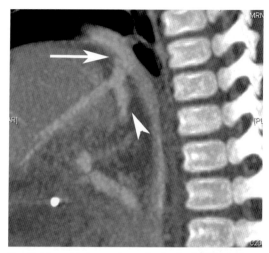

Fig. 8. Piggy-back anastomosis. Sagittal MIP contrast-enhanced CT image shows typical appearance of a piggy-back IVC anastomosis (*arrow*) with blind-ending donor IVC distally (*arrowhead*).

intrahepatic portal veins (**Fig. 10**), the hepatic veins, and IVC, including the respective anastomoses,[30] with attention to the peak systolic velocity and waveform morphology. The resistive index (RI), calculated as (peak systolic velocity - end diastolic velocity)/peak systolic velocity of the main, right, and left hepatic arteries should also be measured. The hepatic artery RI is often transiently elevated in the immediate postoperative period, up

---

Box 3
Imaging techniques

Doppler ultrasound
- Gray-scale imaging of the entire liver transplant
- Color and spectral Doppler evaluation of liver inflow and outflow: Hepatic arteries, portal veins, hepatic veins, IVC including all anastomoses

CT
- Axial, coronal, and sagittal reformatted images obtained after the administration of oral and intravenous contrast
- CTA if indicated with multiplanar thin-cut and maximum-intensity-projection (MIP) images as well as 3-dimensional (3D) volume-rendered images of vascular structures

MR
- Multiplanar T1- and T2-weighted images
- MRA if indicated with 2-dimensional or 3D time-of-flight images

---

to 0.95,[31] thought to be related to older donor age and prolonged ischemic time.[32,33] In addition, a tardus parvus waveform may be seen within the hepatic arteries due to edema at the anastomosis up to 72 hours after transplantation.[34]

CT and MR imaging are typically reserved for problem-solving. CTA or MRA may be useful when a suspected thrombosis of the hepatic artery or portal vein cannot be visualized by Doppler sonogram due to technical factors such as bowel gas. MR cholangiopancreatography (MRCP) is more sensitive than ultrasound in evaluating the biliary tree.[35]

Imaging Findings/Pathology

Hepatic artery thrombosis and stenosis
Early hepatic arterial thrombosis (**Fig. 11**), occurring within the first month after transplantation, is a serious complication that can result in graft loss and death. The reported risk of hepatic arterial thrombosis is higher in pediatric liver transplantation than in adults, ranging in incidence between 4.9% and 8.3%.[36–38] Late hepatic arterial thrombosis, occurring after the first month after transplant, occurs in up to 44% of pediatric patients.[39] Factors that are associated with an increased risk of early hepatic arterial thrombosis include cytomegalovirus mismatch (seropositive donor liver in seronegative recipient), retransplantation, prolonged operation time, low recipient weight, variant arterial anatomy, low-volume transplantation centers, arterial conduits, and prolonged ischemic time.[36,40] Sanchez and colleagues[41] found an increased risk of hepatic artery thrombosis in pediatric patients transplanted for malignancy. Late hepatic arterial thrombosis was associated with a higher donor/recipient weight ratio.[39]

Gu and colleagues[42] found that intraoperative Doppler sonogram could predict hepatic artery thrombosis using parameters of a hepatic artery diameter less than 2 mm, hepatic artery peak systolic velocity of less than 40 cm/s, and a hepatic artery RI of less than 0.60. In the postoperative period, hepatic artery thrombosis should be suspected when common hepatic artery flow is absent or slower than 50 cm/s (**Table 1**), or when the RI is less than 0.50.[31] A filling defect within the common hepatic artery on CTA or MRA is diagnostic. Regarding hepatic artery stenosis (**Fig. 12**), a focal 3- to 4-fold increase in peak systolic velocity within the common hepatic artery is diagnostic of a hemodynamically significant stenosis.[34] The most common location of hepatic artery stenosis is at the anastomosis.

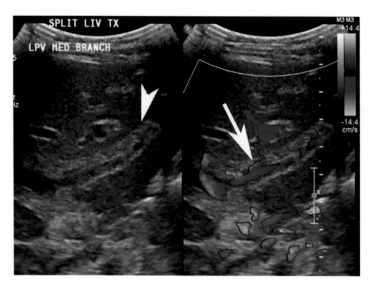

Fig. 9. Normal postoperative edema. Transverse gray-scale image demonstrates increased echogenicity of the portal triads (*left, arrowhead*). The hepatic artery (*right, arrow*) and adjacent portal vein show appropriate color flow on color Doppler imaging.

Portal vein thrombosis and stenosis

Portal vein complications can result in graft dysfunction or loss. There is a reported incidence of portal vein thrombosis of 1% to 5.5% and of portal vein stenosis of 2.7% to 5.6%.[31,43–45] On gray-scale imaging, portal vein thrombosis (**Fig. 13**) appears as a filling defect within the portal vein with absent color, spectral, or power Doppler flow. On CTA and MRA, a filling defect can similarly be seen within the portal vein. With respect to portal vein stenosis (**Fig. 14**), a portal vein caliber of less than 3 to 3.5 mm should suggest the diagnosis.[43,46] Additional findings that suggest portal vein stenosis include a stenotic ratio (prestenotic diameter−stenotic diameter/prestenotic diameter) of greater than 50% and a velocity ratio (peak velocity at stenosis/velocity at the prestenotic site) of greater than 3:1.[43] Splenomegaly, thrombocytopenia, and ascites may also be present in the setting of portal vein stenosis.[43,47,48] Graft rotation of left-sided grafts has been identified as a contributing factor to portal vein complications in pediatric living donor liver transplants.[49]

Hepatic vein outflow obstruction

Hepatic vein outflow obstruction (**Fig. 15**) is another potential vascular complication after liver transplantation that can cause graft dysfunction or loss. The incidence of hepatic vein stenosis is higher in children than adults, at 2.3% to 8.6%[50–52] and 1.8%,[53] respectively. The highest rates of hepatic vein stenosis in children are in the setting of living donor liver transplantation, in which the hepatic veins are individually anastomosed to the IVC.[54] With hepatic vein thrombosis, a filling defect and absent color, spectral, or power Doppler flow is seen within the hepatic veins, which can be confirmed by conventional venogram. Diagnostic criterion for hepatic vein stenosis is a hepatic vein velocity ratio (velocity at the anastomosis/velocity at the main trunk 1–2 cm proximal to the anastomosis) of greater than 4.1 to yield a sensitivity of 83% and specificity of 76%.[55] Although a monophasic waveform may be seen in the absence of hepatic vein stenosis, the identification of a triphasic waveform excludes the diagnosis.[54,55] On conventional venography, a pressure gradient of greater than 10 mm Hg between the hepatic vein and IVC suggests a substantial stenosis.[54]

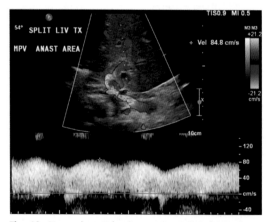

Fig. 10. Normal portal vein anastomotic edema. Spectral waveform analysis of the portal vein anastomosis shows expected mild turbulence and increased velocity at the anastomosis secondary to postoperative edema.

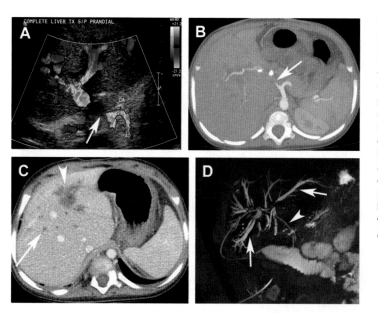

Fig. 11. Hepatic artery thrombosis. (A) Doppler sonogram shows no color Doppler flow in the expected location of the common hepatic artery (arrow). (B) Axial MIP image from a CT angiogram shows a corresponding filling defect in the expected location of the common hepatic artery (arrow). (C) Axial contrast-enhanced CT image shows biliary ductal dilatation (arrow) and a geographic region of low density (arrowhead), suggesting infarct. (D) Subsequent MRCP shows biliary ductal dilatation (arrows) with biliary drain in place (arrowhead). AO, aorta; CA, celiac axis.

Biliary complications

The more common biliary complications following liver transplantation include bile leaks (Fig. 16), strictures, and sludge or stone formation. The reported incidence of biliary complications in children following liver transplantation is 14% to 15%,[56,57] and as high as 38% in pediatric living related liver transplant recipients.[58] On cross-sectional imaging, bile leaks may appear as a nonspecific fluid collection. The diagnosis of a bile leak can be more definitively made by nuclear medicine biliary imaging, which shows progressive accumulation of activity external to bowel. With biliary strictures, biliary ductal dilatation may be seen proximal to the site of obstruction, although ultrasound and CT are relatively insensitive.[35,57,59,60] In contrast, MRCP

(see Fig. 11D) has been shown to be sensitive to subtle focal and diffuse changes in biliary caliber.[35] On MRCP, intrahepatic ducts may be considered dilated at a caliber of greater than 4 mm.[35] Various patterns of abnormalities have been described at MRCP, including global dilatation with or without stricture, focal intrahepatic dilatation with or without bile lakes, and beading of ducts with or without bile lakes.[35]

Rare biliary complications include dysfunction of the sphincter of Oddi and cystic duct remnant mucocele. On imaging, dysfunction of the sphincter of Oddi manifests as dilatation of both the donor and the native bile duct, without evidence of stenosis.[61] Cystic duct remnant mucocele presents on imaging as a cystic mass,

Table 1		
Diagnostic criteria for pediatric liver transplantation vascular complications		
Complication	**Modality**	**Criteria**
Hepatic artery thrombosis	Doppler ultrasound CTA or MRA	Absent or slow flow <50 cm/s; RI <0.50 Filling defect within the common hepatic artery
Hepatic artery stenosis	Doppler ultrasound	3 to 4-fold increase in peak systolic velocity within the common hepatic artery
Portal vein thrombosis	Doppler ultrasound CTA or MRA	Filling defect within the portal vein with absent color, spectral, or power Doppler flow Filling defect within the portal vein
Portal vein stenosis	Ultrasound or CT	Portal vein caliber <3–3.5 mm
Hepatic vein stenosis	Doppler ultrasound	Velocity at anastomosis/velocity at main trunk 1–2 cm proximal to anastomosis >4.1

A

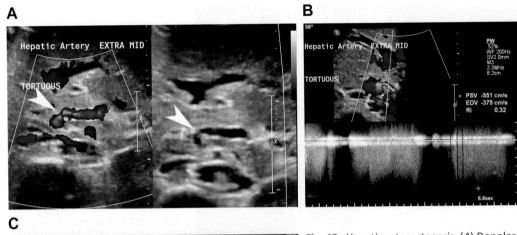

B

C

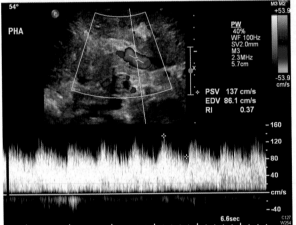

Fig. 12. Hepatic artery stenosis. (*A*) Doppler sonogram shows color aliasing (*left, arrowhead*) corresponding to a curved segment of the hepatic artery (*right, arrowhead*). (*B*) Spectral waveform analysis of the area of color aliasing shows elevated peak systolic velocity of 551 cm/s. (*C*) Spectral waveform analysis more distally in the hepatic artery shows a tardus parvus waveform, characteristic of a proximal stenosis.

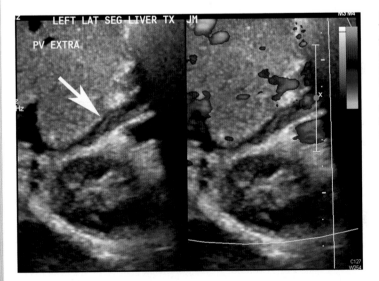

Fig. 13. Portal vein thrombosis. Transverse gray-scale sonogram of the left lobe transplant shows echogenic material within the extrahepatic portion of the portal vein (*left, arrow*). Corresponding transverse color Doppler image (*right*) confirms corresponding lack of color Doppler flow, consistent with thrombosis.

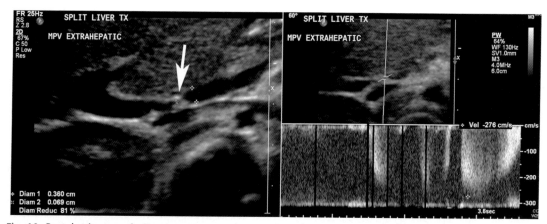

Fig. 14. Portal vein stenosis. Transverse gray-scale sonogram shows pronounced narrowing of the portal vein at the anastomosis (*left, arrow*) with estimated caliber of 0.6 mm. Spectral waveform analysis of this location (*right*) shows turbulent flow with velocity of 276 cm/s.

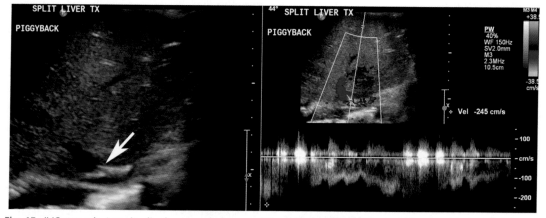

Fig. 15. IVC stenosis. Longitudinal gray-scale image of the IVC piggy-back anastomosis suggests narrowing (*left, arrow*). Doppler interrogation of the anastomosis (*right*) shows turbulent flow with peak velocity of 245 cm/s, confirming stenosis.

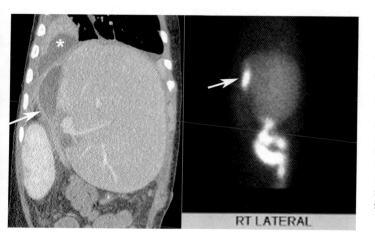

Fig. 16. Bile leak. Sagittal contrast-enhanced CT image shows a rim-enhancing fluid collection posterior to the liver transplant (*left, arrow*). A small right pleural effusion (*left, asterisk*) and adjacent atelectatic lung are also noted. Nuclear medicine hepatobiliary iminodiacetic acid scan (HIDA) study shows focal accumulation of activity posterior to the liver (*right, arrow*) on a static lateral image obtained at 90 minutes, confirming bile leak corresponding to the fluid collection seen on CT.

representing a dilated donor remnant cystic duct, compressing and obstructing the biliary system at the porta hepatis.[62]

Postoperative fluid collections

Hematomas (**Fig. 17**) are common in the 2 weeks following liver transplantation and often resolve spontaneously.[63] On gray-scale imaging, hematomas are usually hyperechoic fluid collections, often occurring in the perihepatic region and lesser sac[63] and are hyperdense on CT.[64] Bilomas often appear as simple fluid collections on sonography.[64] Abscesses may contain internal echoes or septations on sonography, although they may also appear as simple-appearing fluid collections.[65]

Pearls, Pitfalls, Variants

- Intrahepatic arterial flow may be seen in the setting of hepatic artery thrombosis due to collateral vessels, with an abnormal, tardus parvus waveform.
- The finding of a biliary stricture should raise concern for hepatic artery stenosis or thrombosis.
- Ultrasound and CT are relatively insensitive in the evaluation of biliary stricture.
- Splenomegaly, thrombocytopenia, and ascites should raise the possibility of portal vein thrombosis.
- Monophasic waveform of the hepatic veins can be seen in the absence of stenosis. Documentation of triphasic waveforms within the hepatic veins excludes stenosis.

What the Referring Physician Needs to Know

- Are there any focal or diffuse gray-scale abnormalities of the liver transplant parenchyma?
- Is there biliary ductal dilatation to suggest biliary complication?
- Are there any focal fluid collections to suggest hematoma, bile leak, or abscess?
- Are there any abnormalities of liver inflow or outflow to suggest vascular complication?

MULTIVICERAL TRANSPLANTATION
Introduction

In the pediatric population, intestinal and multivisceral transplantation are potential treatments for several surgical and nonsurgical conditions that compromise intestinal function. Unlike adult patients, who commonly receive these complex transplants for portomesenteric thrombosis, Crohn disease, or familial polyposis syndromes with desmoid tumors, the children treated by intestinal or multivisceral transplantation most commonly have underlying medical problems, including gastroschisis (25%), midgut volvulus (24%), or pseudo-obstruction (10%).[66] The choice of graft type is based on the specific nature of the patient's intestinal failure. Isolated intestinal transplant (IIT) can be performed in pediatric patients without associated liver disease, whereas combined liver-pancreas-small bowel transplants (Liv-SB) are commonly used for pediatric patients with intestinal failure–associated liver disease.[67] Multivisceral transplants (MVT), which include the stomach, liver, pancreatoduodenal complex, and small bowel, may be performed for pediatric patients with extensive congenital anomalies or a history of pseudo-obstruction.[67]

Normal Anatomy and Imaging Techniques

Although surgical technique varies among centers, IIT typically involves an arterial end-to-side anastomosis with the native aorta and a venous, end-to-end anastomosis with the native SMV. A proximal intestinal anastomosis is established with the native bowel, and an end ileostomy is usually created, as is the case in the later described Liv-SB and MVT, to facilitate surveillance of the transplant in the postoperative period. With Liv-SB, the transplant comprises the liver, pancreas, and small bowel harvested en bloc with an aortic segment, including the donor celiac axis and superior mesenteric artery, so that an aortic conduit may be fashioned, allowing for a single arterial anastomosis. A portocaval anastomosis is necessary to maintain venous drainage of the native

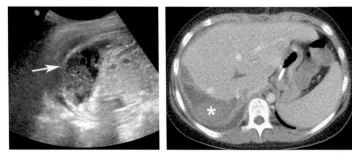

Fig. 17. Hematoma. Transverse gray-scale sonogram shows a fluid collection containing internal echoes posterolateral to the liver transplant (*left, arrow*). Subsequent axial contrast-enhanced CT image shows a corresponding mildly hyperdense fluid collection without rim enhancement (*right, asterisk*).

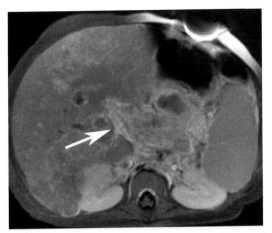

Fig. 18. Axial T1-weighted postcontrast MR image of a 22-month-old girl with multifocal hepatoblastoma demonstrates extensive tumor thrombus occluding the portal venous system (*arrow*). Because of the extent of tumor invasion, she received a MVT.

and thrombocytosis. However, when the donor spleen is included, higher rates of graft-versus-host disease (GVHD) are observed.[68,69] One group has proposed preservation of the native spleen to avoid the asplenic state and the higher rates of GVHD associated with a donor spleen.[70]

Preoperative Assessment

Preoperative imaging in pediatric patients receiving MVT is varied, but is usually tailored to the underlying clinical conditions necessitating the transplant. Pretransplant imaging may also play a role in determining a patient's suitability for a certain type of graft (**Fig. 18**). Fluoroscopic evaluation is typically performed of the native bowel to delineate anatomy. Cross-sectional imaging is valuable for assessing the native vasculature to confirm feasibility of transplantation.

Postoperative Assessment

As postoperative anatomy can be confusing and challenging, with multiple different types of arterial anastomoses and conduits reported in the literature, the authors recommend close consultation with the surgical team to document the precise anatomy in the patient to be imaged.[71] Early postoperative imaging will serve to define the patient's anatomy and provide a guide for future studies (**Fig. 19**).

In the immediate postoperative period, ultrasound is essential for documenting the patency of the graft vasculature and the surgical anastomoses. Ultrasound is also useful in rapidly assessing pediatric patients with additional postoperative concerns, including intra-abdominal bleeding, abscess, or vascular thrombosis. However, in many cases, CT may be necessary for full evaluation of these complex conditions.[72] Because of the lack

bowel. A piggy-back or end-to-end IVC anastomosis is created. An MVT includes the stomach (foregut), intestine, and sometimes portions of the hindgut; if necessary, the liver or potentially other organs may be included in the transplant. An end-to-end gastric anastomosis is performed. The arterial and venous anastomoses are similar to those of the IIT or Liv-SB, depending on whether the liver is included in the transplant specimen. Of note, a biliary anastomosis is not required with Liv-Sb or MVT, because the pancreas is included in the transplant, leaving the donor biliary system intact. One area of controversy is whether to perform a splenectomy with Liv-SB and MVT, and whether to include the spleen with the transplant specimen. In the setting of splenectomy, the patient is susceptible to encapsulated bacteria

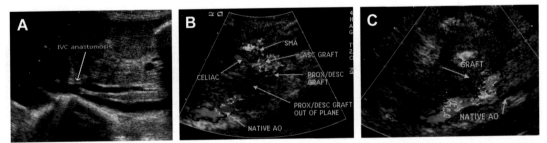

Fig. 19. (*A*) Longitudinal ultrasound imaging after MVT for hepatoblastoma demonstrates a patent IVC anastomosis (*arrow*). (*B*) Postoperative Doppler imaging of the arterial anastomoses demonstrates a patent superior mesenteric artery (SMA) and celiac axis (CELIAC) with connection to a vascular graft (labels on figure). Because of the complex nature of this anatomy, the anastomosis between the aorta and the graft cannot be imaged in the same plane. ASC GRAFT, ascending portion of the vascular graft; PROX/DESC GRAFT, proximal and descending portion of the vascular graft; PROX/DESC GRAFT OUT OF PLANE, the region of the proximal and descending vascular graft that was not well visualized due to location out of plane; AO, aorta. (*C*) Postoperative Doppler imaging of the arterial anastomoses (*longer arrow*) demonstrated a patent connection between the arterial graft (GRAFT) and the patient's aorta (*shorter arrow*).

of ionizing radiation, MR imaging is currently the preferred cross-sectional imaging modality for most nonurgent imaging questions, including assessment for postoperative fungal infections or neoplasm. Mild distention of the transplanted bowel is commonly seen in the first 2 months after transplantation, in combination with mild bowel wall thickening of 3 to 5 mm.[73]

Imaging Findings/Pathology

In the acute setting, clinical concerns center on the status of the transplanted bowel, which may undergo ischemia and reperfusion injury, leading to edema and third spacing of fluid.[67] Acute rejection of the graft is also an important early complication and may require aggressive immunosuppression. Concerns for GVHD and rejection also continue through the subacute period. Typically, these are both evaluated through endoscopy and biopsy (Table 2), with imaging playing an ancillary role.[67] Postoperative fluid collections commonly occur after intestinal transplantation and may be evaluated similar to those occurring after liver transplantation, described above.

Infection

Despite prophylaxis with broad-spectrum antibiotics,[67] infection is a nearly universal complication, with 97% of patients in one series developing an infection following transplant.[74] In this series, 50% of infections occurred in the first 3 months, whereas 25% occurred between 3 and 12 months, and 25% occurred after 1 year.[74] Because infection is a significant cause of morbidity in these patients, aggressive management is paramount. Imaging for this indication follows standard imaging protocols for imaging intrathoracic or intraabdominal bacterial or fungal infections (Fig. 20).

Vascular Complications

Vascular complications such as thrombosis are a substantial cause of mortality and graft loss in the intestinal transplant population, occurring in approximately 20%,[75] most commonly in the immediate postoperative period. Late thrombosis is less common, but may be seen in the setting of infection or chronic rejection.[44] Characteristic findings on Doppler evaluation are the absence of both color Doppler flow and arterial spectral waveform within the thrombosed arterial segment. CTA may be performed for confirmation, which shows a filling defect in the thrombosed vessel. Arterial or venous stenosis is also a possible complication, with similar diagnostic criteria to those described above for renal and liver transplantation (Fig. 21).

Intestinal Complications

The main intestinal complications following intestinal transplant include intestinal perforation, bowel obstruction, and abdominal compartment syndrome.[76] Intestinal perforation has been described at the donor duodenal stump as well as less commonly at the recipient duodenum.[76] Spontaneous bowel perforation as well as wound dehiscence related to an anastomotic site leak has also been reported.[76] CT is considered more sensitive than conventional contrast studies when a leak is strongly suspected.[72] Mechanical dysfunction of the graft can be evaluated by water-soluble gastrointestinal studies, with abnormalities ranging from dysmotility, which is common in the immediate postoperative period, to bowel obstruction (Fig. 22).[77] Acute compartment syndrome occurs primarily with primary closure and can be avoided with staged closure.[76]

Table 2
Diagnostic criteria for pediatric intestinal transplantation complications

Complication	Modality	Criteria
Rejection	Endoscopy, biopsy	Imaging plays an ancillary role
GVHD	Endoscopy, biopsy	Imaging plays an ancillary role
Vascular complications	Doppler ultrasound CTA or MRA	Similar diagnostic criteria to liver transplantation (see Table 1)
Intestinal complications	Water-soluble gastrointestinal series or CT	Prolonged transit time suggests dysmotility Identification of a transition zone suggests partial or complete bowel obstruction Extraluminal contrast suggests leak
PTLD	Ultrasound, CT, or MR	Mass arising from the neck, chest, abdomen or pelvis; lymphadenopathy; pulmonary nodules

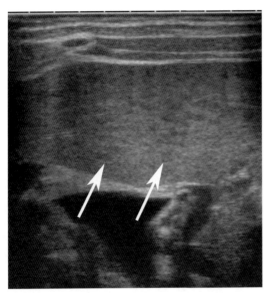

Fig. 20. Splenic ultrasound shows multiple hypodense splenic lesions (*arrows*), compatible with fungal disease. Use of a high-frequency linear transducer provides adequate resolution to visualize these small lesions.

Posttransplant Neoplasms

Posttransplant neoplasms pose a substantial concern in the long-term management of pediatric patients receiving MVT. Most of these neoplasms are associated with the Epstein-Barr virus (EBV) and include both posttransplant lymphoproliferative disorder (PTLD) and EBV-associated smooth muscle tumors.[78] PTLD may present as a mass or lymphadenopathy of the neck, chest, abdomen, or pelvis. EBV-associated smooth muscle tumors demonstrate a characteristic peripheral rim enhancement.[78] Although there are no existing follow-up guidelines to direct clinicians in assessing for these neoplasms, imaging may play a role in determining the extent of disease and monitoring a patient's response to therapy (**Fig. 23**). In particular, fluorodeoxyglucose-PET/CT or MR imaging may provide important information on sites of disease and response to treatment, and it is anticipated that its indications in this clinical setting will expand in the future.[79]

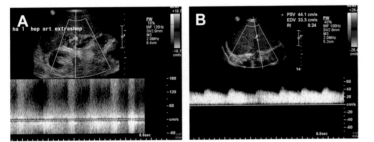

Fig. 21. Hepatic artery stenosis. (*A*) Aliasing in the celiac arm of the aortic conduit. (*B*) Interrogation of the hepatic artery shows tardus parvus waveform distal to the stenosis. (*Adapted from* Phillips GS, Bhargava P, Stanescu L, et al. Pediatric intestinal transplantation: normal radiographic appearance and complications. Pediatr Radiol 2011;41(8):1038; with permission.)

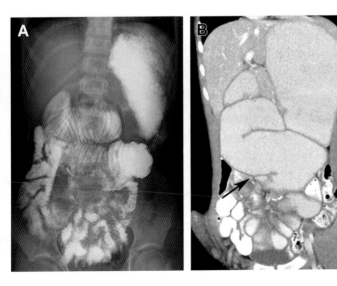

Fig. 22. Partial small bowel obstruction. (*A*) Upper gastrointestinal series shows a transition zone between dilated proximal and normal-caliber distal small bowel loops, suggesting partial small bowel obstruction. (*B*) Correlative coronal contrast-enhanced CT image shows markedly dilated proximal small bowel loops with a transition zone (*arrow*) in the right lower abdomen. Pathologic diagnosis of the enterectomy specimen was consistent with sclerosing peritonitis, a rare late complication of small bowel transplantation. (*Adapted from* Phillips GS, Bhargava P, Stanescu L, et al. Pediatric intestinal transplantation: normal radiographic appearance and complications. Pediatr Radiol 2011;41(8):1037; with permission.)

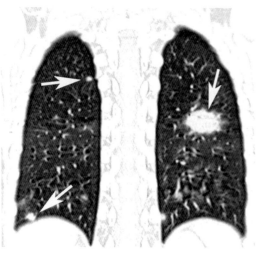

Fig. 23. Coronal chest CT image demonstrates multiple pulmonary parenchymal masses (*arrows*) suspicious for PTLD. These responded to a reduction of immunosuppression.

Pearls, Pitfalls, Variants

- As postoperative anatomy can be confusing and challenging, with multiple different types of arterial anastomoses and conduits reported in the literature, the authors recommend close consultation with the surgical team to document the precise anatomy in the patient to be imaged.
- GVHD and rejection are frequent complications that are both evaluated through endoscopy and biopsy, with imaging playing an ancillary role.
- Infection is a nearly universal complication.
- Color Doppler ultrasound findings suggesting thrombosis need spectral waveform confirmation to exclude slow flow.

What the Referring Physician Needs to Know

- What are the size, location, and imaging characteristics of any postoperative fluid collections?
- Are the arterial and venous anastomoses patent?
- Is there any evidence of dysmotility, bowel obstruction, or leak?
- Are there any unexpected masses or lymphadenopathy to suggest PTLD?

REFERENCES

1. United States Renal Data System. 2014 annual report. vol. 2. Pediatric endstage renal disease. 2014. [Chapter 7]. Available at: http://www.usrds.org/2014/view/v2_07.aspx. Accessed May 12, 2015.

2. Dharnidharka VR, Fiorina P, Harmon WE. Kidney transplantation in children. N Engl J Med 2014; 371(6):549–58.
3. Gillen DL, Stehman-Breen CO, Smith JM, et al. Survival advantage of pediatric recipients of a first kidney transplant among children awaiting kidney transplantation. Am J Transplant 2008;8(12):2600–6.
4. Rianthavorn P, Al-Akash SI, Ettinger RB, et al. Kidney transplantation in children, Chapter 14. Philadelphia: Lippincott, William and Wilkins; 2005. p. 198–230.
5. Horslen S, Barr ML, Christensen LL, et al. Pediatric transplantation in the United States, 1996-2005. Am J Transplant 2007;7(5 Pt 2):1339–58.
6. David Hatch SMG. Pediatric kidney transplantation. Available at: http://emedicine.medscape.com/article/1012654-overview. Accessed May 15, 2015.
7. Ruth A, McDonald M. General principles of renal transplantation in children. Available at: http://www.uptodate.com/contents/general-principles-of-renal-transplantation-in-children. Accessed May 15, 2015.
8. Brown ED, Chen MY, Wolfman NT, et al. Complications of renal transplantation: evaluation with US and radionuclide imaging. Radiographics 2000;20(3):607–22.
9. Nixon JN, Biyyam DR, Stanescu L, et al. Imaging of pediatric renal transplants and their complications: a pictorial review. Radiographics 2013;33(5):1227–51.
10. Schwenger V, Hankel V, Seckinger J, et al. Contrast-enhanced ultrasonography in the early period after kidney transplantation predicts long-term allograft function. Transplant Proc 2014;46(10):3352–7.
11. Schwenger V, Korosoglou G, Hinkel UP, et al. Real-time contrast-enhanced sonography of renal transplant recipients predicts chronic allograft nephropathy. Am J Transplant 2006;6(3):609–15.
12. Yamamoto A, Zhang JL, Rusinek H, et al. Quantitative evaluation of acute renal transplant dysfunction with low-dose three-dimensional MR renography. Radiology 2011;260(3):781–9.
13. Zhang JL, Rusinek H, Chandarana H, et al. Functional MRI of the kidneys. J Magn Reson Imaging 2013;37(2):282–93.
14. Ruiz E, Ferraris J. 25 years of live related renal transplantation in children: the Buenos Aires experience. Indian J Urol 2007;23(4):443–51.
15. Gulati A, Sarwal MM. Pediatric renal transplantation: an overview and update. Curr Opin Pediatr 2010; 22(2):189–96.
16. Shapiro R, Sarwal MM. Pediatric kidney transplantation. Pediatr Clin North Am 2010;57(2):393–400.
17. Heap SL, Webb NJ, Kirkman MA, et al. Extraperitoneal renal transplantation in small children results in a transient improvement in early graft function. Pediatr Transplant 2011;15(4):362–6.
18. Routh JC, Yu RN, Kozinn SI, et al. Urological complications and vesicoureteral reflux following pediatric kidney transplantation. J Urol 2013;189(3):1071–6.

19. Veroux MVP. Kidney transplantation: challenging the future. Bentham Science Publishers; 2012. Available at: http://ebooks.benthamscience.com/book/9781608051441/. Accessed June 01, 2015.

20. Tublin ME, Dodd GD 3rd. Sonography of renal transplantation. Radiol Clin North Am 1995;33(3):447–59.

21. Sharfuddin A. Renal relevant radiology: imaging in kidney transplantation. Clin J Am Soc Nephrol 2014;9(2):416–29.

22. El Atat R, Derouiche A, Guellouz S, et al. Surgical complications in pediatric and adolescent renal transplantation. Saudi J kidney Dis Transpl 2010; 21(2):251–7.

23. Gargah T, Abidi K, Rajhi H, et al. Vascular complications after pediatric kidney transplantation. Tunis Med 2011;89(5):458–61.

24. Kolofousi C, Stefanidis K, Cokkinos DD, et al. Ultrasonographic features of kidney transplants and their complications: an imaging review. ISRN Radiol 2013;2013:480862.

25. Surratt JT, Siegel MJ, Middleton WD. Sonography of complications in pediatric renal allografts. Radiographics 1990;10(4):687–99.

26. Shokeir AA, Osman Y, Ali-El-Dein B, et al. Surgical complications in live-donor pediatric and adolescent renal transplantation: study of risk factors. Pediatr Transplant 2005;9(1):33–8.

27. Paltiel H. Pediatric ultrasound, an issue of ultrasound clinics, vol. 8. Philadelphia: Elsevier. Elsevier Health Sciences; 2013. p. 381. Issue 3 of The Clinics: Radiology.

28. Network report. Available at: http://optn. transplant.hrsa.gov/converge/latestData/rptData.asp. Accessed June 30, 2015.

29. Rodriguez-Davalos MI, Arvelakis A, Umman V, et al. Segmental grafts in adult and pediatric liver transplantation: improving outcomes by minimizing vascular complications. JAMA Surg 2014;149(1):63–70.

30. American College of Radiology (ACR), Society for Pediatric Radiology (SPR), Society of Radiologists in Ultrasound (SRU), et al. AIUM practice guideline for the performance of an ultrasound examination of solid-organ transplants. J Ultrasound Med 2014; 33(7):1309–20.

31. Jamieson LH, Arys B, Low G, et al. Doppler ultrasound velocities and resistive indexes immediately after pediatric liver transplantation: normal ranges and predictors of failure. AJR Am J Roentgenol 2014;203(1):W110–6.

32. Garcia-Criado A, Gilabert R, Salmeron JM, et al. Significance of and contributing factors for a high resistive index on Doppler sonography of the hepatic artery immediately after surgery: prognostic implications for liver transplant recipients. AJR Am J Roentgenol 2003;181(3):831–8.

33. Garcia-Criado A, Gilabert R, Berzigotti A, et al. Doppler ultrasound findings in the hepatic artery shortly after liver transplantation. AJR Am J Roentgenol 2009;193(1):128–35.

34. Babyn PS. Imaging of the transplant liver. Pediatr Radiol 2010;40(4):442–6.

35. Norton KI, Lee JS, Kogan D, et al. The role of magnetic resonance cholangiography in the management of children and young adults after liver transplantation. Pediatr Transplant 2001;5(6):410–8.

36. Bekker J, Ploem S, de Jong KP. Early hepatic artery thrombosis after liver transplantation: a systematic review of the incidence, outcome and risk factors. Am J Transplant 2009;9(4):746–57.

37. Mali VP, Aw M, Quak SH, et al. Vascular complications in pediatric liver transplantation; single-center experience from Singapore. Transplant Proc 2012; 44(5):1373–8.

38. Uchida Y, Sakamoto S, Egawa H, et al. The impact of meticulous management for hepatic artery thrombosis on long-term outcome after pediatric living donor liver transplantation. Clin Transplant 2009; 23(3):392–9.

39. Kivela JM, Kosola S, Kalajoki-Helmio T, et al. Late hepatic artery thrombosis after pediatric liver transplantation: a cross-sectional study of 34 patients. Liver Transplant 2014;20(5):591–600.

40. Orlandini M, Feier FH, Jaeger B, et al. Frequency of and factors associated with vascular complications after pediatric liver transplantation. J Pediatr (Rio J) 2014;90(2):169–75.

41. Sanchez SE, Javid PJ, Lao OB, et al. Hepatic artery thrombosis and liver malignancy in pediatric liver transplantation. J Pediatr Surg 2012;47(6):1255–60.

42. Gu LH, Fang H, Li FH, et al. Prediction of early hepatic artery thrombosis by intraoperative color Doppler ultrasound in pediatric segmental liver transplantation. Clin Transplant 2012;26(4):571–6.

43. Huang TL, Chen TY, Tsang LL, et al. Hemodynamics of portal venous stenosis before and after treatment in pediatric liver transplantation: evaluation with Doppler ultrasound. Transplant Proc 2012;44(2):481–3.

44. Low G, Crockett AM, Leung K, et al. Imaging of vascular complications and their consequences following transplantation in the abdomen. Radiographics 2013;33(3):633–52.

45. Berrocal T, Parron M, Alvarez-Luque A, et al. Pediatric liver transplantation: a pictorial essay of early and late complications. Radiographics 2006;26(4):1187–209.

46. Suzuki L, de Oliveira IR, Widman A, et al. Real-time and Doppler US after pediatric segmental liver transplantation: I. Portal vein stenosis. Pediatr Radiol 2008;38(4):403–8.

47. Karakayali H, Sevmis S, Boyvat F, et al. Diagnosis and treatment of late-onset portal vein stenosis after pediatric living-donor liver transplantation. Transplant Proc 2011;43(2):601–4.

48. Schneider N, Scanga A, Stokes L, et al. Portal vein stenosis: a rare yet clinically important cause of

delayed-onset ascites after adult deceased donor liver transplantation: two case reports. Transplant Proc 2011;43(10):3829–34.

49. Moon SB, Moon JI, Kwon CH, et al. Graft rotation and late portal vein complications in pediatric living donor liver transplantation using left-sided grafts: long-term computed tomography observations. Liver Transpl 2011;17(6):717–22.

50. Westra SJ, Zaninovic AC, Hall TR, et al. Imaging in pediatric liver transplantation. Radiographics 1993; 13(5):1081–99.

51. Buell JF, Funaki B, Cronin DC, et al. Long-term venous complications after full-size and segmental pediatric liver transplantation. Ann Surg 2002; 236(5):658–66.

52. Sommovilla J, Doyle MM, Vachharajani N, et al. Hepatic venous outflow obstruction in pediatric liver transplantation: technical considerations in prevention, diagnosis, and management. Pediatr Transplant 2014;18(5):497–502.

53. Settmacher U, Nussler NC, Glanemann M, et al. Venous complications after orthotopic liver transplantation. Clin Transplant 2000;14(3):235–41.

54. Ko EY, Kim TK, Kim PN, et al. Hepatic vein stenosis after living donor liver transplantation: evaluation with Doppler US. Radiology 2003;229(3):806–10.

55. Suzuki L, de Oliveira IR, Widman A, et al. Real-time and Doppler US after pediatric segmental liver transplantation: II. Hepatic vein stenosis. Pediatr Radiol 2008;38(4):409–14.

56. Feier FH, Chapchap P, Pugliese R, et al. Diagnosis and management of biliary complications in pediatric living donor liver transplant recipients. Liver Transpl 2014;20(8):882–92.

57. Pariente D, Bihet MH, Tammam S, et al. Biliary complications after transplantation in children: role of imaging modalities. Pediatr Radiol 1991;21(3):175–8.

58. Kling K, Lau H, Colombani P. Biliary complications of living related pediatric liver transplant patients. Pediatr Transplant 2004;8(2):178–84.

59. Laor T, Hoffer FA, Vacanti JP, et al. MR cholangiography in children after liver transplantation from living related donors. AJR Am J Roentgenol 1998; 170(3):683–7.

60. Griffith JF, John PR. Imaging of biliary complications following paediatric liver transplantation. Pediatr Radiol 1996;26(6):388–94.

61. Keogan MT, McDermott VG, Price SK, et al. The role of imaging in the diagnosis and management of biliary complications after liver transplantation. AJR Am J Roentgenol 1999;173(1):215–9.

62. Ahlawat SK, Fishbien TM, Haddad NG. Cystic duct remnant mucocele in a liver transplant recipient. Pediatr Radiol 2008;38(8):884–6.

63. Quiroga S, Sebastia MC, Margarit C, et al. Complications of orthotopic liver transplantation: spectrum of findings with helical CT. Radiographics 2001; 21(5):1085–102.

64. Caiado AH, Blasbalg R, Marcelino AS, et al. Complications of liver transplantation: multimodality imaging approach. Radiographics 2007;27(5):1401–17.

65. Crossin JD, Muradali D, Wilson SR. US of liver transplants: normal and abnormal. Radiographics 2003; 23(5):1093–114.

66. Mazariegos GV, Squires RH, Sindhi RK. Current perspectives on pediatric intestinal transplantation. Curr Gastroenterol Rep 2009;11(3):226–33.

67. Bhamidimarri KR, Beduschi T, Vianna R. Multivisceral transplantation: where do we stand? Clin Liver Dis 2014;18(3):661–74.

68. Kato T, Kleiner G, David A, et al. Inclusion of spleen in pediatric multivisceral transplantation. Transplant Proc 2006;38(6):1709–10.

69. Kato T, Tzakis AG, Selvaggi G, et al. Transplantation of the spleen: effect of splenic allograft in human multivisceral transplantation. Ann Surg 2007; 246(3):436–44 [discussion: 445–6].

70. Hernandez F, Andres AM, Encinas JL, et al. Preservation of the native spleen in multivisceral transplantation. Pediatr Transplant 2013;17(6):556–60.

71. Kato T, Ruiz P, Thompson JF, et al. Intestinal and multivisceral transplantation. World J Surg 2002; 26(2):226–37.

72. Pecchi A, De Santis M, Torricelli P, et al. Radiologic imaging of the transplanted bowel. Abdom Imaging 2005;30(5):548–63.

73. Sandrasegaran K, Lall C, Ramaswamy R, et al. Intestinal and multivisceral transplantation. Abdom Imaging 2011;36(4):382–9.

74. Tzakis AG, Kato T, Levi DM, et al. 100 multivisceral transplants at a single center. Ann Surg 2005; 242(4):480–90 [discussion: 491–3].

75. Grant D, Abu-Elmagd K, Reyes J, et al. 2003 report of the intestine transplant registry: a new era has dawned. Ann Surg 2005;241(4):607–13.

76. Gupte GL, Haghighi KS, Sharif K, et al. Surgical complications after intestinal transplantation in infants and children–UK experience. J Pediatr Surg 2010;45(7):1473–8.

77. Phillips GS, Bhargava P, Stanescu L, et al. Pediatric intestinal transplantation: normal radiographic appearance and complications. Pediatr Radiol 2011;41(8):1028–39.

78. Hryhorczuk AL, Kim HB, Harris MH, et al. Imaging findings in children with proliferative disorders following multivisceral transplantation. Pediatr Radiol 2015;45(8):1138–45.

79. von Falck C, Maecker B, Schirg E, et al. Post transplant lymphoproliferative disease in pediatric solid organ transplant patients: a possible role for [18F]-FDG-PET(/CT) in initial staging and therapy monitoring. Eur J Radiol 2007;63(3):427–35.

Complications of Immunosuppressive Therapy in Solid Organ Transplantation

Venkata Katabathina, MD[a], Christine O. Menias, MD[b],
Perry Pickhardt, MD[c], Meghan Lubner, MD[c], Srinivasa R. Prasad, MD[d],*

KEYWORDS

- Immunosuppression • Complications • Transplantation • Infections • Malignancy
- Computed tomography • Posttransplant lymphoproliferative disorder (PTLD) • MR imaging

KEY POINTS

- Three drugs are commonly used in clinical practice to achieve immunosuppression (corticosteroids, mycophenolate mofetil, and tacrolimus/cyclosporine); mammalian target of rapamycin inhibitors and other novel drugs with more favorable adverse effect profiles and increased potency are increasingly being used.
- Drug-related metabolic side effects are commonly diagnosed from clinical and laboratory findings; imaging is pivotal in the detection and management of posttransplant infections and malignancies.
- A wide spectrum of opportunistic infections occurs in transplant cohorts because of associated immunosuppression. A high index of clinical suspicion, supportive laboratory findings, and imaging features, as well as imaging-guided biopsy/aspiration are invaluable in establishing the correct diagnosis and instituting timely treatment.
- There is an increased tendency for transplant cohorts to develop unique de novo malignancies, including human papillomavirus–associated squamous cell carcinomas and anogenital carcinomas, Epstein-Barr virus–related posttransplant lymphoproliferative disorder, and other virally induced cancers. Transplant cancers are generally associated with aggressive biology, poor response to chemotherapy, and resultant poor prognosis.
- Recent advances in immunology, virology, molecular genetics, and therapeutics have enabled better understanding of complications of immunosuppression, and have also facilitated development of so-called designer drugs to achieve adequate graft function and decrease the risks associated with lifelong immunosuppression.

INTRODUCTION

Solid organ transplantation (SOT) is the treatment of choice for patients with end-stage organ failure. More than 29,000 transplants are performed in the United States each year, with kidney being the most commonly transplanted organ, followed by liver, heart, and lung.[1] The ongoing success of transplantation, with graft survival rates approaching 90% at 1 year and 75% at 5 years, is mainly

Disclosures: The authors have no financial disclosures.
[a] Department of Radiology, University of Texas Health Science Center, 7703 Floyd Curl Drive, San Antonio, TX 78229, USA; [b] Department of Radiology, Mayo Clinic, 13400 E Shea Blvd, Scottsdale, AZ 85259, USA; [c] Department of Radiology, University of Wisconsin, G3/310 600 Highland Avenue, Madison, WI 53792, USA; [d] Department of Radiology, University of Texas MD Anderson Cancer Center, 1400 Pressler Street, Houston, TX 77030, USA
* Corresponding author.
E-mail address: sprasad2@mdanderson.org

Radiol Clin N Am 54 (2016) 303–319
http://dx.doi.org/10.1016/j.rcl.2015.09.009

attributable to the availability of potent immuno-suppressive drugs that prevent allograft rejection. However, long-term survivals following SOT have not improved because of several factors, including chronic rejection, cardiovascular diseases, and complications of chronic immunosuppression, such as infections and malignancies. The chronic use of immunosuppressive drugs in this cohort of patients leads to 2 categories of complications: (1) drug-related adverse effects such as renal dysfunction, hypertension, hyperlipidemia, and diabetes mellitus; and (2) infections and malig-nancies.[2] Common posttransplant opportunistic infections secondary to depressed immune system include viral (cytomegalovirus [CMV], herpes simplex virus [HSV], varicella-zoster virus [VZV], and Epstein-Barr virus [EBV]), fungal (Candida species, Aspergillus species, Pneumo-cystis jiroveci, Cryptococcus neoformans, and mu-cormycosis), bacterial (Nocardia species, Legionella pneumophila, Listeria monocytogenes, and mycobacteria), and parasitic (Toxoplasma gondii and strongyloidiasis). Nonmelanoma skin cancer, posttransplant lymphoproliferative disor-der (PTLD), Kaposi sarcoma, anogenital cancer, lung cancer, renal cell carcinoma (RCC), and he-patocellular carcinoma (HCC) are the most com-mon malignancies that develop secondary to chronic immunosuppression (**Box 1**). Although clinical features and laboratory findings are essen-tial in diagnosing most drug-related metabolic side effects, cross-sectional imaging techniques such as ultrasonography, computed tomography (CT), 18-fluorodeoxyglucose (FDG) PET, and MR imaging play important roles in the initial diagnosis, treatment follow-up, and long-term surveillance of posttransplant infections and malignancies.

This article first describes mechanisms of ac-tion and side effects of commonly used immuno-suppressive drugs in SOT. It then reviews the pathogenesis and cross-sectional imaging find-ings of common posttransplant infections and cancers and discusses the role of imaging in screening, diagnosis, and surveillance of these conditions.

IMMUNOSUPPRESSIVE DRUGS IN SOLID ORGAN TRANSPLANTATION

Antigen-presenting cells (APCs) such as B lym-phocytes, macrophages, and dendritic cells, along with T lymphocytes, play a central role in the process of alloimmune response and trans-plant rejection.[3] Initiation of immune response is triggered by T-cell recognition of foreign antigens presented by APCs. This recognition

---

> **Box 1**
> **Complications of immunosuppressive therapy in SOT**
>
> *Drug-related side effects*
>
> Renal dysfunction
>
> Hypertension
>
> Hyperlipidemia
>
> Diabetes mellitus
>
> *Infections*
>
> Viral: CMV, HSV, VZV, and EBV
>
> Fungal: *Candida* species, *Aspergillus* species, *P jiroveci*, *C neoformans*, and mucormycosis
>
> Bacterial: *Nocardia* species, *L pneumophila*, *L monocytogenes*, and mycobacteria.
>
> Parasitic: *T gondii* and strongyloidiasis.
>
> *Malignancies*
>
> RCC
>
> HCC
>
> Skin cancers
>
> Posttransplant lymphoproliferative disorder
>
> Anogenital cancer
>
> Lung carcinoma

leads to activation of multiple signal transduction pathways in the T cells, including the calcium-calcineurin pathway.[2,3] These pathways stimu-late production of new molecules, including interleukin (IL)-2, which is a major stimulator of T-cell proliferation. IL-2 binds to CD 25 (IL-2 re-ceptor) present on the surface of the activated T cells, which leads to proliferation and differen-tiation of effector T cells, resulting in tissue rejec-tion (**Fig. 1**).[3] In addition, activated B cells synthesize alloantibodies against donor anti-gens.[3,4] Several immunosuppressive drug com-binations are used in SOT with the goal of providing adequate immunosuppression with minimum side effects (**Box 2**).[4,5] Given the crit-ical role of T cells in the rejection process, most available drugs target T-cell activation and proliferation, thereby affecting overall pro-duction of T cells. However, drugs targeting B lymphocytes with downstream effects on alloan-tibody production and components of the innate immune system (complement and macrophages) are also being investigated (see **Fig. 1**).[5] Current regimens include at least 3 drugs that work at different parts of the immune system; this allows dose optimization of each drug with lower side effect profiles while increasing synergistic

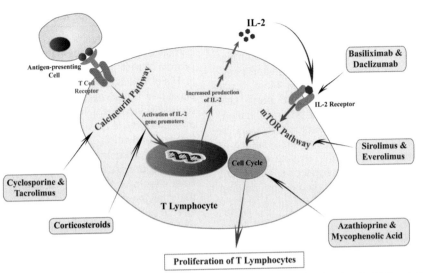

Fig. 1. Intracellular mechanisms of the T lymphocytes responsible for allograft rejection in SOT and sites of action of commonly used immunosuppressive medication. mTOR, mammalian target of rapamycin.

Box 2
Immunosuppressive agents commonly used in SOT

Antibodies

Antithymocyte globulin

Alemtuzumab

Basiliximab

Daclizumab

Corticosteroids

Methylprednisolone

Prednisone

Calcineurin inhibitors

Cyclosporine

Tacrolimus

Antimetabolites

Azathioprine

Mycophenolic acid

Mammalian target of rapamycin inhibitors

Sirolimus

Everolimus

Novel Immunosuppressive Agents

Belatacept

Rituximab

Infliximab

Bortezomib

---

efficacy.[2,5] Transplant immunosuppression can be divided into 2 phases: induction and maintenance. Drugs that are used in the first few days to weeks after transplantation are referred to as induction agents, whereas maintenance agents are used in later stages of transplantation.[5]

Antibodies

Antibodies are commonly used as induction agents in most kidney and pancreas transplant recipients and less frequently in liver transplant patients. In addition, they are also useful in severe and/or steroid-resistant rejections. Polyclonal antithymocyte globulin, monoclonal antibodies including alemtuzumab (anti-CD52 receptors), and muromonab (OKT3; anti-CD3 receptors) are depleting types of antibodies that act by reducing the number of circulating T cells and B cells.[4] Nondepleting antibodies include basiliximab and daclizumab, which bind to IL-2 receptors on T cells and block the proliferative response of T cells to circulating IL-2.[2,3] Side effects of antibodies include allergic reactions; serum sickness; cytokine release phenomena secondary to severe cytolysis; seizures; thrombocytopenia; arthralgias; and, importantly, increased risk of infections and PTLD development.[5]

Corticosteroids

Corticosteroids have been the mainstay of immunosuppression since the beginning of SOT.[5] They exert immune-modulatory effects by downregulating cytokine gene expression in lymphocytes leading to decreased serum IL-2 levels, inhibiting macrophage differentiation, and suppressing neutrophil functions.[2,6] Corticosteroids are thus very effective in the prevention and treatment of acute allograft rejections. Most acute rejection episodes are treated with pulse steroids.[5] Weight gain, impaired wound healing, increased risk of infection, osteoporosis, avascular necrosis of bone, hypertension, hyperglycemia, and cataracts are common side effects of steroids; among them, osteoporosis and avascular bone necrosis can be detected on imaging studies.[7,8]

Calcineurin Inhibitors

Cyclosporine and tacrolimus are the two most commonly used calcineurin inhibitors (CNIs) in clinical practice. These drugs act by inhibiting calcineurin (intracellular calcium/calmodulin-activated phosphatase), which in turn inhibits translocation and activation of nuclear factors of activated T cells, resulting in decreased production of T-cell growth factors such as IL-2, and subsequent proliferation of T cells.[2,5] Nephrotoxicity resulting from endothelial damage and interstitial fibrosis is a major universal side effect of CNIs; up to 20% may progress to renal failure requiring renal transplantation.[4] Other adverse effects of CNIs include infections, malignancies, hypertension, hyperglycemia, neurotoxicity, and hyperlipidemia.[6] Tacrolimus is more potent than cyclosporine with less severe side effects and is frequently used in transplant regimens.[3]

Antimetabolites

Azathioprine and mycophenolic acid (MPA) are well-known examples of antimetabolites that interfere with DNA and RNA replication by blocking de novo purine synthesis, resulting in the prevention of proliferation and clonal expansion of T and B cells.[2] MPA blocks the action of the inosine monophosphate dehydrogenase enzyme, a rate-limiting step in the biosynthesis of purines that is crucial to cell cycling of lymphocytes.[4] Azathioprine has been replaced by mycophenolate mofetil (MMF) and mycophenolate sodium, two preparations of MPA, in many transplant regimens. The main side effects of MPA include abdominal pain, diarrhea, nausea, bone marrow suppression, and increased risk of CMV infections, especially at high doses.[4] MMF does not seem to be associated with an increased risk of posttransplant cancers; a slight protective effect of MMF against PTLD has been reported.[9]

Mammalian Target of Rapamycin Inhibitors

Sirolimus and everolimus are recently introduced immunosuppressive agents in SOT that inhibit a protein called mammalian target of rapamycin (mTOR). This action results in inhibition of synthesis of new ribosomal proteins that are essential for progression of cells from the G1 to the S phase during cell cycle and ultimately block the proliferation and activation of T cells and B cells.[3,4] In addition, they also inhibit fibroblast growth factors required for tissue repair. This feature has 2 beneficial effects on transplant recipients: reduction of the malignancy risk because of antiangiogenic effects and halting progression of fibrosis in liver transplant patients.[10] The common side effects include impaired wound healing that can result in the development of incisional hernias and lymphoceles, hyperlipidemia, oral ulcers, thrombosis, leukopenia, thrombocytopenia, and arthralgias.[5] Increased incidences of delayed graft function, pneumonia, and herpes virus infection have also been reported with sirolimus.[2]

Novel Immunosuppressive Agents

Efforts are underway to develop novel immunosuppressive therapy with improved efficacy and decreased adverse effects. These drugs target both T-cell and B-cell surface receptors and intracellular pathways.[4] Belatacept is a fusion protein that prevents T-cell activation by selectively blocking T-cell costimulation molecules.[4,5] Rituximab, a monoclonal antibody directed against CD20 antigen on B cells, is being tried in antibody-mediated rejection and as part of desensitization protocols in highly sensitive recipients.[4] Bortezomib is a protease inhibitor that induces apoptosis in rapidly dividing cells with active protein synthesis, such as plasma cells.[4] Infliximab is a monoclonal antibody against tumor necrosis factor that prevents cytokines from binding to their receptors.[4]

COMPLICATIONS OF CHRONIC IMMUNOSUPPRESSION: INFECTIONS

Infectious complications are the most common cause of mortality and morbidity in transplant recipients who are on long-term immunosuppression.[11] Because clinical signs and symptoms of infection are often subtle, atypical, or absent in these patients, diagnosis is mainly established by comprehensive testing, including laboratory work-up and imaging evaluation. In addition, invasive diagnostic procedures such as imaging-guided aspiration may be critical in identifying the causative organism.[12] The patient's risk of infection is mainly based on the net state of immunosuppression, which is a complex function determined by several factors, with dose, duration, and sequence of immunosuppressive agents being major determinants.[11] Infections occur in a predictable pattern in organ recipients. Posttransplant timelines can be divided into 3 time periods related to risks of infection by specific pathogens: early posttransplantation (first month), intermediate period (1–6 months), and the late period (after 6 months).[11] Because immunosuppression is not fully effective during the first month, infections related to technical complications of surgery are common during this period. Immunosuppression is tapered after 6 months in recipients with satisfactory graft function, because the risk of infection is similar to that of the general population, with community-acquired pathogens being most common.[11]

Immunosuppression is at its peak during the intermediate period and SOT patients carry the greatest risk of infection during this time, especially with opportunistic pathogens; additionally, there is significant risk of reactivation of latent infections.[13] Most immunosuppressive agents depress cell-mediated immunity because of T-cell dysfunction that leads to increased susceptibility of intracellular pathogens and herpes viruses.[14] The common viral, fungal, bacterial, mycobacterial, and parasitic infections that develop secondary to chronic immunodeficiency in patients with SOT are summarized in Box 1.

VIRAL INFECTIONS
Cytomegalovirus

CMV is the most common opportunistic pathogen in organ recipients and can be seen in up to 70% of patients. Half of these infections are associated with symptomatic disease.[15,16] CMV can occur either as primary infection or reactivation of latent infection. CMV typically has 3 major pathologic effects in immunocompromised patients: presentation with invasive disease in multiple organs by direct involvement, predisposing infections with other opportunistic organisms, and increased allograft rejection.[14,16]

Depending on the severity of immunosuppression, CMV can either affect the allograft, resulting in localized inflammation, or cause disseminated disease, with the lungs and the gastrointestinal tract being the common target sites.[11,13] On imaging, gastrointestinal involvement is characterized by diffuse, irregular bowel thickening with adjacent fat stranding. The esophagus and colon are more frequently involved more than other parts of the gastrointestinal tract and may show multiple ulcers or plaques on barium studies and endoscopy (Fig. 2).[17,18] Radiographic findings of CMV pneumonitis include diffuse haziness, reticulonodular opacities, and dense areas of consolidation. On CT, bilateral, mixed areas of ground-glass opacities, poorly defined centrilobular nodules, and consolidations are common findings (Fig. 3).[19,20] Ganciclovir is commonly used for treatment and prophylaxis of CMV infections.

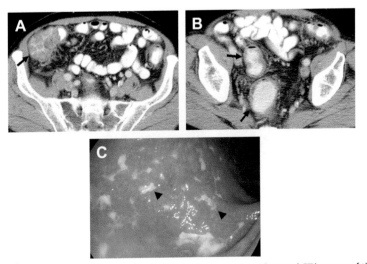

Fig. 2. CMV colitis in a post–liver transplant patient. (A, B) Axial contrast-enhanced CT images of the abdomen show diffuse, irregular wall thickening of the colon, predominantly involving the cecum and ascending colon with associated pericolonic fat stranding (arrows). (C) Flexible sigmoidoscopy shows friable mucosa with purulent exudative plaques (arrowheads) and acute CMV colitis was proved on biopsy.

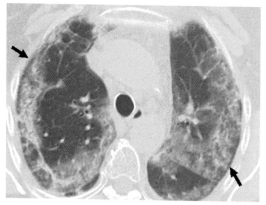

Fig. 3. CMV lung infection in a post–lung transplant patient. Axial unenhanced CT image of the chest (lung windows) shows mixed areas of centrilobular nodules and ground-glass opacities, predominantly involving the periphery of the bilateral lung parenchyma (*arrows*). Lung biopsy findings are consistent with CMV infection.

Other Herpes Virus Infections

HSV, VZV, EBV, and human herpes virus (HHV) 6-8, and 8 are other herpes serotypes that develop in organ recipients because of reactivation of latent infection.[16] Although oral or genital mucocutaneous ulcers are the usual clinical manifestations of HSV, severe disease can cause pneumonitis, esophagitis, hepatitis, encephalitis, and disseminated visceral disease.[14,15] VZV and HHV-6 infections, if severe, may also cause encephalitis, pneumonitis, and hemorrhagic rash; additionally, VZV may cause cerebellitis, cerebritis, vasculopathy, and meningitis (**Fig. 4**).[14] EBV infection is discussed later.

FUNGAL INFECTIONS

Fungal infections are responsible for significant posttransplant mortality and morbidity. They may be seen in 5% to 40% of patients, with liver transplant recipients carrying the greatest risk of invasive disease.[15] Large doses of immunosuppressive drugs (especially steroids), hyperglycemia, immunomodulatory viral infections, multiple rejection episodes, environmental factors, poor transplant function, technical or anatomic abnormalities, and old age are important risk factors for fungal infections.[14,21] Candida and *Aspergillus* are the most common invasive fungal infections; additionally, *Pneumocystis*, *Cryptococcus*, mucormycosis, and *Actinomyces* are also seen. Amphotericin B and voriconazole are commonly used antifungal agents in treatment and prophylaxis.

Candida Species

Invasive candidiasis accounts for 80% of all fungal infections; *Candida albicans* remains the most common species. Liver transplant recipients are at greatest risk of candidiasis; gastrointestinal colonization in liver/pancreas transplants and tracheobronchial colonization in lung transplant patients are the common sources.[15,22] Mucosal disease of the oral cavity (ie, thrush) is the most common clinical presentation. Candidal esophagitis appears as multiple, whitish exudates, plaques, nodules, and ulcers on endoscopy. On double-contrast esophagogram, multiple, discrete, longitudinally oriented, plaquelike nodules separated by normal mucosa; multiple small oval/round ulcers; and a grossly distorted shaggy appearance

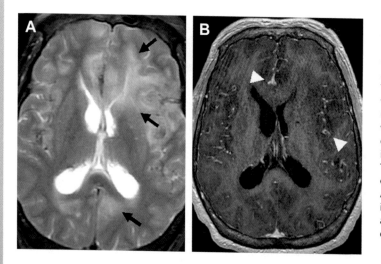

Fig. 4. VZV encephalitis in a 60-year-old woman following renal transplant. Axial T2-weighted (*A*) and gadolinium-enhanced (*B*) MR images of the brain show multifocal T2 hyperintensities involving the white matter of the frontal, temporal, and occipital lobes (*arrows*) with superimposed leptomeningeal enhancement (*arrowheads*). There is associated susceptibility on the T2* sequence (not shown here) indicating a hemorrhagic component. Although these MR imaging findings are not specific for VZV encephalitis, the same diagnosis was proved on laboratory analysis.

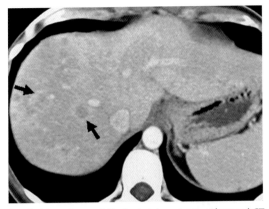

Fig. 5. Hepatic candidiasis. Axial contrast-enhanced CT of the abdomen shows ill-defined hypodensities in the liver with peripheral enhancement (*arrows*), which were proved on pathology to be microabscesses caused by *C albicans*.

of the esophagus are characteristic findings of candida esophagitis.[23]

Disseminated candidiasis with involvement of the chest and abdomen is common, especially with intense immunosuppression. Pulmonary disease is seen with lung transplants and presents as patchy consolidations, diffuse reticulonodular opacities, and pleural effusions on radiographs.[24] Multiple intra-abdominal abscesses, diffuse peritonitis, ill-defined focal abscesses involving the liver and spleen, cystitis with or without fungal balls, and renal lesions are the usual abdominal findings (**Fig. 5**).[25]

Aspergillus Species

Invasive aspergillosis (IA) is responsible for about 15% to 20 % of fungal infections in organ recipients and is associated with mortalities ranging from 65% to 92%. The highest incidence of IA is seen in lung transplants, and *Aspergillus fumigatus* is the most common species.[21,26] Pulmonary disease, tracheobronchitis, sinusitis, and central nervous system (CNS) abscesses are common

manifestations of IA.[27,28] Although pulmonary parenchymal and airway disease is frequently seen in lung transplants, CNS involvement may be seen in up to 50% of patients with disseminated IA.[15]

Multiple nodules with or without a peripheral ground-glass halo (indicating hemorrhage secondary to angioinvasiveness), ill-defined consolidations, and multiple masses are the common imaging features of pulmonary disease (**Fig. 6**).[29] Irregular wall thickening and enhancement involving the trachea and major bronchi resulting in luminal narrowing, typically at the anastomotic site in lung transplants, is suggestive of tracheobronchitis.[21,27,30] IA of the CNS appears either as multiple, nonenhancing, hemorrhagic foci involving the cerebral parenchyma or as enhancing soft tissue thickening at the orbital apex, extending into the cranial cavity and resulting in cavernous sinus thrombosis (**Fig. 7**).[28,31,32]

Pneumocystis jirovecii

P jiroveci pneumonia (PJP) can affect up to 15% of organ recipients, usually in the first 6 months following SOT, and is associated with an aggressive course and significant mortality in the absence of trimethoprim-sulfamethoxazole prophylaxis.[15,33] A recent study by Wang and colleagues[34] showed a late presentation of PJP, especially after an acute rejection episode or CMV and stressed the importance of prolonged PJP prophylaxis under special circumstances. Patients with PJP typically present with fever, dyspnea, nonproductive cough, and hypoxemia out of proportion to the radiographic and physical findings. PJP manifests as interstitial infiltrates on radiographs (**Fig. 8**).[13,14] On high-resolution chest CT, extensive ground-glass opacities with upper lobe predominance is the characteristic feature; additionally, patchy consolidations, nodules, cysts, and spontaneous pneumothorax may also be seen (see **Fig. 8**).[35]

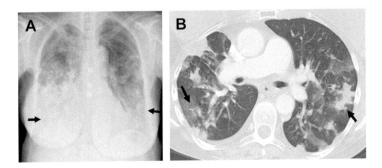

Fig. 6. Pulmonary aspergillosis in a post–lung transplant patient. Supine chest radiograph (*A*) and axial chest CT image (lung windows) (*B*) show ill-defined areas of parenchymal consolidations and masses with surrounding areas of ground glassing involving the bilateral lung parenchyma (*arrows*). Infection with *A fumigatus* was proved on lung biopsy.

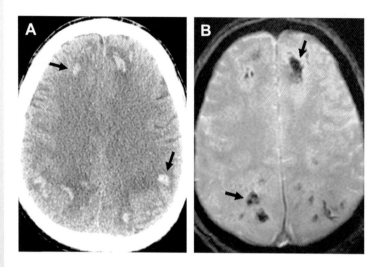

Fig. 7. IA of the CNS in a 34-year-old man status post–renal transplant. Axial contrast-enhanced CT (A) and T2* MR imaging (B) images of the brain show multifocal regions of hemorrhage within the subcortical regions throughout the brain (arrows). The diagnosis of the aspergillosis was confirmed by identifying septated hyphae in the cerebrospinal fluid.

Cryptococcus neoformans

C neoformans infection has been reported in up to 5% of organ transplant recipients; inhalation of the organisms is the primary mode of transmission with the development of pulmonary disease.[13,14,21] Hematogenous dissemination, most frequently to the CNS, bones, and skin, can occur, mainly secondary to intense immunosuppression. Multiple ill-defined tiny nodules, large masses, diffuse interstitial infiltrates, and cavitary nodules are common chest CT findings (Fig. 9).[36] Hydrocephalus, dilated Virchow-Robin spaces, diffuse meningeal enhancement, cystlike structures, and granulomas of the choroid plexuses are typically seen CNS features.[37]

Mucormycosis

Mucormycosis accounts for 2% of invasive fungal infections in solid organ recipients; Rhizopus species and Mucor species are the most frequently isolated organisms.[38] Diabetic ketoacidosis, steroid use, and bicarbonate leak in pancreatic transplants are risk factors; infection commonly occurs by inhalation, ingestion, or direct traumatic inoculation of fungal spores.[14] Rhinocerebral, pulmonary, renal, gastrointestinal, and disseminated disease are common; paranasal sinuses and orbital disease followed by rapid and progressive involvement of the cavernous sinus, vascular structures, and intracranial contents are characteristic MR imaging findings of rhinocerebral mucormycosis.[39] Single or multiple lung masses surrounded by ground-glass opacities are commonly seen on chest CT. Necrotic areas involving multiple intra-abdominal organs, including the kidneys and gastrointestinal tract, can present on imaging (Fig. 10).[40,41]

BACTERIAL INFECTIONS

Opportunistic bacterial infections that commonly occur between 2 to 6 months after SOT include

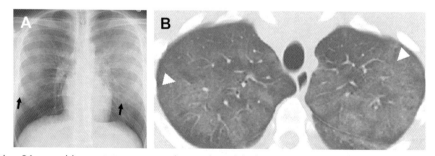

Fig. 8. PJP in a 34-year-old man status post–renal transplant. (A) Chest radiograph shows diffuse, ill-defined interstitial prominence and ground-glass appearance (arrows). (B) Axial unenhanced CT of the chest (lung windows) shows extensive ground-glass opacities involving bilateral lung parenchyma with upper lobe predominance (arrowheads). These findings are strongly suggestive of PJP, which was subsequently proved on pathologic examination.

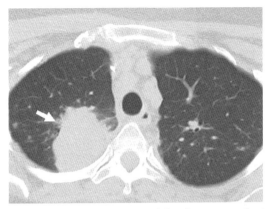

Fig. 9. Pulmonary cryptococcosis in a heart transplant recipient who was treated with high-dose steroids for an episode of rejection. Axial contrast-enhanced CT of the chest (lung windows) shows a large parenchymal mass in the right upper lobe (*arrow*), which was proved to be secondary to *C neoformans* infection on pathology.

Nocardia species, *L monocytogenes*, and *L pneumophila*.

Nocardiosis

Nocardial infections are rare, with a reported incidence of 0.7% to 3.5% in solid organ recipients, with *Nocardia asteroides* being the most common species; high-dose steroids, CMV, and high levels of CNIs are independent risk factors.[42] Pulmonary involvement is the most common presentation, although meningitis and brain abscess may also be seen.[14] CT features of pulmonary disease are nonspecific and mimic other infections and tumors, and include multiple nodules, masses, consolidation, and pleural effusions, as well as chest wall involvement (Fig. 11).[43,44]

Mycobacterial Infections

Solid organ recipients are at an increased risk of developing tubercular and nontubercular mycobacterial infections. The incidence of *Mycobacterium tuberculosis* infection (tuberculosis [TB]) is 20 to 75 times higher than in the general population and this disease may occur in up to 15% of these patients.[14,45] In one series, about 50% of TB involved the lungs, whereas 33% presented as disseminated disease, and 16% of patients had extrapulmonary involvement.[46] Reactivation of latent TB is the most common cause; active TB is associated with 30% mortality. There is also significant morbidity caused by alterations of metabolism of immunosuppressive drugs by antituberculosis chemotherapy resulting in increased infection and rejection.[45] On imaging, lung parenchymal infiltrates and cavitary nodules/masses with preferential upper lobe involvement are common findings; hepatosplenic TB is characterized by multiple, ill-defined, hypoattenuating nodules and masses (Fig. 12).[47] *Mycobacterium avium* complex infections have also been rarely reported in SOT patients.

Other Bacterial Infections

Although *L monocytogenes* commonly involves the CNS and causes meningitis and encephalitis, pneumonia with or without abscess formation and cavitation is the common presentation for *L pneumophila*.[13,14] Disseminated infections involving multiple organs may occur during the state of severe immunosuppression.

PARASITIC INFECTIONS

T gondii poses a significant risk in heart transplant recipients because there is a predilection of cysts for muscle tissue.[48] Reactivation of latent infection in the myocardium is a common cause of toxoplasmosis and carries a mortality of up to 100%.[13] Meningoencephalitis, brain abscess, myocarditis, and pneumonia are common imaging findings.[14] *Strongyloides stercoralis* infection presents either with gastrointestinal disease (small bowel obstruction and ileus) or pulmonary disease (alveolar or interstitial infiltrates).[14,48]

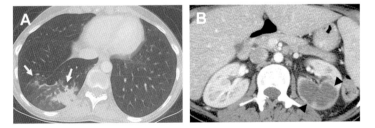

Fig. 10. Mucormycosis infection involving the lungs and the left kidney in a post–heart transplant recipient. (*A*) Axial contrast-enhanced CT of the chest (lung windows) shows ill-defined parenchymal opacities in the right lung parenchyma surrounded by ground-glass opacities (*arrows*). (*B*) Axial contrast-enhanced CT of the abdomen shows a large necrotic focal lesion in the left kidney (*arrowheads*). The diagnosis of disseminated mucormycosis was made on biopsy from the kidney lesion.

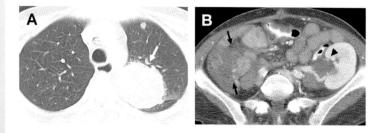

Fig. 11. Disseminated nocardia infection in a combined kidney-pancreas transplant recipient. (A) Axial contrast-enhanced CT image of the chest show a large left upper lobe pulmonary mass (*white arrow*). (B) Axial contrast-enhanced CT of the abdomen shows multiple, low attenuation lesions in the left lower quadrant kidney transplant (*arrowheads*) and low attenuating infiltrative soft tissue surrounding the right lower quadrant pancreas graft (*black arrows*). This patient was found to have disseminated nocardia infection on biopsy.

COMPLICATIONS OF CHRONIC IMMUNOSUPPRESSION: MALIGNANCIES

Solid organ transplant recipients carry an overall 2-fold to 3-fold increased risk of developing a wide range of cancers compared with the general population.[49] Moreover, the cancer risk is substantial with long-term immunosuppression; it is estimated that there is a 20% cancer incidence after 10 years of immunosuppression; the risk of posttransplant lymphoma is increased 20% to 120% compared with normal cohorts.[50,51] Posttransplant cancers can be arbitrarily divided into 3 categories based on origin and pathogenesis: de novo (new cancers that develop away from the transplanted organ), donor related (either transmitted from donor organs inadvertently or originating within the transplant), and recurrent cancers (recurrence of pretransplant cancers).[52] Nonmelanoma skin cancer, PTLD, and anogenital cancers are the most common de novo malignancies. Although RCC and malignant melanoma are commonly donor related, HCC and cholangiocarcinoma are malignancies that commonly recur.[52,53]

A complex interaction of several factors predisposes patients to posttransplant malignances. Important risk factors include the type of organ transplanted, underlying medical conditions, and exposure to oncogenic viral infections, immunosuppressive therapy, and environmental factors.[54,55] Long-term immunosuppressive therapy plays a central role in the pathogenesis of all 3 categories of posttransplant cancers[9,49]; the type, total dosage, duration, and intensity of drug regimens influence the risk of malignancy. Increasing intensity of immunosuppression after cancer development may result in more aggressive tumor progression manifesting as accelerated growth and metastases.[9] There are at least 3 oncogenic mechanisms through which chronic immunosuppression can increase the cancer risk: (1) direct pro-oncogenic properties of select immunosuppressive agents; (2) increased risk of oncoviral-driven malignancy, and (3) impaired immunosurveillance of neoplastic cells.[9,56]

It has been shown that cyclosporine, tacrolimus, and azathioprine exert direct effects on the cells that can promote cancers, because there is an increased production of transforming growth factor-beta (TGF-β) and vascular endothelial growth factor (VEGF), and decreased production of IL-2 from helper T cells. Inhibition of apoptosis and DNA repair mechanisms from CNIs may stimulate cancer growth.[9,55] Although TGF-β regulates tumor cell invasion and metastatic potential, VEGF increases angiogenesis. Azathioprine can alter postreplicative DNA mismatch repair systems and thus result in carcinogenesis.[9] mTOR inhibitors and MMF show antiproliferative effects and decrease cancer risk.[57]

The increased risk of oncoviral infections such as EBV, human papilloma virus (HPV), and HHV-8 in organ recipients is mainly attributed to

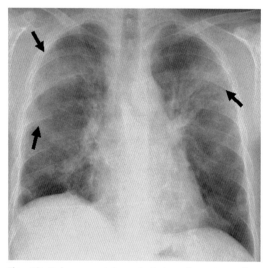

Fig. 12. Pulmonary tuberculosis in a lung transplant recipient. Chest radiograph shows ill-defined air space opacities associated with interstitial thickening predominantly involving the bilateral upper lobe lung parenchyma (*arrows*), suggestive of pulmonary tuberculosis.

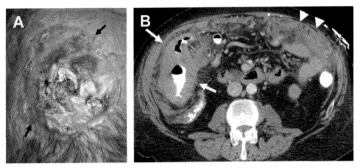

Fig. 13. Multiple BCCs and PTLD in a 68-year-old man, who is a heart and kidney transplant recipient. (*A*) The scalp shows a large ulcerating mass (*black arrows*), which was proved to be BCC on pathologic examination. In addition, few similar-appearing lesions are noted in the facial region (not shown here), consistent with multiple BCCs. (*B*) Axial contrast-enhanced CT image shows irregular wall thickening of the colon (*white arrows*) and diffuse omental nodularity (*arrowheads*). The diagnosis of PTLD was made on biopsy from the omentum.

chronic immunosuppression.[52] Oncogenic viruses act on subcellular pathways that lead to the disruption of mitotic check points (blocking of apoptosis and immune evasion) and activate oncogenes, suppress tumor suppressor genes, and activate cell proliferation, resulting in carcinogenesis.[58]

Cancer immunosurveillance is the function carried by potent innate and adaptive immune systems and plays an important role in the in the identification and elimination of cancer cells.[59] Impairment of this function in organ recipients caused by chronic immunosuppression predisposes the recipients to high cancer risk and aggressive progression of malignancies; in addition, the immune system also fails to eliminate virus-infected and mutated cells that can progress to malignancy.[59] Abnormal cancer immunosurveillance is also a promoting factor in donor-related malignancies and the recurrence of posttransplant malignancies. For example, cancer cells, when present in the immunocompetent donor's body, can be quiescent, and those same cells when transferred to the recipient may proliferate and metastasize under an immunosuppressed state.[9,52,59]

Nonmelanoma Skin Cancer

Nonmelanoma skin cancers are the most common posttransplant malignancies, presenting in more than half of all transplant recipients.[60] SOT recipients are up to 250 times more likely to develop skin cancers than controls. Immunosuppressive drugs, particularly azathioprine and CNIs, promote carcinogenesis by exacerbating ultraviolet radiation–induced DNA damage and by other mechanisms described earlier. Squamous cell carcinoma (SCC) is the most common subtype, followed by basal cell carcinoma (BCC), Merkel cell carcinoma, and Kaposi sarcoma. SCCs and BCCs together account for greater than 90% of skin cancers; the ratio of BCC/SCC of 4:1 in the general population is reversed in transplant patients.[60] Although HHV-8–associated Kaposi sarcoma occurs within 1 to 2 years after SOT, HPV-associated SCC presents several years after SOT. The risk for SCCs in heart transplant patients is greater than with liver/kidney transplant recipients.[60]

SCCs frequently coexist with premalignant conditions such as warts, Bowen disease, and keratoacanthomas. HPV DNA is found in up to 90%

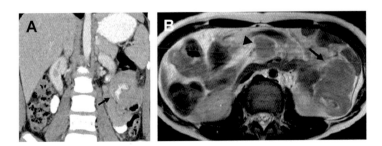

Fig. 14. Small bowel PTLD in a 13-year-old girl with a history of heart transplantation. Coronal contrast-enhanced CT (*A*) and axial T2-weighted MR (*B*) images of the abdomen show irregular wall thickening of the multiple small bowel loops (*arrows*) and mesenteric lymphadenopathy (*arrowhead*). PTLD was diagnosed on mesenteric biopsy.

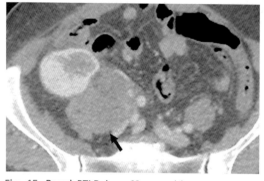

Fig. 15. Renal PTLD in a 62-year-old woman, status deceased-donor renal transplant. Axial contrast-enhanced CT image shows a heterogeneously enhancing soft tissue attenuating mass arising from the transplanted kidney (*arrow*). This was proved to be PTLD on biopsy.

of SCCs in transplant cohorts. Approximately 30% to 50% of patients with SCCs also develop BCCs. Although 80% of SCCs occur in the dorsum of hands and forearms in young patients (<40 years at SOT), 80% of cancers in older patients present with head and neck tumors.[60] Posttransplant SCCs are biologically aggressive, frequently multi-centric, recur locally in greater than 10% of patients, and metastasize in 5% to 8% of patients, thus contributing to significant morbidity and mortality.[60] Most of these skin cancers are diagnosed by clinical examination; imaging studies such as contrast-enhanced CT or 18-FDG-PET/CT may help in the assessment of deep tissue involvement, nodal staging, and evaluating for distant metastatic disease (**Fig. 13**).[61]

Posttransplant Lymphoproliferative Disorder

PTLD refers to a spectrum of lymphoproliferative disorders that present after stem cell transplantation or SOT. PTLD is the most common malignancy in pediatric patients after organ transplantation and the second most common malignancy after skin cancer in adults. PTLD is predominantly B cell in origin in 85% to 90% of cases; 10% to 15% of cases are of T-cell or natural killer cell origin. Although 60% to 70% of B-cell PTLDs are associated with EBV infection, 60% to 90% of T-cell PTLDs are EBV negative.[62–64]

The greatest risk of development of PTLD is in the first year after transplantation.[65] The risk factors for PTLD include host genetic factors, degree of immunosuppression, viral infections (EBV, human T-cell lymphotropic virus type 1), recipient age (patients aged <10 years and >60 years show greater risk), and type of allograft.[66] The risk of PTLD is highest (20%) for intestinal and multivisceral transplantation, intermediate (2%–10%) in heart and lung transplants recipients, and lowest (1%–5%) in patients with liver/kidney transplants. The spectrum of PTLD ranges from indolent polyclonal proliferations to highly

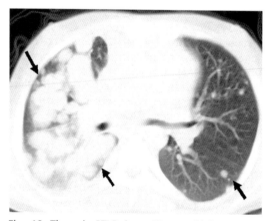

Fig. 16. Thoracic PTLD in a 17-year-old boy, status post–heart transplant with fevers. Axial CT image of the chest (lung windows) shows multiple alveolar masses involving bilateral lung parenchyma (*arrows*), more severe on the right side. Pathology confirmed diffuse large B-cell lymphoma.

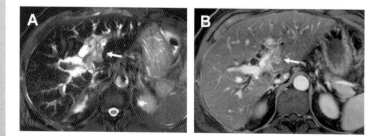

Fig. 17. Perihepatic PTLD in a 67-year-old man, status post–liver transplant. Axial T2-weighted (*A*) and axial contrast-enhanced T1-weighted (*B*) MR images show infiltrating periportal and perihilar soft tissue masses (*arrows*). The diagnosis of lymphoma was made on pathologic examination.

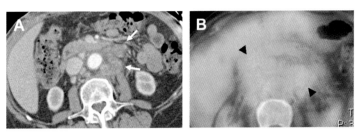

Fig. 18. Retroperitoneal PTLD in a 67-year-old man, status post–renal transplant. (*A*) Axial contrast-enhanced CT of the abdomen shows multiple enlarged retroperitoneal lymph nodes (*arrows*). (*B*) Axial 18-FDG-PET/CT image shows increased uptake (*arrowheads*). The diagnosis of lymphoma was made on pathologic examination.

aggressive lymphomas. The 2008 World Health Organization scheme recognizes 4 types of PTLD: benign/polyclonal early lesions, polymorphic, monomorphic, and classic Hodgkin lymphoma–like PTLD.[67]

The disease presentation is frequently nonspecific, thus delaying the diagnosis. Imaging plays a pivotal role in the initial detection, guiding percutaneous biopsy, follow-up, and long-term surveillance (see **Fig. 13**).[68,69] CT imaging is the most commonly used modality, whereas MR imaging can be useful in assessing bone marrow, CNS, and hepatic involvement.[69] On imaging, PTLD appears as space-occupying lesions at multiple extranodal sites, such as the gastrointestinal tract, lungs, bone marrow, and the CNS, or as bulky lymphadenopathy (**Figs. 14–16**).[51,68–70] PTLD needs to be excluded in any new mass or lymph node developing in transplant patients; PTLD may involve the transplanted organ in approximately half the cases (**Fig. 17**).[66] PTLD shows increased uptake on 18-FDG-PET/CT and occult lesions involving extranodal sites can be identified (**Fig. 18**).[69]

The treatment strategies for PTLD are type/stage and disease specific and include reduction of immunosuppressive drugs, systemic chemotherapy, antivirals, rituximab, and external beam radiation therapy (for CNS PTLD).[66] Current mortalities associated with PTLD are in the range of 30% to 60%.

Anogenital Cancers

The incidence of HPV-associated anogenital cancers in transplant recipients is 100 times greater than in the general population; they comprise less than 3% of all cancers.[60] The mean latency is approximately 7 years, with a distinct female predilection (female/male = 2:1). The lesions are usually large, multicentric, and refractory to treatment. HPV-related female genital tract tumors present in liver/kidney transplant recipients as early as

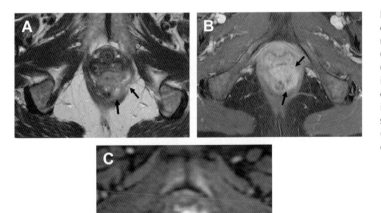

Fig. 19. Anal carcinoma in a 61-year-old woman, status post–liver and renal transplant. Axial T2-weighted (*A*), contrast-enhanced T1-weighted (*B*), and diffusion-weighted (*C*) MR images of the anal canal show a heterogeneously enhancing anal mass infiltrating into the left external sphincter and posterior vaginal wall (*arrows*). This mass shows restricted diffusion (*arrowhead*).

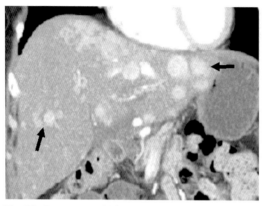

Fig. 20. Recurrent HCC in a 61-year-old woman, status post–liver transplant who presented with increased alpha fetoprotein levels. Coronal contrast-enhanced CT image of the liver during arterial phase shows multiple hypervascular hepatic masses (*arrows*), which were confirmed to be recurrent, multifocal HCC on biopsy.

6 months posttransplantation despite pretransplant HPV-negative status. HPV-positive renal transplant recipients have a 14-fold greater risk for cervical cancer, 50-fold greater risk for vulvar cancer, and 100-fold greater risk for anal carcinoma.[71] Periodic evaluation of the anogenital region is thus recommended in high-risk transplant patients. Imaging is important in local staging, detecting lymph nodal and distant metastatic disease, treatment follow-up, and long-term surveillance (**Fig. 19**).

Cancers Caused by Predisposing Chronic Disorders

The risk of development of HCC in the setting of chronic hepatitis infection is approximately

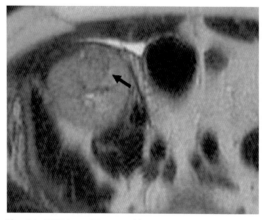

Fig. 21. RCC in a 65-year-old man, status post–kidney transplant. Axial T2-weighted MR image shows a mildly hypointense renal mass (*arrow*) in the transplanted kidney, which was proved to be clear cell RCC on pathology.

0.05% per year. A substantial number of liver transplants are performed for cirrhosis secondary to chronic hepatitis infection; thus a significant proportion of liver transplant recipients are at risk for development of HCC (**Fig. 20**). HCCs may recur in liver transplant recipients in approximately 3.5% to 21% of cases; they portend a poor prognosis in this cohort.[52,72] In addition, patients with primary sclerosing cholangitis with associated ulcerative colitis receiving liver transplants are at increased risk for development of both cholangiocarcinoma and colon cancer.[73]

Similarly, there is a greater risk of development of RCCs in renal transplant recipients; the incidence of RCCs in end-stage renal disease is approximately 4.2%. In addition, there is risk of transplanting organs (liver/kidney) with microscopic malignancy that may grow into macroscopic cancers because of associated immunosuppression in transplant cohorts (donor-related transmission). The risk of RCCs is also increased in kidney, liver, and heart transplant recipients. RCCs in the transplant cohorts are generally small and asymptomatic as well as of lower grade/stage, with resultant favorable prognosis following surgery (**Fig. 21**).[52] Cross-sectional imaging studies play an important role in periodic surveillance, early diagnosis, and management of cancers in patients with greater risk of carcinogenesis caused by predisposing chronic conditions.

SUMMARY

Adequate transplant function depends on lifelong immunosuppression. Chronic immunosuppression is a double-edged sword in SOT; although it ensures prevention of organ rejection, it places transplant recipients at an increased risk of developing a wide spectrum of opportunistic infections and cancers, which leads to increased morbidity and mortality. Cross-sectional imaging plays an important role in the diagnosis and management of infectious and neoplastic complications of chronic immunosuppression.

REFERENCES

1. Organ Procurement and Transplantation Network (OPTN). Available at: http://optn.transplant.hrsa. gov/. Accessed June 18, 2015.
2. Girlanda R. Complications of post-transplant immunosuppression. In: Andrades JA, editor. Regenerative medicine and tissue engineering. InTech; 2013. http://dx.doi.org/10.5772/55614. ISBN: 978-953-51-1108-5. Available at: http://www.intechopen.com/ books/regenerative-medicine-and-tissue-engineering/ complications-of-post-transplant-immunosuppression.

3. Halloran PF. Immunosuppressive drugs for kidney transplantation. N Engl J Med 2004;351(26):2715–29.

4. Girlanda R, Matsumoto CS, Melancon KJ, et al. Current immunosuppression in abdominal organ transplantation, immunosuppression - role in health and diseases. In: Kapur S, editor. InTech; 2012. http://dx.doi.org/10.5772/26683. ISBN: 978-953-51-0152-9. Available at: http://www.intechopen.com/books/immunosuppression-role-in-health-and-diseases/currentimmunosuppression-in-abdominal-organ-transplantation.

5. Moini M, Schilsky ML, Tichy EM. Review on immunosuppression in liver transplantation. World J Hepatol 2015;7(10):1355–68.

6. van Sandwijk MS, Bemelman FJ, Ten Berge IJ. Immunosuppressive drugs after solid organ transplantation. Neth J Med 2013;71(6):281–9.

7. Hedri H, Cherif M, Zouaghi K, et al. Avascular osteonecrosis after renal transplantation. Transplant Proc 2007;39(4):1036–8.

8. Maalouf NM, Shane E. Osteoporosis after solid organ transplantation. J Clin Endocrinol Metab 2005;90(4):2456–65.

9. Gutierrez-Dalmau A, Campistol JM. Immunosuppressive therapy and malignancy in organ transplant recipients: a systematic review. Drugs 2007;67(8):1167–98.

10. Geissler EK, Schlitt HJ. The potential benefits of rapamycin on renal function, tolerance, fibrosis, and malignancy following transplantation. Kidney Int 2010;78(11):1075–9.

11. Fishman JA. Infection in solid-organ transplant recipients. N Engl J Med 2007;357(25):2601–14.

12. Pagalilauan GL, Limaye AP. Infections in transplant patients. Med Clin North Am 2013;97(4):581–600, x.

13. Fischer SA. Infections complicating solid organ transplantation. Surg Clin North Am 2006;86(5):1127–45, v–vi.

14. Patel R, Paya CV. Infections in solid-organ transplant recipients. Clin Microbiol Rev 1997;10(1):86–124.

15. Singh N. Infections in solid-organ transplant recipients. Am J Infect Control 1997;25(5):409–17.

16. Jenkins FJ, Rowe DT, Rinaldo CR Jr. Herpesvirus infections in organ transplant recipients. Clin Diagn Lab Immunol 2003;10(1):1–7.

17. Murray JG, Evans SJ, Jeffrey PB, et al. Cytomegalovirus colitis in AIDS: CT features. AJR Am J Roentgenol 1995;165(1):67–71.

18. Poghosyan T, Ackerman SJ, Ravenel JG. Infectious complications of solid organ transplantation. Semin Roentgenol 2007;42(1):11–22.

19. Moon JH, Kim EA, Lee KS, et al. Cytomegalovirus pneumonia: high-resolution CT findings in ten non-AIDS immunocompromised patients. Korean J Radiol 2000;1(2):73–8.

20. Franquet T, Lee KS, Muller NL. Thin-section CT findings in 32 immunocompromised patients with cytomegalovirus pneumonia who do not have AIDS. AJR Am J Roentgenol 2003;181(4):1059–63.

21. Silveira FP, Husain S. Fungal infections in solid organ transplantation. Med Mycol 2007;45(4):305–20.

22. Silveira FP, Kusne S, AST Infectious Diseases Community of Practice. Candida infections in solid organ transplantation. Am J Transplant 2013;13(Suppl 4):220–7.

23. Levine MS, Rubesin SE. Diseases of the esophagus: diagnosis with esophagography. Radiology 2005;237(2):414–27.

24. Buff SJ, McLelland R, Gallis HA, et al. Candida albicans pneumonia: radiographic appearance. AJR Am J Roentgenol 1982;138(4):645–8.

25. Pastakia B, Shawker TH, Thaler M, et al. Hepatosplenic candidiasis: wheels within wheels. Radiology 1988;166(2):417–21.

26. Singh N, Husain S, AST Infectious Diseases Community of Practice. Invasive aspergillosis in solid organ transplant recipients. Am J Transplant 2009;9(Suppl 4):S180–91.

27. Singh N, Paterson DL. Aspergillus infections in transplant recipients. Clin Microbiol Rev 2005;18(1):44–69.

28. Ruhnke M, Kofla G, Otto K, et al. CNS aspergillosis: recognition, diagnosis and management. CNS drugs 2007;21(8):659–76.

29. Qin J, Fang Y, Dong Y, et al. Radiological and clinical findings of 25 patients with invasive pulmonary aspergillosis: retrospective analysis of 2150 liver transplantation cases. Br J Radiol 2012;85(1016):e429–35.

30. Franquet T, Muller NL, Gimenez A, et al. Spectrum of pulmonary aspergillosis: histologic, clinical, and radiologic findings. Radiographics 2001;21(4):825–37.

31. Almutairi BM, Nguyen TB, Jansen GH, et al. Invasive aspergillosis of the brain: radiologic-pathologic correlation. Radiographics 2009;29(2):375–9.

32. Starkey J, Moritani T, Kirby P. MRI of CNS fungal infections: review of aspergillosis to histoplasmosis and everything in between. Clin Neuroradiol 2014;24(3):217–30.

33. Martin SI, Fishman JA, AST Infectious Diseases Community of Practice. Pneumocystis pneumonia in solid organ transplantation. Am J Transplant 2013;13(Suppl 4):272–9.

34. Wang EH, Partovi N, Levy RD, et al. Pneumocystis pneumonia in solid organ transplant recipients: not yet an infection of the past. Transpl Infect Dis 2012;14(5):519–25.

35. Kanne JP, Yandow DR, Meyer CA. Pneumocystis jiroveci pneumonia: high-resolution CT findings in patients with and without HIV infection. AJR Am J Roentgenol 2012;198(6):W555–61.

36. Nicod LP, Pache JC, Howarth N. Fungal infections in transplant recipients. Eur Respir J 2001;17(1):133–40.

37. Andreula CF, Burdi N, Carella A. CNS cryptococcosis in AIDS: spectrum of MR findings. J Comput Assist Tomogr 1993;17(3):438–41.

38. Lanternier F, Sun HY, Ribaud P, et al. Mucormycosis in organ and stem cell transplant recipients. Clin Infect Dis 2012;54(11):1629–36.

39. Herrera DA, Dublin AB, Ormsby EL, et al. Imaging findings of rhinocerebral mucormycosis. Skull Base 2009;19(2):117–25.

40. Hamdi A, Mulanovich VE, Matin SF, et al. Isolated renal mucormycosis in a transplantation recipient. J Clin Oncol 2015;33(10):e50–1.

41. Spellberg B. Gastrointestinal mucormycosis: an evolving disease. Gastroenterol Hepatol 2012;8(2):140–2.

42. Peleg AY, Husain S, Qureshi ZA, et al. Risk factors, clinical characteristics, and outcome of Nocardia infection in organ transplant recipients: a matched case-control study. Clin Infect Dis 2007;44(10):1307–14.

43. Kanne JP, Yandow DR, Mohammed TL, et al. CT findings of pulmonary nocardiosis. AJR Am J Roentgenol 2011;197(2):W266–72.

44. Raby N, Forbes G, Williams R. Nocardia infection in patients with liver transplants or chronic liver disease: radiologic findings. Radiology 1990;174(3 Pt 1):713–6.

45. Munoz P, Rodriguez C, Bouza E. Mycobacterium tuberculosis infection in recipients of solid organ transplants. Clin Infect Dis 2005;40(4):581–7.

46. Singh N, Paterson DL. Mycobacterium tuberculosis infection in solid-organ transplant recipients: impact and implications for management. Clin Infect Dis 1998;27(5):1266–77.

47. Burrill J, Williams CJ, Bain G, et al. Tuberculosis: a radiologic review. Radiographics 2007;27(5):1255–73.

48. Barsoum RS. Parasitic infections in transplant recipients. Nat Clin Pract Nephrol 2006;2(9):490–503.

49. Engels EA, Pfeiffer RM, Fraumeni JF Jr, et al. Spectrum of cancer risk among US solid organ transplant recipients. JAMA 2011;306(17):1891–901.

50. Opelz G, Henderson R. Incidence of non-Hodgkin lymphoma in kidney and heart transplant recipients. Lancet 1993;342(8886–8887):1514–6.

51. Pickhardt PJ, Siegel MJ. Posttransplantation lymphoproliferative disorder of the abdomen: CT evaluation in 51 patients. Radiology 1999;213(1):73–8.

52. Campistol JM, Cuervas-Mons V, Manito N, et al. New concepts and best practices for management of pre- and post-transplantation cancer. Transplant Rev 2012;26(4):261–79.

53. Martinez OM, de Gruijl FR. Molecular and immunologic mechanisms of cancer pathogenesis in solid organ transplant recipients. Am J Transplant 2008;8(11):2205–11.

54. Hall EC, Pfeiffer RM, Segev DL, et al. Cumulative incidence of cancer after solid organ transplantation. Cancer 2013;119(12):2300–8.

55. Chapman JR, Webster AC, Wong G. Cancer in the transplant recipient. Cold Spring Harb Perspect Med 2013;3(7):1–15.

56. Sherston SN, Carroll RP, Harden PN, et al. Predictors of cancer risk in the long-term solid-organ transplant recipient. Transplantation 2014;97(6):605–11.

57. Knoll GA, Kokolo MB, Mallick R, et al. Effect of sirolimus on malignancy and survival after kidney transplantation: systematic review and meta-analysis of individual patient data. BMJ 2014;349:g6679.

58. Saha A, Kaul R, Murakami M, et al. Tumor viruses and cancer biology: modulating signaling pathways for therapeutic intervention. Cancer Biol Ther 2010;10(10):961–78.

59. Swann JB, Smyth MJ. Immune surveillance of tumors. J Clin Invest 2007;117(5):1137–46.

60. Euvrard S, Kanitakis J, Claudy A. Skin cancers after organ transplantation. N Engl J Med 2003;348(17):1681–91.

61. Jennings L, Schmults CD. Management of high-risk cutaneous squamous cell carcinoma. J Clin Aesthet Dermatol 2010;3(4):39–48.

62. Swerdlow SH. T-cell and NK-cell posttransplantation lymphoproliferative disorders. Am J Clin Pathol 2007;127(6):887–95.

63. Pickhardt PJ, Siegel MJ. Abdominal manifestations of posttransplantation lymphoproliferative disorder. AJR Am J Roentgenol 1998;171(4):1007–13.

64. Pickhardt PJ, Siegel MJ, Anderson DC, et al. Chest radiography as a predictor of outcome in posttransplantation lymphoproliferative disorder in lung allograft recipients. AJR Am J Roentgenol 1998;171(2):375–82.

65. Pickhardt PJ, Siegel MJ, Hayashi RJ, et al. Posttransplantation lymphoproliferative disorder in children: clinical, histopathologic, and imaging features. Radiology 2000;217(1):16–25.

66. Al-Mansour Z, Nelson BP, Evens AM. Posttransplant lymphoproliferative disease (PTLD): risk factors, diagnosis, and current treatment strategies. Curr Hematol Malig Rep 2013;8(3):173–83.

67. Campo E, Swerdlow SH, Harris NL, et al. The 2008 WHO classification of lymphoid neoplasms and beyond: evolving concepts and practical applications. Blood 2011;117(19):5019–32.

68. Camacho JC, Moreno CC, Harri PA, et al. Posttransplantation lymphoproliferative disease: proposed imaging classification. Radiographics 2014;34(7):2025–38.

69. Borhani AA, Hosseinzadeh K, Almusa O, et al. Imaging of posttransplantation lymphoproliferative disorder after solid organ transplantation. Radiographics 2009;29(4):981–1000 [discussion: 2].

70. Pickhardt PJ, Wippold FJ 2nd. Neuroimaging in posttransplantation lymphoproliferative disorder. AJR Am J Roentgenol 1999;172(4):1117–21.

71. Hinten F, Meeuwis KA, van Rossum MM, et al. HPV-related (pre)malignancies of the female anogenital tract in renal transplant recipients. Crit Rev Oncol Hematol 2012;84(2):161–80.

72. Castroagudin JF, Molina E, Bustamante M, et al. Orthotopic liver transplantation for hepatocellular carcinoma: a thirteen-year single-center experience. Transplant Proc 2008;40(9):2975–7.

73. Khorsandi SE, Salvans S, Zen Y, et al. Cholangiocarcinoma complicating recurrent primary sclerosing cholangitis after liver transplantation. Transpl Int 2011;24(10):e93–6.

Pediatric Thoracic Organ Transplantation
Current Indications, Techniques, and Imaging Findings

 CrossMark

Patricia T. Chang, MD[a], Jamie Frost, DO[a],
A. Luana Stanescu, MD[b], Grace S. Phillips, MD[b],
Edward Y. Lee, MD, MPH[c],*

KEYWORDS

- Pediatric lung transplantation • Heart transplantation • Acute rejection • Chronic rejection
- Infection • Posttransplant lymphoproliferative disorder (PTLD)

KEY POINTS

- Accurate and timely radiologic diagnosis of transplant complications facilitates appropriate treatment and minimizes morbidity and mortality.
- As in adults, the major complication affecting long-term survival in pediatric lung transplant recipients is bronchiolitis obliterans from chronic lung rejection.
- The clinical and imaging features of post–lung transplant complications can overlap. Thus, knowledge of the time point at which the complication occurs is essential to distinguish the different entities.
- Allograft rejection in post–heart transplant patients remains one of the main complications limiting long-term graft survival and is the primary cause of death during the first 3 years posttransplant.
- Cardiac magnetic resonance (MR) imaging can be useful as a less invasive alternative to endomyocardial biopsy in the surveillance of acute cellular rejection after orthotopic heart transplant in conjunction with clinical and laboratory findings.

INTRODUCTION

Since the initial use of lung and heart transplantation for end-stage cardiopulmonary disease in the 1980s, substantial advancements have been made in surgical technique, immunosuppressive regimens, recognition and treatment of allograft rejection, and multidisciplinary long-term care.[1] Imaging is an essential component in the evaluation of pretransplant and posttransplant pediatric patients for initial diagnosis, follow-up, assessment, and detection of complications. Clear knowledge of the spectrum of disease patterns and their relation to the time course from transplantation is essential for the appropriate management of these pediatric patients, particularly those presenting with acute rejection. Furthermore, recognition of characteristic imaging

Disclosure: The authors have nothing to disclose.
[a] Department of Radiology, Boston Children's Hospital, Harvard Medical School, 300 Longwood Avenue, Boston, MA 02115, USA; [b] Department of Radiology, Seattle Children's Hospital, University of Washington School of Medicine, Seattle, 4800 Sand Point Way NE, WA 98105, USA; [c] Thoracic Imaging Division, Department of Radiology, Boston Children's Hospital, Harvard Medical School, 300 Longwood Avenue, Boston, MA 02115, USA
* Corresponding author.
E-mail address: Edward.Lee@childrens.harvard.edu

Radiol Clin N Am 54 (2016) 321–338
http://dx.doi.org/10.1016/j.rcl.2015.09.005
0033-8389/16/$ – see front matter © 2016 Elsevier Inc. All rights reserved.

radiologic.theclinics.com

features is important because it can guide treatment and may obviate unnecessary additional imaging studies or invasive procedures such as biopsy or surgery. This article reviews the current indications and up-to-date imaging techniques for evaluating children both before and after thoracic organ transplantation and the spectrum of imaging findings that can occur in this patient population.

LUNG TRANSPLANTATION
Current Indications

Lung transplantation in the pediatric population should be considered in carefully selected patients who present with untreatable end-stage or progressively worsening advanced lung disease or pulmonary vascular disease for which there is no further available medical therapy. The common indications for lung transplant in children vary by age group (**Table 1**). Most pediatric patients who receive lung transplants are those with severe advanced cystic fibrosis. Another common diagnosis leading to lung transplantation in children is pulmonary hypertension, either idiopathic or related to congenital heart disease (CHD). In addition, less frequent but also important indications for transplant unique to children include pediatric interstitial lung diseases (eg, congenital surfactant deficiency syndrome and chronic lung disease of

infancy), congenital cardiac diseases involving the pulmonary vasculature, and primary pulmonary vascular conditions.

Bilateral lung transplantation is the most common surgical technique in children, especially in patients with cystic fibrosis, and is preferable in children with pulmonary hypertension.[2] Absolute contraindications for lung transplantation are mostly derived from experiences with the adult population and include active malignancy, sepsis, active infection such as tuberculosis, severe neuromuscular disease, refractory nonadherence, multiorgan dysfunction, and hepatitis C infection with histologic liver disease.[3] Relative contraindications for lung transplantation include congenital or acquired immunodeficiency syndromes, renal insufficiency, poorly controlled diabetes mellitus, active collagen vascular disease, and severe scoliosis.[3]

Although short-term (1 year) survival rates for pediatric lung transplantation recipients have improved, long-term outcomes for children receiving lung transplantation have not. At present, survival in pediatric patients at 1 year after lung transplantation is approximately 80% and at 5 years approximately 50%.[4] The most common cause of early mortality is related to primary graft failure, whereas the most common cause of death within the first year is infection.[5] As in adults, the major complication affecting long-term survival is bronchiolitis obliterans (BO) from chronic lung rejection.[5]

Imaging Techniques

Imaging evaluation is essential in assessing the degree of existing lung disease and potentially ascertaining the underlying cause of the patient's respiratory dysfunction. It also plays an important role in managing the other stages of pediatric lung transplant patients, including assessing donor quality and size, and posttransplant monitoring.

The preoperative assessment of potential lung transplant recipients includes posteroanterior and lateral chest radiographs and computed tomography (CT) angiogram with two-dimensional (2D) and three-dimensional (3D) reconstructions of the airway and vascular structures. The combination of these imaging modalities is helpful in the assessment of the extent of the lung disorder, chest and lung size, mediastinal vessels, and large airways. Chest CT with multiplanar and 3D reformats is useful in detailing the anatomy of the airway and vascular structures before surgery. Ventilation-perfusion (V/Q) scans can provide information on lung function. V/Q scans also aid in

Table 1	
Common indications for pediatric lung transplantation by age	
Age Group (y)	**Indication for Transplant**
<1 (infants)	• Surfactant protein B deficiency • Congenital heart disease • IPAH
1–5	• IPAH • IPF • Pulmonary fibrosis (other) • Retransplant
6–10	• CF • IPAH • Bronchiolitis obliterans, nonretransplant • Retransplant • IPF
11–17	• CF • IPAH • Retransplant

Abbreviations: CF, cystic fibrosis; IPAH, idiopathic pulmonary arterial hypertension; IPF, idiopathic pulmonary fibrosis.

the decision of which lung to transplant in the setting of single-lung transplantation and in determining which lung should be replaced first in a bilateral sequential lung transplantation procedure. In addition, bone densitometry, which can provide information for accurately assessing risk for fractures in patients with end-stage lung disease, may be needed because these patients often have a history of steroid use and are at increased risk for fracture.

Standard donor evaluation typically includes chest radiographs, CT, and pulmonary function tests. Ideally, the donor should have clear lungs without evidence of underlying lung disorder. The lung volume can be precisely measured on 3D volume rendered CT images for the size compatibility in advance of surgery (**Fig. 1**). Other parameters include a PaO_2 of greater than 300 mm Hg on fraction of inspired oxygen (FiO_2) of 1.0 and a normal bronchoscopy.[6]

The imaging algorithm for pediatric patients after lung transplantation used at our institution is outlined in **Box 1**. Patients undergo a frontal chest radiograph every day during hospitalization and on discharge. A chest radiograph and CT angiogram (with 2D and 3D reconstructions of the airway and vascular structures) are typically obtained on the patient's 1-month follow-up visit (**Fig. 2**). Subsequently, an enhanced chest CT scan with expiratory cuts is performed to evaluate the patient at 3 and 6 months and yearly thereafter. Administration of intravenous contrast when performing chest CT examinations in this population after lung transplantation is helpful for the complete evaluation of mediastinal and hilar structures, including lymph nodes,

---

Box 1
Lung transplant imaging protocol

Pre–lung transplant imaging evaluation

- Posteroanterior (PA) and lateral chest radiographs
- CT angiogram (with 2D and 3D reconstruction of airway and vascular structures)

Post–lung transplant imaging evaluation

- Anteroposterior chest radiographs every day during hospitalization
- PA and lateral chest radiographs on the day of discharge from the hospital
- PA and lateral chest radiograph at 1-month follow-up clinic visit
- CT angiogram (with 2D and 3D reconstructions of airway and vascular structures) at 1-month follow-up clinic visit
- Chest CT with expiratory cuts at 3-month and 6-month follow-up clinic visits
- Chest CT with expiratory cuts at yearly follow-up

---

which can be enlarged in the setting of posttransplant lymphoproliferative disorder (PTLD). Expiratory CT imaging is valuable for detecting air trapping, which is characteristic of posttransplant BO.

Postoperative Imaging Findings

The clinical and imaging features of post–lung transplant complications can overlap. Thus, knowledge of the time point at which the complication occurs is essential to distinguish the different entities. In addition, because imaging features can be nonspecific, caution is needed in basing clinical decisions solely on radiographic presentation without clinical and histopathologic correlation.

Post–lung transplant complications can be broadly categorized based on time of occurrence: (1) immediate (<24 hours), (2) early (>24 hours to 1 week), (3) intermediate (8 days to 2 months) to primary late (2–4 months), and (4) secondary late (>4 months), as discussed later (**Table 2**).

Immediate complications (<24 hours)

Donor-recipient size mismatch A size discrepancy between the donor lung and the recipient thoracic cage can result in mechanical complications manifesting as atelectasis and impaired ventilation. Distortion of the airways and atelectasis from lungs that are too large may progress to

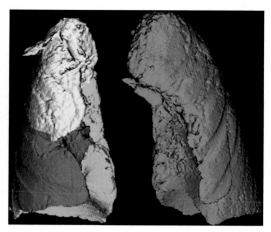

Fig. 1. A 20-year-old female lung transplant donor. 3D volume rendered CT image of the lungs with color-coded volumetric measurement for preoperative assessment.

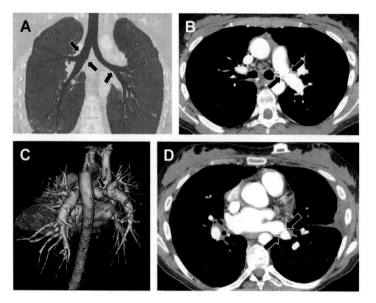

Fig. 2. Expected postsurgical changes after lung transplant. (A) CT image in an oblique coronal minimal intensity projection shows both the right and left main stem bronchi anastomoses (arrows) following bilateral lung transplant. (B) Contrast-enhanced axial CT image shows focal caliber change at the level of left main pulmonary artery anastomosis (arrows). Note surgical clips in the hilum. (C) 3D rendered image shows expected postsurgical narrowing (arrow) of the left pulmonary artery. (D) Contrast-enhanced axial CT image shows focal caliber change at the level of left lower pulmonary vein anastomosis (arrows). Note minimal residual left pleural thickening and fluid.

scarring. Lungs that are too small may lead to hemodynamic compromise, exercise limitations, and pulmonary hypertension from inadequate pulmonary vascular circulation. An acceptable size difference between the donor lung and the recipient thoracic cage is reported to be about 10% to 25%.[7] Before lung transplantation, 3D volumetric measurement of the donor lung based on CT study can be obtained for the size compatibility (see **Fig. 1**).

Table 2
Complications occurring post–lung transplant based on time of occurrence

Time Period Posttransplantation	Complications
Immediate (<24 h)	• Donor-recipient size mismatch • Hyperacute rejection
Early (>24 h to 1 wk)	• Primary graft dysfunction • Pleural complications
Intermediate (8 d to 2 mo) to primary late (2–4 mo)	• Acute rejection • Anastomotic complications • Pulmonary thromboembolic events
Secondary late (>4 mo)	• Chronic rejection • Upper-lobe fibrosis • Cryptogenic organizing pneumonia • PTLD

Hyperacute rejection Hyperacute rejection is an uncommon complication nowadays. Virtual crossmatching performed preoperatively in patients with a high reactive panel can prospectively identify any possible incompatibility that could develop between the recipient and donor. When hyperacute rejection does occur, it is within minutes to hours after transplantation as a result of a recipient antibody response to donor vascular endothelium. It manifests clinically as respiratory failure and radiographically as diffusely dense homogeneous opacification throughout the allograft. Treatment consists of plasmapheresis in the operating room and should be started immediately during the postoperative period. However, this complication is associated with very poor prognosis.[5]

Early complications (>24 hours to 1 week)
Primary graft dysfunction Primary graft dysfunction is a noncardiogenic pulmonary edema that typically appears within the first 48 to 72 hours. Clinically, it is characterized by a low relationship between Pao_2 and Fio_2.[5] It generally improves by the end of the first week and eventually resolves within 3 weeks. Primary graft dysfunction is caused by an ischemic vascular injury that results in increased capillary permeability and alveolar damage. The radiographic and CT features of primary graft dysfunction are nonspecific but most frequently appear as reticular interstitial or airspace opacities predominantly in the middle and lower lobes, accompanied by peribronchial and perivascular thickening (**Fig. 3**).

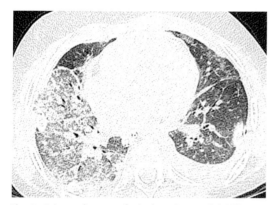

Fig. 3. Primary lung graft dysfunction. Axial CT image obtained on postoperative day 6 from bilateral lung transplantation for pulmonary artery stenosis shows bilateral lower lobe ground-glass opacities, interstitial thickening, bronchovascular thickening, and pleural effusions. Bilateral chest tubes and an enteric tube are also present. These findings completely resolved on a CT scan obtained at 3 months (not shown).

Pleural complications Pleural abnormalities occur in approximately 22% of patients after lung transplantation[8] as a result of the transplant procedure, and include pneumothorax, hemothorax, pleural effusion, empyema, and persistent or temporary air leaks (**Fig. 4**). Development of pleural effusion early on is thought to be secondary to increased capillary permeability and impaired lymphatic clearance. Postoperative effusion usually resolves by 2 weeks. Persistent or delayed effusions should raise the suspicion of underlying empyema, rejection, or vascular abnormalities (**Fig. 5**). A persistent air leak can be caused by several factors, including bronchial anastomotic dehiscence, and is associated with increased mortality.

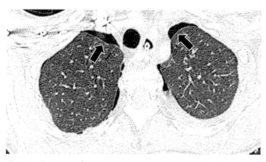

Fig. 4. Expected postoperative pneumothorax. Axial CT image obtained 10 days following combined whole-liver and bilateral lung transplant for cystic fibrosis shows bilateral pneumothoraces (*arrows*), with air predominantly in the antidependent portions of the chest.

Intermediate (8 days to 2 months) and primary late (2–4 months) complications

Acute rejection Acute rejection can occur anytime from within the first week through the first year after lung transplantation but most often occurs with the first 3 to 6 months. It is caused by a cell-mediated immune response. Definitive diagnosis is made using histologic findings via transbronchial lung biopsy that show perivascular mononuclear cell infiltrate. Recurrent acute rejection is a risk factor for the development of chronic rejection or BO syndrome (BOS). Imaging characteristics are similar to those of primary graft dysfunction with ground-glass opacities often in a basal distribution, interlobar and intralobular septal thickening, peribronchial cuffing, and pleural effusions (**Fig. 6**). Absence of ground-glass opacities makes acute rejection unlikely.[9] Substantial improvement in the radiologic abnormalities within 48 hours following intravenous steroid administration favors a diagnosis of acute rejection.

Anastomotic complications Complications can occur at the 3 main anastomoses after lung transplant, which include airway, pulmonary arterial, and pulmonary vein to left atrium.

Airway anastomotic complications include infection, dehiscence, and stenosis, which are rare in the pediatric population. Infection and dehiscence are typically seen earlier than stenosis after lung transplantation. Because the native bronchial circulation is disrupted and not reconnected with the transplant procedure, the airway circulation depends on retrograde perfusion through the pulmonary circulation, which can result in donor bronchus ischemia. CT best detects partial bronchial dehiscence with the presence of extraluminal air around the anastomotic site and an enlarging ipsilateral pneumothorax or pneumomediastinum.

Anastomotic stenosis is more common than dehiscence and is typically diagnosed within 4 months of lung transplantation. Although diagnosis of bronchial stenosis can be made with conventional bronchoscopy, CT with 2D and 3D reconstructions of the central airway is a useful noninvasive imaging modality for accurately detecting the stenosis and precisely assessing the degree of narrowing and extent. Bronchial stenosis after the lung transplantation is typically located at the site of surgical anastomosis and focal in its distribution (**Fig. 7**).[10]

Vascular anastomotic complications after lung transplantation are also rare and include pulmonary artery and vein stenosis at the surgical anastomosis. CT with 2D and 3D reconstructions can show narrowing or occlusion. Vascular

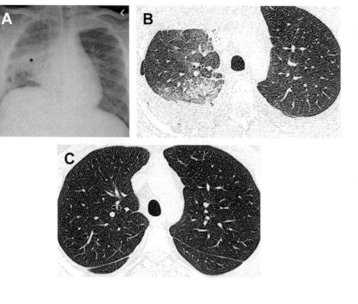

Fig. 5. Postoperative hematoma and primary graft dysfunction. (*A*) Chest radiograph shows a left apical hematoma (*asterisk*) and right perihilar opacities with right pleural effusion 10 days following bilateral lung transplant. (*B*) Same day axial CT image in lung window shows right upper-lobe ground-glass opacities, interstitial thickening, and pleural fluid. Note minimal residual right-sided pleural gas. (*C*) On 2-month follow-up CT examination, the lungs are clear and pleural fluid has resolved.

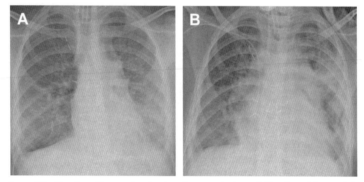

Fig. 6. Acute rejection. (*A*) Chest radiograph obtained several days following bilateral lung transplant in a 14-year-old girl shows expected postsurgical changes, including mediastinal clips, sternal wires, bibasilar edema, left lower lobe atelectasis, and small pleural effusions. (*B*) Several months later in the setting of an acute respiratory decompensation, chest radiograph shows pulmonary edema, perihilar opacities, and pleural effusion. Lung biopsy was consistent with acute rejection.

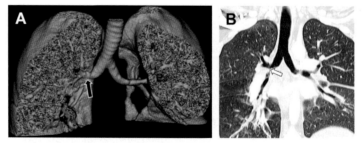

Fig. 7. Spectrum of bronchial findings post–lung transplant. (*A*) Expected postsurgical findings. 3D rendered image of the large airways and lungs shows discrete caliber change (*arrow*) of the right main stem bronchus. (*B*) Severe stenosis. Coronal reformatted CT image of a 19-year-old woman 6 months after bilateral lung transplant shows a short segment of severe stenosis (*arrow*) of the bronchus intermedius at the site of anastomosis.

dehiscence is rare but can manifest as an acute and massive hemothorax with resultant sudden death (**Fig. 8**).

Pulmonary infections Pulmonary infection is one type of complication that can occur during the entire posttransplant follow-up period. The incidence of pulmonary infection after lung transplantation is high, and more frequent than in other organ transplant procedures.[11] Bacterial and fungal infections are most frequent in the first month after lung transplant. Viral infections typically occur in the second to third months after lung transplant.

Gram-negative bacteria such as *Pseudomonas* and *Klebsiella*, as well as *Staphylococcus aureus*, are the most common causes of bacterial infections in pediatric patients with lung transplantation.[9] On CT, patchy and confluent consolidation, ground-glass opacity, tree-in-bud nodular opacities, and pleural effusions can be seen (**Fig. 9**).

Fungal infections are most often caused by *Aspergillus* and *Candida albicans* in pediatric patients with lung transplantation. Typical imaging features of aspergillus infection include focal nodular and masslike regions of consolidation, cavitation, nodules with a surrounding rim of ground-glass opacity (the halo sign), and pleural thickening (**Fig. 10**). Radiologic findings of candida infection include patchy and confluent areas of consolidation as well as typically multiple nodules (**Fig. 11**).

Long-term treatment of aspergillus and candida infections with voriconazole, a powerful second-generation antifungal agent, can lead to periostitis deformans from possible medication-induced fluoride toxicity. Fluffy periosteal new bone formation in a distribution atypical for hypertrophic osteoarthropathy, such as the ribs, clavicle, and proximal medial humerus, can be seen on radiographs. In addition, unlike the smooth and single-layer periostitis in hypertrophic osteoarthropathy, the osseous changes in voriconazole-induced periostitis have been reported as dense and irregular periosteal reaction with diffuse involvement (**Fig. 12**).[12] Bone scans show diffuse multifocal intense radiotracer uptake. Affected pediatric patients typically present with severe bone pain, absence of clubbing, and increased alkaline phosphatase levels.[13] Discontinuation of voriconazole results in complete resolution of the radiographically dramatic periostitis as well as in improved pain and reduction in alkaline phosphatase and fluoride levels.[13]

Cytomegalovirus (CMV) pneumonitis is the most common viral infection in children with lung transplantation, followed in frequency by herpes simplex and Epstein-Barr virus (EBV) infections.[14] Imaging features include geographic ground-glass opacities in a crazy-paving pattern, centrilobular nodules, interlobular septal thickening, and pleural effusions (**Fig. 13**).

Pulmonary thromboembolic events The incidences of pulmonary embolism and pulmonary infarction have been reported to be as high as 27% and 40%, respectively, in patients with lung transplant, with most occurring in the allograft.[15] Increased perfusion of the allograft and arterial anastomosis can lead to increased thrombogenesis. CT pulmonary angiography can aid in the diagnosis of suspected thromboembolic disease. Central arterial filling defects, abrupt arterial occlusion, peripheral wedge-shaped opacities representing pulmonary infarction, and oligemia can be visualized.

Secondary late complications (>4 months)
Chronic rejection Chronic rejection usually begins 6 months after lung transplantation and is the main limiting factor in long-term survival.[16] It is characterized by bronchiolitis obliterans (BO), which involves scarring of the smaller distal airways.[17] Bronchiolitis obliterans syndrome (BOS) is the clinical correlate, in which there is an unexplained reduction in lung function from the posttransplantation baseline. It is diagnosed when there is a 20% decrease in the forced expiratory volume in 1 second (FEV_1) value compared with the patient's baseline.[18]

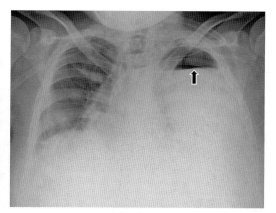

Fig. 8. Postoperative hydropneumothorax. Chest radiograph in this 17-year-old girl after bilateral lung transplant shows left hemithorax opacification with an air-fluid level (*arrow*) compatible with a hydropneumothorax on postoperative day 22. The patient returned to the operating room emergently and was found to have active bleeding from the left internal mammary artery.

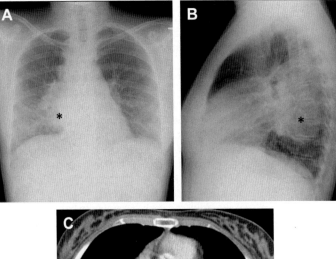

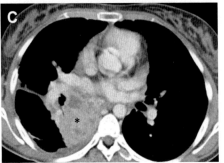

Fig. 9. Pseudomonas infection. Frontal (A) and lateral (B) radiographs of a 17-year-old girl with cystic fibrosis after bilateral lung transplant shows a right lower lobe opacity (asterisk). CT performed on the same patient shows a large complex heterogeneous right perihilar consolidation (asterisk) and a small right pleural effusion. Biopsy confirmed necrotic abscess from pseudomonas infection, which ultimately required a right pneumonectomy.

For imaging evaluation of BO, CT is more sensitive than chest radiography in showing mosaic attenuation, bronchial dilatation, and bronchial wall thickening associated with BO. If there is clinical suspicion for chronic rejection, paired inspiratory and end-expiratory CT images should be obtained in order to look for air trapping, which most strongly indicates chronic rejection (Fig. 14).[19] The previously published study, which investigated the usefulness of thin-section expiratory CT compared with that of thin-section inspiratory CT in detecting air trapping in pediatric lung transplant recipients with BOS, showed that expiratory CT can provide more accurate diagnosis of small airway obstruction (ie, BO) than inspiratory CT in this population. Expiratory CT for the diagnosis of BO has a sensitivity of 100%, a specificity of 71%, a positive predictive value of 64%, and a negative predictive value of 100% in pediatric lung transplant recipients.[20] CT can be also helpful for evaluating and excluding other potential causes of FEV_1 decline, which can mimic BOS, such as surgical anastomotic stenosis of the bronchus or respiratory infections.

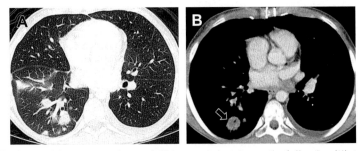

Fig. 10. Fungal infection. Axial contrast-enhanced CT images taken 2 months following bilateral lung transplant in lung (A) and soft tissue (B) windows show right lower lobe nodules of varying sizes, some with hazy surrounding ground-glass opacities and air bronchograms versus early cavitation (arrow), which was found to be aspergillus infection. Small residual left pleural effusion and anterior mediastinal postsurgical changes are also evident.

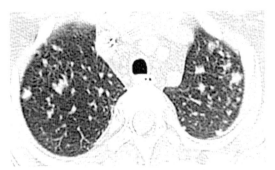

Fig. 11. Fungal infection. *C albicans* infection in 11-year-old girl with lung transplantation. Axial lung window CT image shows multiple pulmonary nodules in both lungs.

Upper-lobe fibrosis Progressive upper-lobe fibrosis can occur 1 to 4 years after transplantation.[21] Upper-lobe fibrosis is a unique presentation of chronic allograft dysfunction in lung transplant recipients and can be differentiated from BOS from radiologic findings.[22] Its imaging features include interlobular septal thickening, reticular opacities, traction bronchiectasis, honeycombing, architectural distortion, and volume loss in the upper lobes.

Cryptogenic organizing pneumonia Cryptogenic organizing pneumonia (COP) can be associated with both acute and chronic rejection, which are characterized by airway inflammation and fibrosis involving the distal airways, particularly the alveolar ducts and alveoli.[23] It manifests on imaging as reticular or ground-glass opacities, airspace consolidation, and architectural distortion (**Fig. 15**). When associated with acute rejection, it responds rapidly to high-dose corticosteroid therapy with dramatic improvement in the pulmonary opacities.

Posttransplant lymphoproliferative disorder The prevalence of PTLD within 1 year of lung transplantation ranges from 2% to 10%.[24,25] It occurs in less than 6% of patients, with the most common risk factors being immunosuppression with cyclosporine and EBV.[26,27] PTLD refers to a spectrum of diseases that are primarily of B-cell origin.[24] Pulmonary nodules and masslike consolidation are the most frequent lung parenchymal findings seen at imaging, along with mediastinal and hilar adenopathy, which may have central low attenuation representing necrosis (**Fig. 16**). Fluorodeoxyglucose (FDG)-PET/CT can also be performed to define the extent of disease and to select an appropriate site for tissue sampling (**Fig. 17**).

In pediatric lung transplant recipients, PTLD occurs with high frequency in both the chest and abdomen. Therefore, it is also important to assess possible abdominal PTLD when thoracic PTLD is encountered in this patient population. In the abdomen, PTLD typically manifests as extranodal disease and presents as bowel wall thickening, focal mass lesions, and splenomegaly. Pediatric patients with PTLD involvement of both the chest and abdomen tend to have lymphomatous features, resulting in a substantial mortality.[28]

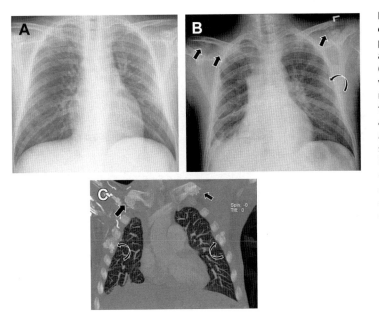

Fig. 12. Voriconazole-induced periostitis. Frontal chest radiographs performed before transplant (*A*) and 3 months following transplant (*B*) in a 17-year-old boy show interval development of multifocal nodular calcifications adjacent to the bilateral clavicles (*straight arrows*) and lateral ribs (*curved arrow*). (*C*) Coronal maximum intensity projection (MIP) CT image better delineates the extent of the diffuse and nodular periostitis along the bilateral clavicles (*straight arrows*) and nodular periostitis along the ribs (*curved arrows*).

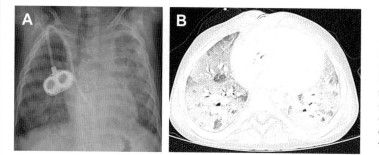

Fig. 13. CMV pneumonitis. (*A*) Chest radiograph in a 7-year-old boy after bilateral lung transplant for severe pulmonary vein stenosis shows hazy opacities in the left lung and right lower lobe with a left pleural effusion. (*B*) Axial lung window CT image of the same patient shows extensive ground-glass opacities with areas of consolidations in both lungs, found to be CMV pneumonitis.

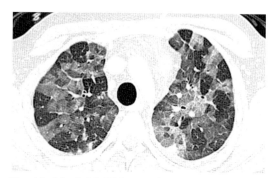

Fig. 14. BO. Axial CT image shows bilateral mosaic ground-glass opacities, bronchiectasis, and bronchial wall thickening, consistent with BO. Biopsy confirmed chronic airway rejection.

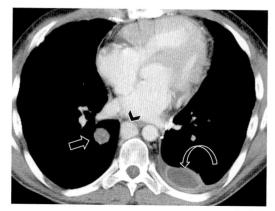

Fig. 16. PTLD. Contrast-enhanced PET-CT image of an 18-year-old man with idiopathic pulmonary hypertension 3 months after bilateral lung transplant. Axial CT image in soft tissue windows shows a 2-cm solid nodule (*straight arrow*) in the right lower lobe. There is also an enhancing left pleural collection (*curved arrow*) that was present postoperatively and had been decreasing. Note the large vessel adjacent to the aorta, consistent with azygous continuation of the inferior vena cava (*arrowhead*).

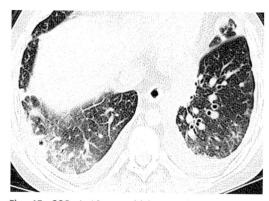

Fig. 15. COP. A 16-year-old boy with bilateral lung transplantation 1 year and 6 months ago who presented with shortness of breath and decreased FEV1 on pulmonary function test. Axial lung window CT image shows reticular and ground-glass opacification with areas of consolidation (*asterisk*). Bilateral pleural effusions are also seen.

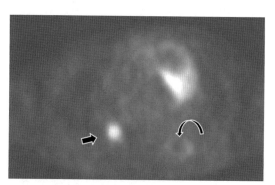

Fig. 17. PTLD. Same patient as in **Fig. 16.** Axial FDG-PET image shows avid focal uptake of the right lower lobe nodule (*straight arrow*) and mild peripheral uptake of the left pleural fluid (*curved arrow*). Biopsy of the right lower lobe nodule was consistent with PTLD. Left pleural effusion was found to be postoperative seroma.

PEARLS AND PITFALLS

- The most common cause of early mortality is related to primary graft failure, whereas the most common cause of death within the first year is infection.
- Administration of intravenous contrast when performing chest CT examinations in post–lung transplant patients is helpful for the complete evaluation of mediastinal and hilar structures, including lymph nodes, which can be enlarged in the setting of PTLD.
- Expiratory CT imaging is valuable for detecting air trapping, which is characteristic of posttransplant BO.
- Because imaging features can be nonspecific for post–lung transplant complications, caution is needed in basing clinical decisions solely on radiographic presentation without clinical and histopathologic correlation.
- Bacterial and fungal infections are most frequent in the first month after lung transplant. Viral infections typically occur in the second to third months after lung transplant.
- In pediatric lung transplant recipients, PTLD occurs with high frequency in both the chest and abdomen. Therefore, it is also important to assess possible abdominal PTLD when thoracic PTLD is encountered in this patient population.

WHAT THE REFERRING PHYSICIAN NEEDS TO KNOW

- Are there any parenchymal or pleural abnormalities?
- Are there any anastomotic complications?
- Are there any typical imaging features that can point to specific type of infection, such as with *Aspergillus*?
- In the setting of chronic rejection, is there air trapping on expiratory CT?
- Is there thoracic lymphadenopathy? Is there extranodal disease in the abdomen?

HEART TRANSPLANTATION
Current Indications

Pediatric heart transplantation is currently performed in more than 100 centers around the world.[29] Pediatric heart transplantation remains the standard of care for children with end-stage heart failure caused by cardiomyopathy or complex CHDs that cannot be repaired and when primary reconstructive procedures or staged long-term palliative procedures have failed.[30] Complex CHD is the main indication for heart transplantation in infants, whereas end-stage cardiomyopathy is the main indication after the first year of life. Dilated cardiomyopathy is the most common form of cardiomyopathy in children.[31]

The most commonly used technique for pediatric heart transplantation is bicaval anastomosis, which preserves normal atrial morphology, sinus node function, and valvular function, thereby decreasing the incidence of atrial arrhythmias and the need for pacemaker implantation.[32] Contraindications to heart transplant in the pediatric population include multisystem organ failure, active underlying malignancy, active untreated infection, and increased pulmonary vascular resistance unresponsive to oxygen and vasodilators with a transpulmonary gradient greater than 15 mm Hg.[30]

Long-term survival of pediatric heart transplant patients has improved dramatically over the past decade. Ten-year survival for patients with CHD is approximately 67% compared with those with cardiomyopathy at 83%.[33] Allograft rejection remains one of the main posttransplant complications limiting long-term graft survival and has been the primary cause of death during the first 3 years after transplant.[34] Allograft posttransplant coronary artery disease is the major cause of late mortality.[35]

Imaging Techniques

Radiologic imaging plays an important role in the preoperative assessment of both donors and recipients for heart transplantation. At present, a combination of various imaging modalities is used to assess the anatomy and function of the heart and great vessels before heart transplantation.

Chest radiography and contrast-enhanced chest CT can be obtained to screen for a contraindication to transplantation, such as active infection or neoplasm. Anatomic variations in the thoracic great vessels can be evaluated with CT for better surgical planning of the aortic, pulmonary arterial, and caval anastomotic sites between the donor and the recipient. Echocardiography can assess structural abnormalities, ventricular function, regional wall motion, and right ventricular contractility in the potential donor heart.

Cardiac magnetic resonance imaging (CMR) can be used in the postoperative follow-up of heart transplant patients. It can be particularly useful as a less invasive alternative to endomyocardial biopsy in the surveillance of acute cellular rejection after orthotopic heart transplant in conjunction with clinical and laboratory findings.[36]

A CMR protocol using a 32-channel coil for posttransplant evaluation is outlined in **Table 3**.

Postoperative Imaging Findings

Pediatric patients who undergo heart transplantation require therapy with potent immunosuppressive agents in order to prevent the onset of allograft complications such as graft failure, rejection, and accelerated coronary atherosclerosis. However, these medications also make transplant recipients highly vulnerable to opportunistic infections and lymphoproliferative disease.

In normal postoperative orthotopic heart transplants, the cardiac silhouette can appear enlarged for the first several months,[37] decreasing in size over time. A double right atrial contour from anastomosis of the donor and recipient right atria can also be seen on postoperative chest radiographs.[38] Pericardial effusions as well as pneumomediastinum, pneumothorax, pneumopericardium, and subcutaneous emphysema are expected and can all be seen in the immediate postoperative period. Mediastinal widening from postoperative mediastinal bleeding can also be seen in the first couple of weeks after surgery (**Fig. 18**).[39] In addition, if mediastinal widening persists, steroid-induced fat deposition may be the cause, which can be confirmed on cross-sectional imaging studies such as CT or MR imaging.[40]

Cross-sectional imaging of normal postoperative cardiac transplants may show vessel redundancy, size discrepancies between the donor and recipient vessels, and caliber changes at the sites of vascular anastomosis (**Fig. 19**).[40]

Anatomic modifications specific to CHD can also be seen.

Complications of cardiac transplantation can be categorized into 3 periods: (1) those that occur immediately in the postoperative period (acute), (2) those that occur within the first year after transplant (subacute), and (3) those that occur after 1 year (chronic).

Acute and subacute complications

Acute allograft rejection Rejection remains one of the main posttransplant complications. Acute allograft rejection is mediated through both cellular and humoral pathways[41] and can occur anywhere from 1 week to 3 months after heart transplantation.[42] Affected pediatric patients usually present with shortness of breath and weakness, indicating worsening heart failure and ventricular decompensation (**Fig. 20**). The definitive diagnosis of acute allograft rejection can be made with endomyocardial biopsy. However, less invasive contrast-enhanced MR imaging can be used to assess early signs of transplant rejection. Myocardial T2 relaxation time from a black-blood MR imaging sequence has been shown to identify most moderate acute rejections documented with biopsy and is a strong predictor of the subsequent occurrence of biopsy-defined acute rejections.[43]

Infection Infection, which accounts for approximately 12% of deaths during the first year following heart transplantation in the pediatric population, remains an important underlying cause of morbidity and mortality.[34] Immunosuppressive therapy given to prevent rejection can also increase susceptibility to infections.[44] Pneumonia is the leading infectious complication and usually occurs within the first 3 to 4 months following heart transplantation because of the high degree of immunosuppression during this period.

In the immediate postoperative period, bacterial and viral pathogens account for most pneumonias. In pediatric heart transplant recipients, bacterial infections, including *Staphylococcus* species, *Pseudomonas* species, and *Enterobacter cloacae*, typically occur in the early posttransplant period.[45] On imaging studies, bacterial infections typically present as either bronchopneumonia or lobar pneumonia, sometimes associated with underlying lung abscess or concomitant pleural infection (**Fig. 21**). As with lung transplant patients, CMV pneumonia is the most common viral infection, with a peak potential 6 to 8 weeks after transplantation,[45] and occurring in up to 10% of cardiac transplant recipients.[46] CMV infection may also increase the risk of rejection, cardiac allograft

---

Table 3
CMR protocol for post–heart transplant evaluation on a 32-channel coil

Analysis	Sequence
Cardiac function	SSFP sequences in short-axis and long-axis planes
Edema	STIR sequences
Perfusion	0.1–0.2 mmol/kg of gadolinium intravenous contrast injected as fast as possible for perfusion imaging in 1 long-axis and 1 short-axis plane[a]
LGE/MDE	LGE/MDE acquired 10–15 min after injection with long-axis and short-axis imaging[a]

Abbreviations: LGE, late gadolinium enhancement; MDE, myocardial delayed enhancement; SSFP, steady-state free precession; STIR, short tau inversion recovery.

[a] Short-axis stack should be through the left ventricle followed by any area of concern.

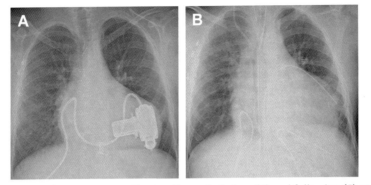

Fig. 18. Expected postoperative appearance. Chest radiographs before (*A*) and following (*B*) cardiac transplantation of an 11-year-old boy with critical aortic stenosis palliated with left ventricular assist device. Supine frontal radiograph following heart transplantation (*B*) reveals an enlarged cardiac silhouette, pulmonary edema, bibasilar atelectasis, and a small right pneumothorax. Bilateral thoracostomy tubes, endotracheal tube, enteric tube, mediastinal drainage catheter, right internal jugular catheter, and intra-atrial catheters are also seen. No sternal wires are seen, because the chest was closed the following day.

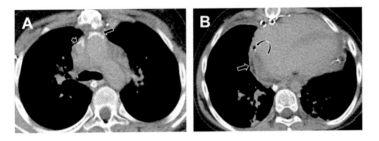

Fig. 19. Expected postoperative appearance. Axial CT image obtained on the same patient 2 days following OHT shows several expected postsurgical findings, including (*A*) dense aortic (*long arrow*) and superior vena cava anastomosis (*short arrow*) suture material. Sternotomy wires are now present. (*B*) Axial CT image at the level of the heart shows a small complex pericardial collection adjacent to the right atrium (*straight arrow*) and pneumomediastinum (*curved arrow*). Partial visualizations of bilateral mediastinal drains are present along the anterior pericardium and left pericardium.

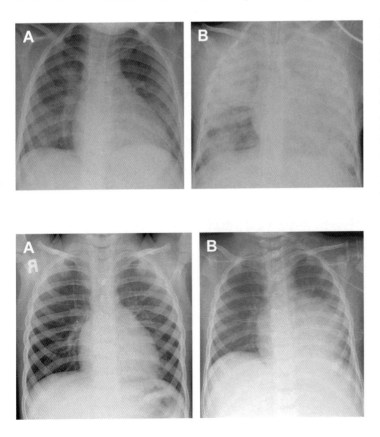

Fig. 20. Heart failure. Chest radiographs performed on a 6.5-year-old girl who presented with acute heart failure 16 months after OHT. (*A*) Chest radiograph obtained on admission shows mild pulmonary edema and cardiomegaly. Left subclavian vein approach peripherally inserted central catheter (PICC) and sternotomy wires are also seen. (*B*) Chest radiograph obtained 1 day later shows marked progression of findings with diffuse patchy airspace consolidations. Autopsy showed evidence of both acute rejection and infarcts.

Fig. 21. Pneumonia and myocarditis. A 2-year-old boy with hypoplastic left heart syndrome 8 months after OHT, who presented with fevers. Chest radiographs performed before discharge from transplantation (*A*) and following presentation for fever (*B*) show mild globular enlargement of the heart, mild pulmonary edema, and retrocardiac and lingular opacities.

vasculopathy, and PTLD.[47] Other common viral infections that can occur in pediatric heart transplant recipients include EBV, herpes simplex virus, varicella zoster virus, and influenza viruses.

Although fungal infection accounts for 6.8% of posttransplant infections in the pediatric population,[48] it is associated with high mortality. It has been reported that invasive fungal infection is associated with a mortality of 49% of all deaths occurring within the first 6 months following transplantation.[48] The 2 most common fungal infections after heart transplantation are *Candida* species and *Aspergillus*. On imaging studies, multiple small pulmonary nodules caused by candida infection and larger nodules with surrounding ground-glass opacification caused by aspergillus infection may be present in pediatric heart transplant recipients.

Cerebral ischemia/infarcts and gastrointestinal complications Cerebral ischemia and infarcts are common in the immediate postoperative period, particularly in patients who required mechanical assist devices before transplantation (**Fig. 22**).[49] Posttransplant patients are also at risk of developing gastrointestinal complications, such as peptic ulcer disease, cholecystitis, and pancreatitis, from the stress of surgery and high-dose corticosteroid and immunosuppressive therapy.

Chronic complications

Cardiac allograft vasculopathy Cardiac allograft vasculopathy (CAV) is a major long-term complication of pediatric heart transplant and is one of the leading causes of mortality. It has been reported that CAV affects approximately 34% of pediatric heart transplant recipients by 10 years after transplantation.[34] Intimal and medial proliferation in CAV causes obliterative distal coronary artery disease and results in diastolic dysfunction and graft

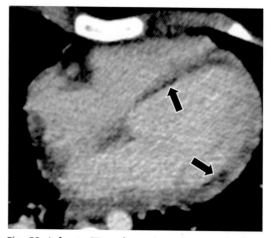

Fig. 23. Infarct. CT performed on the same patient (see **Fig. 22**) shows left ventricular subendocardial hypoattenuation (*arrows*) of the septum and left ventricular free wall. This finding is nonspecific, and the differential includes decreased perfusion, either acute or chronic, as well as subendocardial elastosis or fibrosis. Biopsy confirmed subacute infarction.

failure (**Fig. 23**). The currently known underlying risk factors for developing CAV include (1) patient age between 1 and 18 years (but not infants) at the time of heart transplant, (2) recipient African American race, and (3) retransplantation.[50] The gold standard for diagnosis of CAV is currently coronary angiography. Patients with CAV have 1-year and 3-year survival rates of 66% to 77% and 52% to 60%, respectively.[34]

Neoplasm The second most common long-term complication after CAV in post–cardiac transplant patients is neoplasm, which is thought to be caused by long-term immunosuppression. PTLD accounts for almost all of these neoplasms, ranging from benign lymphoid hyperplasia to aggressive lymphoma (**Fig. 24**). The incidence of

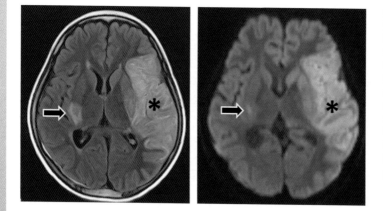

Fig. 22. Extra-thoracic complications. MR imaging of the brain performed 2 weeks following heart transplantation, on extracorporeal membrane oxygenation for acute rejection, T2-weighted fluid-attenuated inversion recovery MR image and diffusion-weighted MR image of the brain show embolic strokes involving the left middle cerebral artery territory infarct (*asterisk*) as well as a smaller right basal ganglion infarct (*arrow*).

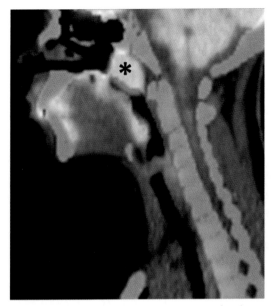

Fig. 24. PTLD. A 12-year-old boy, 10 years after heart transplantation for dilated cardiomyopathy. Sagittal FDG-PET/CT image of the neck shows moderate enlargement of adenoidal tissue (*asterisk*) with marked FDG uptake.

developing PTLD is 6% at 5 years and 10% at 10 years after heart transplantation.[51] On imaging studies, PTLD most commonly affects the lung, presenting as solitary or multiple pulmonary nodules or masses with or without associated mediastinal lymphadenopathy. When PTLD involves the gastrointestinal tract, fusiform dilatation and thickening of bowel loops are often seen (**Figs. 25** and **26**). The current management of PTLD is reduced immunosuppression, which is associated with increased risk of potential rejection. It has been reported that the development of PTLD is associated with poor prognosis, with 75% of affected children surviving 1 year and 67% of affected children surviving 5 years despite treatment.[52] Other frequently observed neoplasms include squamous

cell carcinoma of the skin, adenocarcinoma of the lung and gastrointestinal tract, and Kaposi sarcoma (**Fig. 27**).[53]

Renal dysfunction Renal dysfunction is another long-term complication that can occur as a consequence of nephrotoxicity from calcineurin inhibitors in pediatric heart transplant recipients. At 10 years posttransplantation, severe renal dysfunction, defined as either creatinine level greater than 2.5 mg/dL or requiring dialysis or renal transplantation, is seen in 4% of recipients with heart transplantation performed during infancy and up to 15% of patients who underwent heart transplantation during preadolescence to adolescence.[34] On ultrasonography, nonspecific sonographic findings of decreased corticomedullary differentiation often associated with diffusely increased echogenicity can be seen in the kidneys of pediatric heart transplant recipients who develop renal dysfunction. However, it has been reported that up to 1.4% of these affected pediatric patients eventually need chronic dialysis or renal transplantation.[54]

PEARLS AND PITFALLS

- The most commonly used technique for pediatric heart transplantation is bicaval anastomosis.
- Allograft posttransplant coronary artery disease is the major cause of late mortality.
- In normal postoperative orthotopic heart transplants, the cardiac silhouette can appear enlarged for the first several months, decreasing in size over time.
- If mediastinal widening persists beyond the first couple of weeks after surgery, steroid-induced fat deposition may be the cause, which can be confirmed on cross-sectional imaging studies such as CT or MR imaging.
- Myocardial T2 relaxation time from a black-blood MR imaging sequence has been shown to identify most moderate acute rejections

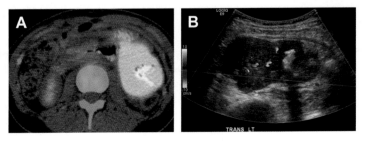

Fig. 25. PTLD. A 17-year-old girl after OHT at 1 year of age for dilated cardiomyopathy presented with chronic and progressive abdominal pain and bloody diarrhea. (*A*) FDG-PET/CT image shows marked left lower quadrant small bowel wall thickening with avid FDG uptake. (*B*) Ultrasonography shows a hypoechoic mass with mild internal color Doppler flow centered within the bowel wall corresponding with the lymphoproliferative infiltration of the jejunum. Note echogenic gas-filled bowel lumen. Pathology confirmed the diagnosis of PTLD.

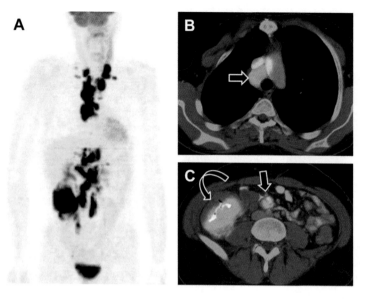

A

B

C

Fig. 26. PTLD. A 24-year-old man 11 years after OHT for dilated cardiomyopathy underwent FDG-PET/CT for evaluation of abdominal pain. Coronal MIP image (*A*) shows marked mediastinal FDG uptake, multiple foci of increased radiotracer uptake centrally within the abdomen, and a focal right lower quadrant focus of increased radiotracer uptake. Selected corresponding images in the chest (*B*) and abdomen (*C*) show that the multifocal uptake correlates with enlarged mediastinal and abdominal lymphadenopathy (*straight arrows*). Right lower quadrant radiotracer uptake corresponds with the markedly thickened cecal wall (*curved arrow*). Biopsy revealed EBV-positive PTLD.

documented with biopsy and is a strong predictor of the subsequent occurrence of biopsy-defined acute rejections.

- CMV infection may increase the risk of rejection, CAV, and PTLD.
- Cerebral ischemia and infarcts are common in the immediate postoperative period, particularly in patients who required mechanical assist devices before transplantation.

- Nephrotoxicity from calcineurin inhibitors in pediatric heart transplant recipients can cause renal dysfunction.

WHAT THE REFERRING PHYSICIAN NEEDS TO KNOW

- Are there any anatomic variations in the donor or recipient?
- Are there any anastomotic complications?
- Are there lung findings to suggest infection?
- Are there associated cerebral infarcts?
- Is there lymphadenopathy to suggest neoplasm?
- Is there increased echogenicity of the kidneys to suggest renal dysfunction?

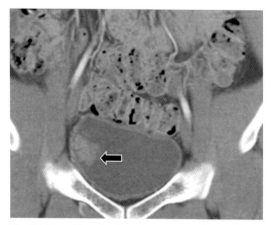

Fig. 27. Transitional cell carcinoma. A 21-year-old man who had 2 heart transplantations, the first performed for restrictive cardiomyopathy at 2 years of age. Contrast-enhanced coronal CT image obtained for evaluation of gross hematuria shows an enhancing irregular mass (*arrow*) along the right urinary bladder wall, which was found to be Polyomavirus hominis 1 (BK) virus positive high-grade invasive transitional cell carcinoma, likely related to the patient's long-standing immunosuppressive therapy.

REFERENCES

1. Benden C, Edwards LB, Kucheryavaya AY, et al. The registry of the International Society for Heart and Lung Transplantation: sixteenth official pediatric lung and heart-lung transplantation report–2013; focus theme: age. J Heart Lung Transplant 2013; 32(10):989–97.
2. Moreno Galdo A, Sole Montserrat J, Roman Broto A. Lung transplantation in children. Specific aspects. Arch Bronconeumol 2013;49(12):523–8.
3. Faro A, Mallory GB, Visner GA, et al. American Society of Transplantation executive summary on pediatric lung transplantation. Am J Transplant 2007;7(2): 285–92.
4. Huddleston CB, Bloch JB, Sweet SC, et al. Lung transplantation in children. Ann Surg 2002;236(3): 270–6.

5. Camargo PC, Pato EZ, Campos SV, et al. Pediatric lung transplantation: 10 years of experience. Clinics (Sao Paulo) 2014;69(Suppl 1):51–4.

6. Van Raemdonck D, Neyrinck A, Verleden GM, et al. Lung donor selection and management. Proc Am Thorac Soc 2009;6(1):28–38.

7. Frost AE. Donor criteria and evaluation. Clin Chest Med 1997;18(2):231–7.

8. Ferrer J, Roldan J, Roman A, et al. Acute and chronic pleural complications in lung transplantation. J Heart Lung Transplant 2003;22(11):1217–25.

9. Krishnam MS, Suh RD, Tomasian A, et al. Postoperative complications of lung transplantation: radiologic findings along a time continuum. Radiographics 2007;27(4):957–74.

10. Kshettry VR, Kroshus TJ, Hertz MI, et al. Early and late airway complications after lung transplantation: incidence and management. Ann Thorac Surg 1997;63(6):1576–83.

11. Collins J, Muller NL, Kazerooni EA, et al. CT findings of pneumonia after lung transplantation. AJR Am J Roentgenol 2000;175(3):811–8.

12. Chen L, Mulligan ME. Medication-induced periostitis in lung transplant patients: periostitis deformans revisited. Skeletal Radiol 2011;40(2):143–8.

13. Wang TF, Wang T, Altman R, et al. Periostitis secondary to prolonged voriconazole therapy in lung transplant recipients. Am J Transplant 2009;9(12):2845–50.

14. Zamora MR. Cytomegalovirus and lung transplantation. Am J Transplant 2004;4(8):1219–26.

15. Burns KE, Iacono AT. Pulmonary embolism on postmortem examination: an under-recognized complication in lung-transplant recipients? Transplantation 2004;77(5):692–8.

16. Ikonen T, Kivisaari L, Taskinen E, et al. High-resolution CT in long-term follow-up after lung transplantation. Chest 1997;111(2):370–6.

17. Morrish WF, Herman SJ, Weisbrod GL, et al. Bronchiolitis obliterans after lung transplantation: findings at chest radiography and high-resolution CT. The Toronto Lung Transplant Group. Radiology 1991;179(2):487–90.

18. Todd JL, Palmer SM. Bronchiolitis obliterans syndrome: the final frontier for lung transplantation. Chest 2011;140(2):502–8.

19. Konen E, Gutierrez C, Chaparro C, et al. Bronchiolitis obliterans syndrome in lung transplant recipients: can thin-section CT findings predict disease before its clinical appearance? Radiology 2004;231(2):467–73.

20. Siegel MJ, Bhalla S, Gutierrez FR, et al. Post-lung transplantation bronchiolitis obliterans syndrome: usefulness of expiratory thin-section CT for diagnosis. Radiology 2001;220(2):455–62.

21. Konen E, Weisbrod GL, Pakhale S, et al. Fibrosis of the upper lobes: a newly identified late-onset complication after lung transplantation? AJR Am J Roentgenol 2003;181(6):1539–43.

22. Pakhale SS, Hadjiliadis D, Howell DN, et al. Upper lobe fibrosis: a novel manifestation of chronic allograft dysfunction in lung transplantation. J Heart Lung Transplant 2005;24(9):1260–8.

23. Chaparro C, Chamberlain D, Maurer J, et al. Bronchiolitis obliterans organizing pneumonia (BOOP) in lung transplant recipients. Chest 1996;110(5):1150–4.

24. Scarsbrook AF, Warakaulle DR, Dattani M, et al. Post-transplantation lymphoproliferative disorder: the spectrum of imaging appearances. Clin Radiol 2005;60(1):47–55.

25. Rappaport DC, Chamberlain DW, Shepherd FA, et al. Lymphoproliferative disorders after lung transplantation: imaging features. Radiology 1998;206(2):519–24.

26. Wudhikarn K, Holman CJ, Linan M, et al. Post-transplant lymphoproliferative disorders in lung transplant recipients: 20-yr experience at the University of Minnesota. Clin Transplant 2011;25(5):705–13.

27. Paranjothi S, Yusen RD, Kraus MD, et al. Lymphoproliferative disease after lung transplantation: comparison of presentation and outcome of early and late cases. J Heart Lung Transplant 2001;20(10):1054–63.

28. Siegel MJ, Lee EY, Sweet SC, et al. CT of posttransplantation lymphoproliferative disorder in pediatric recipients of lung allograft. AJR Am J Roentgenol 2003;181(4):1125–31.

29. Dipchand AI, Kirk R, Edwards LB, et al. The Registry of the International Society for Heart and Lung Transplantation: sixteenth official pediatric heart transplantation report–2013; focus theme: age. J Heart Lung Transplant 2013;32(10):979–88.

30. Canter CE, Shaddy RE, Bernstein D, et al. Indications for heart transplantation in pediatric heart disease: a scientific statement from the American Heart Association Council on Cardiovascular Disease in the Young; the Councils on Clinical Cardiology, Cardiovascular Nursing, and Cardiovascular Surgery and Anesthesia; and the Quality of Care and Outcomes Research Interdisciplinary Working Group. Circulation 2007;115(5):658–76.

31. Lipshultz SE, Sleeper LA, Towbin JA, et al. The incidence of pediatric cardiomyopathy in two regions of the United States. N Engl J Med 2003;348(17):1647–55.

32. Aziz T, Burgess M, Khafagy R, et al. Bicaval and standard techniques in orthotopic heart transplantation: medium-term experience in cardiac performance and survival. J Thorac Cardiovasc Surg 1999;118(1):115–22.

33. Voeller RK, Epstein DJ, Guthrie TJ, et al. Trends in the indications and survival in pediatric heart

transplants: a 24-year single-center experience in 307 patients. Ann Thorac Surg 2012;94(3):807–15 [discussion: 81–6].

34. Dipchand AI, Kirk R, Mahle WT, et al. Ten yr of pediatric heart transplantation: a report from the Pediatric Heart Transplant Study. Pediatr Transplant 2013; 17(2):99–111.

35. Pahl E, Naftel DC, Kuhn MA, et al. The impact and outcome of transplant coronary artery disease in a pediatric population: a 9-year multi-institutional study. J Heart Lung Transplant 2005;24(6):645–51.

36. Krieghoff C, Barten MJ, Hildebrand L, et al. Assessment of sub-clinical acute cellular rejection after heart transplantation: comparison of cardiac magnetic resonance imaging and endomyocardial biopsy. Eur Radiol 2014;24(10):2360–71.

37. Guthaner DF, Schnittger I, Wright A, et al. Diagnostic challenges following cardiac transplantation. Radiol Clin North Am 1987;25(2):367–76.

38. Shirazi KK, Amendola MA, Tisnado J, et al. Radiographic findings in the chest of patients following cardiac transplantation. Cardiovasc Intervent Radiol 1983;6(1):1–6.

39. Florence SH, Hutton LC, McKenzie FN, et al. Cardiac transplantation: postoperative chest radiographs. Can Assoc Radiol J 1988;39(2):115–7.

40. Knisely BL, Mastey LA, Collins J, et al. Imaging of cardiac transplantation complications. Radiographics 1999;19(2):321–39 [discussion: 340–1].

41. Poston RS, Griffith BP. Heart transplantation. J Intensive Care Med 2004;19(1):3–12.

42. Andreone PA, Olivari MT, Ring WS. Clinical considerations of cardiac transplantation in organ transplantation: preoperative and postoperative evaluation. Radiol Clin North Am 1987;25(2): 357–66.

43. Marie PY, Angioi M, Carteaux JP, et al. Detection and prediction of acute heart transplant rejection with the myocardial T2 determination provided by a black-blood magnetic resonance imaging sequence. J Am Coll Cardiol 2001;37(3):825–31.

44. Kulikowska A, Boslaugh SE, Huddleston CB, et al. Infectious, malignant, and autoimmune complications in pediatric heart transplant recipients. J Pediatr 2008;152(5):671–7.

45. Schowengerdt KO, Naftel DC, Seib PM, et al. Infection after pediatric heart transplantation: results of a multiinstitutional study. The Pediatric Heart Transplant Study Group. J Heart Lung Transplant 1997; 16(12):1207–16.

46. Henry DA, Corcoran HL, Lewis TD, et al. Orthotopic cardiac transplantation: evaluation with CT. Radiology 1989;170(2):343–50.

47. Rubin RH. Prevention and treatment of cytomegalovirus disease in heart transplant patients. J Heart Lung Transplant 2000;19(8):731–5.

48. Zaoutis TE, Webber S, Naftel DC, et al. Invasive fungal infections in pediatric heart transplant recipients: incidence, risk factors, and outcomes. Pediatr Transplant 2011;15(5):465–9.

49. Kuhlman JE. Thoracic imaging in heart transplantation. J Thorac Imaging 2002;17(2):113–21.

50. Kobayashi D, Du W, L'Ecuyer TJ. Predictors of cardiac allograft vasculopathy in pediatric heart transplant recipients. Pediatr Transplant 2013;17(5): 436–40.

51. Chinnock R, Webber SA, Dipchand AI, et al, Pediatric Heart Transplant Study. A 16-year multiinstitutional study of the role of age and EBV status on PTLD incidence among pediatric heart transplant recipients. Am J Transplant 2012;12(11):3061–8.

52. Webber SA, Naftel DC, Fricker FJ, et al. Lymphoproliferative disorders after paediatric heart transplantation: a multi-institutional study. Lancet 2006; 367(9506):233–9.

53. Pennock JL, Oyer PE, Reitz BA, et al. Cardiac transplantation in perspective for the future. Survival, complications, rehabilitation, and cost. J Thorac Cardiovasc Surg 1982;83(2):168–77.

54. Chin C, Naftel D, Pahl E, et al. Cardiac retransplantation in pediatrics: a multi-institutional study. J Heart Lung Transplant 2006;25(12):1420–4.

Imaging in Lung Transplantation
Surgical Considerations of Donor and Recipient

Leah M. Backhus, MD, MPH[a],*, Michael S. Mulligan, MD[b],
Richard Ha, MD[a], Jabi E. Shriki, MD[c,d],
Tan-Lucien H. Mohammed, MD[e]

KEYWORDS

- Lung transplant • Transplant evaluation • Transplant surgery • Computed tomography

KEY POINTS

- Imaging is an essential part of the evaluation process for potential lung transplant donors and recipients.
- Extended lung donor criteria and emerging techniques in donor management have become more common as a means of increasing the donor pool.
- Radiologists must be knowledgeable in identifying anatomic abnormalities and medical conditions with implications for surgical techniques in transplantation.

INTRODUCTION

The first lung transplant was performed in 1963 by Hardy and coworkers.[1] Since then, lung transplantation has advanced to become an effective treatment for patients with end-stage lung disease. The medical and ethical complexities and resource use involved in organ transplantation require thorough clinical work-up to ensure maximal benefit for each transplant performed. Imaging plays a critical role in pretransplant assessment for lung transplant recipients and donors. In the recipient, imaging can identify clinical features that require modifications in surgical technique. In the donor, imaging is useful to identify conditions associated with poor clinical outcomes. This article describes the interpretation of radiologic studies in the assessment of lung transplant donors and recipients and implications for work-up and management.

DONOR EVALUATION

Despite the rise in number of lung transplants performed in the United States, availability of suitable donors is the main limitation for continued growth. The number of lungs transplanted per deceased donor has increased from 0.25 in 2000 to 0.39 in 2012, yet 75% of all lung offers are not accepted for transplantation.[2–5] Many potential donors are excluded from donation based on radiographic examinations. Twelve percent of potential lung donors are rejected for findings on chest radiograph alone (Table 1).[6] The most common imaging

Disclosures: The authors have no disclosures.
[a] Department of Cardiothoracic Surgery, Stanford University, Stanford, CA, USA; [b] Division of Cardiothoracic Surgery, Department of Surgery, University of Washington, Seattle, WA, USA; [c] Department of Radiology, University of Washington, Seattle, WA, USA; [d] Diagnostic Imaging Service, VA Puget Sound Health Care System, Seattle, WA, USA; [e] Department of Radiology, University of Florida College of Medicine, Gainesville, FL, USA
* Corresponding author. Department of Cardiothoracic Surgery, Stanford University, 300 Pasteur Drive, Falk Building, Stanford, CA 94304.
E-mail address: lbackhus@stanford.edu

Radiol Clin N Am 54 (2016) 339–353
http://dx.doi.org/10.1016/j.rcl.2015.09.013
0033-8389/16/$ – see front matter Published by Elsevier Inc.

Table 1 Reasons for declining potential lung donors	
Low Pao_2/Fio_2 ratio	11%
Abnormal chest radiograph	12%
Abnormal bronchoscopy	16%
Abnormal intraoperative examination	18%
Postharvest assessment	2%

Abbreviation: Fio_2, fraction of inspired oxygen.
From Alvarez A, Moreno P, Espinosa D, et al. Assessment of lungs for transplantation: a stepwise analysis of 476 donors. Eur J Cardiothorac Surg 2010;37(2):435.

findings for rejection are pulmonary consolidation or contusion (**Table 2**). It is estimated that many more organs might be suitable for transplant with a missed opportunity rate of 200 organs per year. Many of these missed opportunities represent donors who fail to meet strict donation. As such, extended donor criteria have been developed to liberalize selection without compromising clinical outcomes (**Table 3**).[2,7–9]

Donor Management

Protocols that address clinical conditions associated with worse outcomes following lung transplant show promise for increasing the organ donor pool. Lung management protocols in brain-dead donors using protective ventilation strategies, fluid restriction, and hormonal resuscitation have been shown to increase the rate of donor use.[10,11] Although not yet universal, new ventilation modes have also been developed with the goal of resuscitating marginal organs and have yielded lung retrieval rates four times higher than historic controls.[12] The newest, innovative tool for optimizing marginal donors for lung transplant is the ex vivo lung perfusion system. This

Table 2 Chest radiograph findings for rejected lung donors	
Normal	82%
Infiltrate/contusion	9%
Pleural effusion/ pneumothorax	4%
Extensive atelectasis	3%
Pulmonary edema	1%
Not available	1%

From Alvarez A, Moreno P, Espinosa D, et al. Assessment of lungs for transplantation: a stepwise analysis of 476 donors. Eur J Cardiothorac Surg 2010;37(2):434.

Table 3 Lung donor criteria	
Standard Donor Criteria	**Extended Donor Criteria**
Age >55 y	Age >55 y
Pao_2/Fio_2 (Fio_2, 1.0; PEEP, 5 cm H_2O) >300 mm Hg	Pao_2/Fio_2 (Fio_2, 1.0; PEEP, 5 cm H_2O) <300 mm Hg
Clear chest radiograph	Abnormalities on chest radiograph
Smoking history <20 pack-years	Smoking history >20 pack-years
Absence of aspiration	Aspiration
Absence of chest trauma	Chest trauma
Absence of overt lung infection	Donation after circulatory death
—	Ischemic time >6 h (single lung transplant)

Abbreviations: Fio_2, fraction of inspired oxygen; PEEP, positive end-expiratory pressure.

technique was originally developed to assess donors after circulatory death and has since been used in clinical trials to extend cold ischemic time and resuscitation of marginal donors. Results from the ex vivo system demonstrate safety, high rates of successful transplantation, and short-term recipient outcomes similar to recipients from conventional donors.[13–16]

Pulmonary Complications Following Brain Death

Brain-deceased donors comprise 99% of all lung transplant donors.[17] Brain death is associated with major systemic changes with direct impact on suitability for organ donation. The most common physiologic changes associated with brain death include need for vasopressor support (97%), coagulopathy (55%), thrombocytopenia (54%), diabetes insipidus (46%), cardiac ischemia (30%), lactic acidosis (25%), and renal failure (20%).[18] Neurogenic pulmonary edema is a common complication of significant central nervous system injury. Development of pulmonary edema after neurologic insult is abrupt, but the cause is incompletely understood. Blast injury, which results in a catecholamine-induced capillary leak, is one proposed mechanism for its development.[19,20] Pulmonary edema leads to poor gas exchange, resulting in low Pao_2/fraction of inspired oxygen ratios and reduced lung compliance. Aggressive diuresis, recruitment maneuvers, and resuscitation strategies favoring vasopressor support over volume expansion for hemodynamic stability leads to marked improvement in clinical and radiographic results (**Fig. 1**).

Pulmonary Complications Associated with Trauma

Historically, trauma patients have been deemed less desirable if not totally unacceptable for organ donation. This is primarily because of the morbidity of thoracic trauma in the setting of traumatic cardiopulmonary arrest.[21] Today, with aggressive donor management protocols, trauma patients routinely serve as organ donors.[22] Pneumothorax, hemothorax, and pulmonary contusion are commonly encountered in this setting. Pneumothorax may be a direct result of chest injury or a secondary result from chest trauma during cardiopulmonary resuscitation or ventilator-associated barotrauma. Pneumothorax or hemothorax do not preclude lung donation, provided that complete lung expansion and evacuation of the chest cavity has been achieved by tube thoracostomy. Associated lung contusion must be carefully evaluated to determine extent of parenchymal injury and potential impact on gas exchange. Severe pulmonary contusion with respiratory derangement or parenchymal hemorrhage is associated with poor transplant outcomes (**Fig. 2**).[3]

Other Donor Considerations

Atelectasis is frequently observed in lung transplant donors regardless of mechanism of death. Care must be taken to distinguish between dependent (gravitational) atelectasis and underlying pneumonia. Lung transplant donors are prone to aspiration that may have been present since the prehospital period or developed during hospitalization (**Fig. 3**).

Another frequent imaging finding in the setting of young donors is the presence of subpleural blebs. Young donors do not routinely receive a computed tomography (CT) scan during donor evaluation. However, subpleural blebs may be detected incidentally among young donors.[23] Subpleural blebs do not preclude organ donation, with the exception of an extended criteria donor of advanced age or smoking history, where blebs may indicate early chronic obstructive pulmonary disease (**Fig. 4**). Pulmonary nodules must also be fully characterized in a potential lung donor considering the risk of occult malignancy or endemic fungal infections. Although exceedingly rare, there are documented cases of lung cancer developing in the transplanted lung allograft. Donor-origin malignancies account for 8% of all posttransplant primary lung cancers.[24]

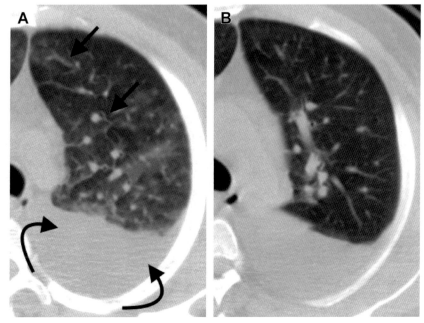

Fig. 1. A 44-year-old man with pulmonary edema. (*A*) Coned down axial computed tomography (CT) of left upper lung shows smooth interlobular septal thickening (*straight arrows*) and ground-glass. Moderate pleural effusion (*curved arrows*). (*B*) Following diuresis, edema resolved.

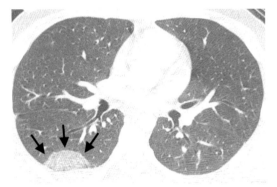

Fig. 2. A 39-year-old man with high-resolution axial CT demonstrating subpleural ground-glass attenuation in the superior segment of the right lower lobe representing pulmonary contusion (*arrows*).

RECIPIENT EVALUATION

Criteria for lung transplant vary based on the cause of underlying lung disease, yet there are common relative contraindications. Exclusion criteria often include age greater than 65 years, mechanical ventilation, extracorporeal membrane oxygenation, severely limited functional status, body mass index greater than 30, severe or symptomatic osteoporosis, or other systemic diseases with end-organ damage including cancer.[25] Although the use of extended donor criteria has been demonstrated as a safe means of increasing the lung donor pool, extended recipient criteria or the combination thereof has been less studied. For the most part, lung transplantation in critically ill recipients is associated with poor outcomes independent of donor selection criteria.[7]

Diaphragm

Chronic lung disease, thoracic surgical procedures, and other comorbid conditions are all risk factors for diaphragm dysfunction (**Fig. 5**). Unlike patients without underlying lung disease where unilateral diaphragm paralysis is well tolerated, diaphragm dysfunction can have a profound impact in the post–lung transplant setting. Diaphragm elevation is common in patients with restrictive lung disease, such as idiopathic pulmonary fibrosis (IPF); however, diaphragm paralysis with paradoxic motion should be confirmed with fluoroscopic examination (Sniff test). Diaphragm plication can be performed at the time of lung transplant to optimize postoperative recovery in the setting of known diaphragm paralysis.[26]

Interstitial Lung Disease

In 2012, there were 1783 lung transplants performed in the United States, of which 49% were for restrictive lung disease.[27] IPF is the most common subtype of interstitial pneumonia, and is characterized by radiographic and pathologic findings of usual interstitial pneumonia, in the absence of a specific causative etiology. When typical features are present, the radiologic diagnosis of a usual interstitial pneumonia–type pattern is highly predictive of pathologic findings. Radiologic features of usual interstitial pneumonia include bibasilar predominant honeycombing, traction bronchiectasis/bronchiolectasis, subpleural reticulation, architectural distortion, and lobar volume loss, with mild or no ground-glass opacities (**Fig. 6**). Mild adenopathy may be present.[28] The degree of fibrosis using a radiographic score is

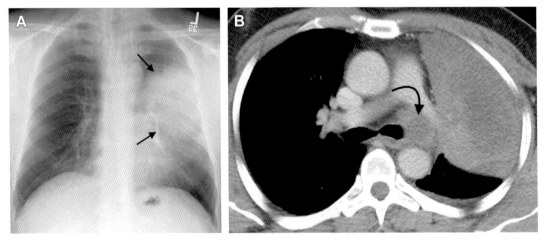

Fig. 3. A 34-year-old man with lobar atelectasis. (*A*) Frontal chest radiograph with round masslike consolidation occupying the left upper chest (*arrows*). (*B*) Axial chest CT reveals complete left upper lobe collapse secondary to hilar obstruction. Note anteroposterior window adenopathy (*curved arrow*).

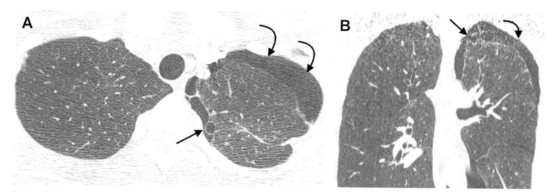

Fig. 4. A 27-year-old woman with moderate left-sided pneumothorax. (*A*) Axial and (*B*) coronal CT demonstrating subpleural blebs (*straight arrow*). *Curved arrows* indicate pneumothorax.

used to correlate with disease severity and thereby predict survival or need for transplantation.[29] Although not validated, radiologic grading of fibrosis offers promise toward improvement in organ allocation based on clinical need.

Sarcoidosis represents a minority of patients undergoing lung transplantation; however, 90% of sarcoid patients have pulmonary involvement, often manifesting as bilateral hilar lymphadenopathy.[30] Lymph node stations most commonly affected are station 7 (subcarinal) (98.6%), right hilar (97.3%), left hilar (86.5%), and right paratracheal (79.7%) (**Fig. 7**).[31] Hilar and mediastinal lymphadenopathy are also commonly encountered in patients with suppurative lung disease and chronic obstructive pulmonary disease. Bulky lymphadenopathy presents several problems for lung transplantation. In recipients, it can complicate hilar dissection, prolong operative time, and increase the risk for chylothorax or hemothorax. In the pretransplant work-up, lymphadenopathy may require further evaluation to rule out occult malignancy delaying transplant listing. PET scan performed to follow-up on suspicious lymph nodes to rule out malignancy is of limited value because granulomatous lymph nodes are usually fluorodeoxyglucose avid (**Fig. 8**).[30]

Nodules

The incidence of pulmonary nodules in interstitial lung disease is 26%, with nodules usually occurring in the lower lobes (**Fig. 9**).[32] Most nodules detected during a pretransplant evaluation are benign; however, patients with interstitial lung disease carry an increased risk of malignancy, with a lifetime incidence of 20% to 30%.[28,33–36] The overall incidence of posttransplant lung cancer ranges from 2.0% to 5.2% with nearly all cases occurring in the native lung identified at the time of explant or in the nontransplanted lung following single lung transplant.[24,35–39] Increased risk of bronchogenic carcinoma in the native lung is likely a result of the cumulative effects of underlying lung disease, prior smoking, and additional risk of posttransplant immunosuppression.

In contrast to lung nodules detected incidentally or through routine lung cancer screening, strict adherence to Fleischner Society Guidelines for timing of follow-up may miss a cancer diagnosis

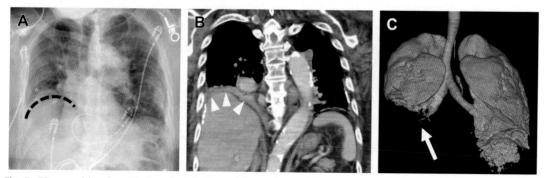

Fig. 5. 72 year-old male with chronic right lower lobe and right basilar atelectasis. The chest radiograph (*A*) shows low lung volumes with asymmetric elevation of the right hemidiaphragm (*dashed black line*). A coronal reformatted CT (*B*) shows dense right basilar atelectasis (*white arrowheads*) as the cause. A volumetric, reformatted CT (*C*) shows decreased volume of the right lung, with abruptly terminating right lower lobe bronchi (*white arrow*).

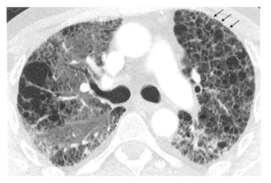

Fig. 6. A 61-year-old woman with rheumatoid arthritis with axial CT image demonstrating extensive honeycombing (*arrows*) from usual interstitial pneumonia.

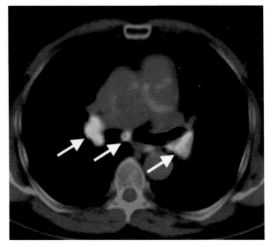

Fig. 8. A 42-year-old man with sarcoidosis. PET/CT shows fluorodeoxyglucose (FDG) avidity in subcarina and bilateral hila (*arrows*).

in the time between pretransplant evaluation and transplantation.[40,41] Standard imaging protocols may be impractical given unpredictable transplant wait list times and the abrupt identification of lung donors. Because posttransplant lung cancer carries a poor prognosis, screening for lung nodules in the pretransplant work-up is critical. One-year posttransplant survival is 43% for those who develop posttransplant lung cancer compared with 86% for non–lung cancer transplant recipients.[24,42] Because of this, bilateral lung transplant is often favored in the setting of a patient with indeterminate lung nodules.[43]

Pleural Space

Often patients with end-stage lung disease have undergone prior therapeutic or diagnostic procedures within the chest. Among patients with cystic

fibrosis (CF), the incidence of prior thoracic surgical procedures is estimated at 12.8%. Most of these consist of pleural procedures.[44] Common prior procedures include median sternotomy for cardiac surgery, pleurodesis, and prior lung resection/lung biopsy. In one of the largest series published on lung transplant following prior cardiothoracic surgery, patients with prior surgery experienced higher rates of re-exploration for bleeding, phrenic nerve injury, prolonged ventilation, renal insufficiency, and intensive care unit length of stay, but without a significant difference in posttransplant survival. Most adverse outcomes were associated with prior noncardiac thoracic or pleural procedures.[45]

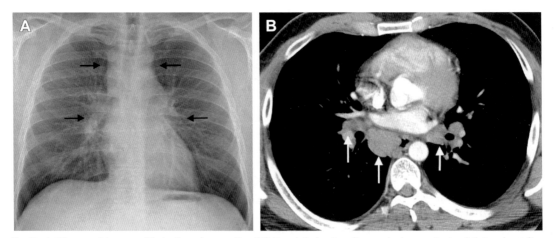

Fig. 7. A 29-year-old man with bulky adenopathy. (*A*) Frontal chest radiograph demonstrates bilateral mediastinal and hilar prominence (*arrows*). (*B*) CT reveals subcarinal and bilateral hilar adenopathy (*arrows*).

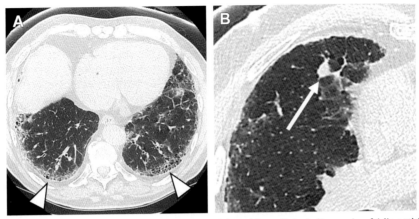

Fig. 9. 62 year-old male with usual interstitial pneumonitis, with a clinical diagnosis of idiopathic pulmonary fibrosis. A high-resolution, transverse image through the chest (*A*) shows typical, peripheral, basilar predominant fibrotic changes with honeycombing (*white arrowheads*). There is also a right middle lobe nodule (*white arrow, B*), which was resected and shown to be bronchogenic carcinoma.

Lung biopsy is still often performed to facilitate diagnosis in interstitial lung disease. It is most often performed via minimally invasive video-assisted thoracoscopic surgery with a stapled wedge resection of each lobe in a single hemithorax. Postoperative adhesions are often benign with minimal impact on technique at the time of transplant. By contrast formal lung volume reduction surgery is performed bilaterally and may involve the use of staple line reinforcement materials, which are associated with intense inflammatory reaction. Lung transplant is done safely in this setting, but is associated with more extensive pleural adhesiolysis, longer operative time, greater need for cardiopulmonary bypass, and increased transfusion requirements.[46,47]

Many lung transplant candidates have had prior tube thoracostomy or pleurodesis procedures for recurrent pneumothoraces. The incidence of pneumothorax among patients with lymphangioleiomyomatosis is 56%.[48] Similarly, 74% of pneumothoraces in patients with CF require pleural intervention.[49] The incidence of re-exploration for hemothorax is 14% to 18% among patients undergoing lung transplant following prior pleurodesis procedure.[45,48] Assessment by CT can help determine the extent of pleural adhesions or pleural symphysis to anticipate technical challenges and provide appropriate preoperative counseling (**Fig. 10**). The accuracy of CT in predicting moderate to severe pleural adhesions following pleurodesis is estimated at 89% sensitivity and 95% specificity.[45]

Preoperative imaging can also be useful for surgical planning in the setting of prior sternotomy. CT can measure the retrosternal distance to coronary

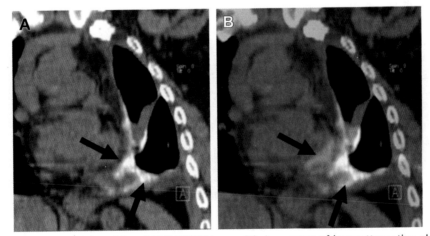

Fig. 10. Coronal CT image (*A*) and fused FDG PET/CT image (*B*) show areas of hyperattenuation along the left pleural surfaces with corresponding increased FDG uptake (*arrows*), in a patient who had previously undergone talc pleurodesis.

grafts or the right ventricle to assess risk for re-entry and need for alternate cardiopulmonary bypass cannulation strategies.

Cystic Fibrosis and Bronchiectasis

Treatment of CF has improved to the point that patients are medically managed into adulthood before need for transplant. Transplant referral is warranted in patients with less than 50% 2-year predicted survival or with severe functional limitations. By this point, most patients with CF are colonized by multidrug-resistant organisms creating a significant challenge to care in the posttransplant period. All patients with chronic bronchiectasis and CF require aggressive perioperative antibiotic regimens with synergy testing to target their pretransplant microbiology.[50] Chronic infection has several consequences that should be taken into account when considering transplant. Chronic inflammation in CF creates dense pleural adhesions requiring tedious dissection during explant. The hilar structures may be contracted and bulky lymphadenopathy may be present, complicating the surgical approach and contributing to difficulty of dissection. This results in increased operative time, need for cardiopulmonary bypass, and risk of postoperative bleeding.

Although treatment of bronchiectasis is largely nonsurgical, cases with focal involvement may undergo surgical resection with implications for subsequent transplant. A rare consequence of this is contraction of the hemithorax ipsilateral to the site of lung resection. Over time, this may result in a marked asymmetry of the hemithorax (**Fig. 11**). Although normally a single lung transplant contralateral to the affected side might circumvent this technical challenge, in the case of bronchiectasis, double lung transplant is routinely performed because of potential contamination of the lung allograft from the colonized native lung. To avoid this potential complication, some have performed single lung transplant on the least affected side and pneumonectomy ipsilateral to the contracted hemithorax. However, this practice carries an increased risk of postpneumonectomy empyema, which is poorly tolerated in the posttransplant setting.[51]

Pulmonary Hypertension

Worldwide, only 2% of all lung transplants are performed for idiopathic pulmonary hypertension; however, many patients undergoing lung transplant have secondary pulmonary hypertension.[52] Pulmonary hypertension is defined as mean pulmonary arterial pressure greater than 25 mm Hg, pulmonary capillary wedge pressure less than 15 mm Hg, and pulmonary vascular resistance greater than or equal to three Woods units. Elevated arterial pressures occur in 5% to 74% of patients with sarcoidosis and 30% to 40% of patients with IPF, and in both diagnoses pulmonary hypertension significantly increases mortality.[28,30,52–54] Because pulmonary hypertension is associated with poor lung transplant outcomes, right heart catheterization is routinely performed as part of the pretransplant work-up. Pulmonary hypertension with right ventricular hypertrophy increases the risk of early postoperative pulmonary edema and primary graft dysfunction. The risk is higher in the setting of single lung transplant compared with double lung transplant.[52] Pulmonary hypertension also requires modifications to the anesthetic plan, consideration of cardiopulmonary bypass, and decision regarding single versus double lung transplant to ensure a safe clinical course.

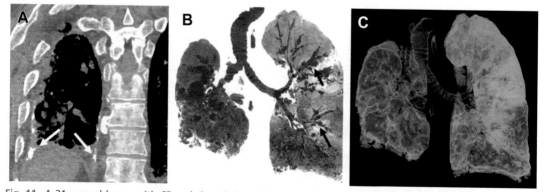

Fig. 11. A 31-year-old man with CF and chronic bronchiectasis who underwent previous pleurodesis. (*A*) Pleural calcifications are noted in the right hemithorax, related to prior pleurodesis (*arrows*). (*B*) Coronal, minimum intensity projection view demonstrates severe bronchiectasis (*arrows*). (*C*) Volumetric reformatting shows severe, asymmetric volume loss on the right with elevation of the hemidiaphragm.

In lieu of repeated invasive and costly testing with right heart catheterization, imaging is a useful adjunct to predict and monitor severity of pulmonary hypertension and right ventricular dysfunction.[55] Chest CT can demonstrate an enlarged pulmonary artery, right atrium, and right ventricle (**Fig. 12**). Although pulmonary hypertension can occur in several fibrotic lung diseases, the degree of fibrosis demonstrated on imaging does not correlate with the degree of pulmonary hypertension.[54]

Anatomic Anomalies

Vascular anatomic variations in either donor or recipient can have significant implications on surgical technique during lung transplantation. Partial anomalous pulmonary venous return is a rare congenital condition in which a portion of the pulmonary venous drainage drains into a systemic vein rather than the left atrium (**Fig. 13**). The discrepancy between donor and recipient anatomy complicates the surgical plan. Lung transplant is normally performed with a single venous anastomosis creating a common venous cuff from superior and inferior pulmonary veins. In the case of a recipient with partial anomalous pulmonary venous return, the donor left atrium contains a single pulmonary vein, requiring reconstruction of the left atrium to accommodate the larger donor venous cuff. Preoperative diagnosis is critical to facilitate safe dissection and explantation. More commonly, accessory pulmonary veins may be encountered in the donor lung draining all or a portion of the upper lobes. Accessory pulmonary veins require modifications in anastomotic technique and can be a source of hemorrhage at the time of transplant if not previously recognized.[56]

The presence of dextrocardia has significant implications for vascular and airway anastomoses. Although uncommon, dextrocardia is associated with lung transplant in the setting of immotile cilia (Kartagener) syndrome with end-stage lung disease (**Fig. 14**). When the recipient has dextrocardia, the lung donor procedure must be modified to maximize the length of donor vascular cuffs used for pulmonary venous and arterial anastomoses. Bronchial anastomoses also present technical challenges. The angulation and length of the recipient bronchi are reversed in dextrocardia, requiring careful technique to avoid posttransplant stenosis or dehiscence.[57]

Vascular anomalies involving the pulmonary arterial tree are uncommon. However, variant pulmonary arterial segmental anatomy is a consideration in living donor lobar transplantation. Living donor lobar transplants are most commonly performed for pediatric lung transplant recipients. In this procedure, two separate donors provide right and left lower lobes for bilateral transplantation in a pediatric recipient. CT angiography has proved useful in visualizing donor pulmonary arterial anatomy to optimize donor selection and planning of vascular anastomoses (**Fig. 15**). The most common surgical modification is sacrifice of the lingular artery or the right middle lobe segmental artery in the donor to provide sufficient arterial length for anastomosis during implantation.[58]

Anatomic variation in bronchial anatomy is rare with an overall incidence of 0.5%. The most common anomaly is a porcine or tracheal bronchus whereby the right upper lobe bronchus arises directly from the trachea at or above the level of the left main stem bronchus (**Fig. 16**). The tracheal bronchus may supply the right upper lobe in its entirety or a lobar segment. A tracheal bronchus in a

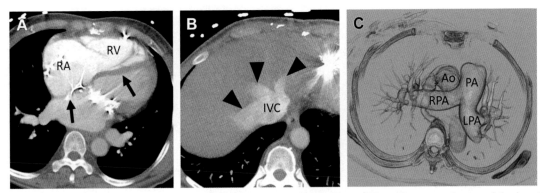

Fig. 12. A 66-year-old man with pulmonary hypertension and right heart failure. Transverse image of the heart (*A*) shows bowing of the interatrial and interventricular septa (*arrows*) toward the left ventricle. (*B*) Enlargement of the inferior vena cava (IVC) with reflux of contrast into enlarged hepatic veins (*arrowheads*). (*C*) Volumetric reconstruction shows enlargement of the main pulmonary artery (PA) and right and left branches, relative to the aorta (Ao). LPA, left pulmonary artery; RA, right atrium; RPA, right pulmonary artery; RV, right ventricle.

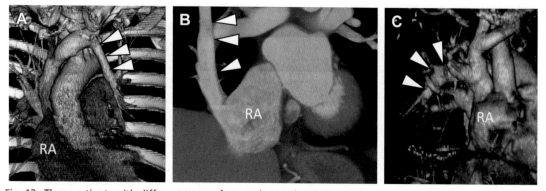

Fig. 13. Three patients with different types of anomalous pulmonary venous return (*arrowheads*). (*A*) A 67-year-old man with left upper lobe vein coursing cranially along the left mediastinum, before joining the brachiocephalic vein. (*B*) A 51-year-old man with a right-sided, scimitar-type anomalous pulmonary venous return, coursing through the lung inferiorly before joining the right atrium. (*C*) A 61-year-old woman with right upper lobe pulmonary venous return joining the superior vena cava. RA, right atrium.

lung transplant recipient has minimal implication. Pneumonectomy can be performed with transection of bronchus intermedius and of the porcine bronchus followed by anastomosis between donor mainstem bronchus and recipient bronchus intermedius.

Tracheomegaly or bronchomegaly represent a rare technical challenge for lung transplantation. Extreme size discrepancy between donor and recipient bronchi must be handled with meticulous surgical anastomotic technique. Suboptimal anastomoses result in poor secretion clearance, repeated infection, and anastomotic dehiscence or stenosis. Extreme tracheal enlargement can also present with mediastinal shift, which requires additional length on the contralateral donor bronchus to accommodate a greater

distance. Anticipation of this possibility is critical for the lung procurement surgery and implantation.

SIZE MATCHING

Matching a given donor to a recipient considers geography and blood type. Thoracic cavity size is also an important component. Acutely, oversized grafts experience compressive atelectasis with impaired ventilation. Chronically, size discrepancy is associated with reduced allograft and patient survival.[59] In general, size differences of 15% to 30% are considered acceptable. There are several methods used for size matching. Most rely on characteristics including body morphometrics, underlying lung diagnosis, and gender.

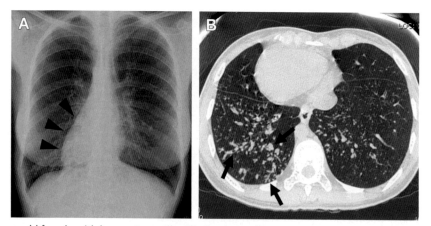

Fig. 14. 32 year old female with known Immotile Cilia Syndrome (Kartagener). Note the fact that there is dextrocardia (*arrowheads*) on the frontal view (*A*). The CT shows areas of basilar right lower lobe (morphologic left lower lobe) predominant bronchial wall thickening and tree-in-bud opacification (*black arrows*).

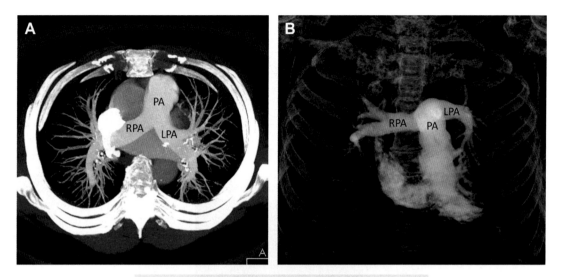

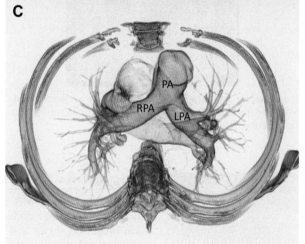

Fig. 15. (*A*) CT with transverse maximum intensity projection demonstrating normal pulmonary arterial anatomy. (*B*) Coronal volume projection. (*C*) Colored-lit projection. LPA, left pulmonary artery; PA, main pulmonary artery; RPA, right pulmonary artery.

Gender mismatch is associated with worse lung transplant outcomes, but it is unclear if this effect is mediated primarily by size mismatch rather than gender itself.[60,61] Size discrepancy in lobar lung transplantation has not been associated with increased complications.[62]

Bedside Morphometrics

Chest wall circumference is one technique used for size matching. It is measured at bedside at the level of the inframammary crease. Optimal donor to recipient circumference ratio is 0.89, which predicts posttransplant forced expiratory volume at 1 second at 3 months posttransplant.[63,64] Sternomanubrial length has also been an accepted means of size matching. The major weaknesses of body morphometric techniques

are that they can be cumbersome to perform in a critically ill patient, may produce inconsistent values, and fail to account for extremes in body habitus or thoracic asymmetry.

Predicted Total Lung Capacity

Height has been the traditional basis for size matching. Increasing donor to recipient height ratio has been associated with reduced risk of death.[65] Matching based on predicted total lung capacity (pTLC) expands on this concept and calculates the predicted value using a mathematical model that incorporates height, sex, and age. The pTLC ratio is defined as pTLC(donor)/pTLC (recipient). A higher ratio is suggestive of an oversized allograft and is associated with improved survival and reduced rates of rejection.[61,66]

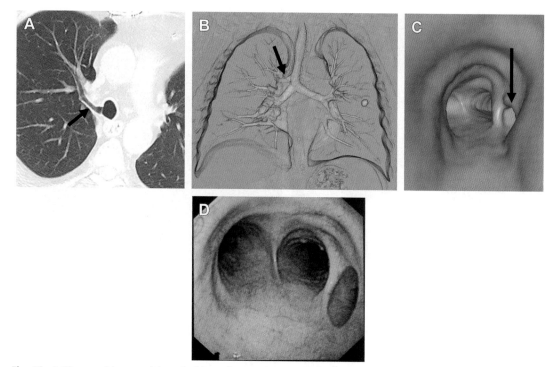

Fig. 16. A 68-year-old man with an incidentally noted tracheal bronchus (*arrow*). (*A*) CT shows right upper lobe bronchus arising directly from the trachea. (*B*) Three-dimensional volume reconstruction of the airways. (*C*) Virtual bronchoscopic CT reconstruction. (*D*) Actual bronchoscopic view.

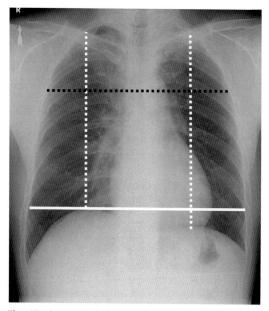

Fig. 17. Annotated chest radiograph in a normal patient demonstrating measurements for lung donor size matching. Coronal chest width measured at the level of the higher hemidiaphragm (*white solid line*) and aortic knob (*black dashed line*). Cranial-caudal dimensions measured at each diaphragm dome to chest apex (*white dashed lines*).

Imaging-Based Size Matching

Imaging can be a reliable and reproducible means of determining size matching. In addition to matching based on donor and recipient height, radiographic chest measurements are performed at four set points on chest radiograph: dome of right and left hemidiaphragm to apex of the chest, width at the level of the aortic knob, and width at the level of the higher hemidiaphragm (**Fig. 17**). Potential donors and recipients are matched within 10% of one another on each parameter. The ideal criteria for size matching are yet to be determined and these methods are imperfect when used in isolation.

SUMMARY

Careful interpretation of imaging studies is critical for evaluating donor and recipient in lung transplantation. The radiologist must be facile in interpreting imaging findings to identify clinical conditions associated with poor outcomes or modifications in surgical technique. Communication between the radiologist and the medical and surgical teams can have significant impact on long-term outcomes.

REFERENCES

1. Hardy JD, Webb WR, Dalton ML Jr, et al. Lung homotransplantation in man. JAMA 1963;186:1065–74.
2. Somers J, Ruttens D, Verleden SE, et al. A decade of extended-criteria lung donors in a single center: was it justified? Transpl Int 2015;28(2):170–9.
3. Van Raemdonck D, Neyrinck A, Verleden GM, et al. Lung donor selection and management. Proc Am Thorac Soc 2009;6(1):28–38.
4. Speicher PJ, Ganapathi AM, Englum BR, et al. Single-lung transplantation in the United States: what happens to the other lung? J Heart Lung Transplant 2015;34(1):36–42.
5. Hornby K, Ross H, Keshavjee S, et al. Non-utilization of hearts and lungs after consent for donation: a Canadian multicentre study. Can J Anaesth 2006;53(8):831–7.
6. Alvarez A, Moreno P, Espinosa D, et al. Assessment of lungs for transplantation: a stepwise analysis of 476 donors. Eur J Cardiothorac Surg 2010;37(2):432–9.
7. Moreno P, Alvarez A, Santos F, et al. Extended recipients but not extended donors are associated with poor outcomes following lung transplantation. Eur J Cardiothorac Surg 2014;45(6):1040–7.
8. Whitson BA, Hertz MI, Kelly RF, et al. Use of the donor lung after asphyxiation or drowning: effect on lung transplant recipients. Ann Thorac Surg 2014;98(4):1145–51.
9. Kawut SM, Reyentovich A, Wilt JS, et al. Outcomes of extended donor lung recipients after lung transplantation. Transplantation 2005;79(3):310–6.
10. Minambres E, Coll E, Duerto J, et al. Effect of an intensive lung donor-management protocol on lung transplantation outcomes. J Heart Lung Transplant 2014;33(2):178–84.
11. Mascia L, Pasero D, Slutsky AS, et al. Effect of a lung protective strategy for organ donors on eligibility and availability of lungs for transplantation: a randomized controlled trial. JAMA 2010;304(23):2620–7.
12. Hanna K, Seder CW, Weinberger JB, et al. Airway pressure release ventilation and successful lung donation. Arch Surg 2011;146(3):325–8.
13. Bennett DT, Reece TB, Smith PD, et al. Ex vivo lung perfusion allows successful transplantation of donor lungs from hanging victims. Ann Thorac Surg 2014;98(3):1051–6.
14. Boffini M, Ricci D, Barbero C, et al. Ex vivo lung perfusion increases the pool of lung grafts: analysis of its potential and real impact on a lung transplant program. Transplant Proc 2013;45(7):2624–6.
15. Cypel M, Yeung JC, Liu M, et al. Normothermic ex vivo lung perfusion in clinical lung transplantation. N Engl J Med 2011;364(15):1431–40.
16. Valenza F, Rosso L, Gatti S, et al. Extracorporeal lung perfusion and ventilation to improve donor lung function and increase the number of organs available for transplantation. Transplant Proc 2012;44(7):1826–9.
17. Israni AK, Zaun D, Rosendale JD, et al. OPTN/SRTR 2012 Annual Data Report: deceased organ donation. Am J Transplant 2014;14(Suppl 1):167–83.
18. Salim A, Martin M, Brown C, et al. Complications of brain death: frequency and impact on organ retrieval. Am Surg 2006;72(5):377–81.
19. Avlonitis VS, Fisher AJ, Kirby JA, et al. Pulmonary transplantation: the role of brain death in donor lung injury. Transplantation 2003;75(12):1928–33.
20. Mascia L, Mastromauro I, Viberti S, et al. Management to optimize organ procurement in brain dead donors. Minerva Anestesiol 2009;75(3):125–33.
21. Raoof M, Joseph BA, Friese RS, et al. Organ donation after traumatic cardiopulmonary arrest. Am J Surg 2011;202(6):701–5 [discussion: 705–6].
22. Straznicka M, Follette DM, Eisner MD, et al. Aggressive management of lung donors classified as unacceptable: excellent recipient survival one year after transplantation. J Thorac Cardiovasc Surg 2002;124(2):250–8.
23. Guimaraes CV, Donnelly LF, Warner BW. CT findings for blebs and bullae in children with spontaneous pneumothorax and comparison with findings in normal age-matched controls. Pediatr Radiol 2007;37(9):879–84.
24. Belli EV, Landolfo K, Keller C, et al. Lung cancer following lung transplant: single institution 10 year experience. Lung Cancer 2013;81(3):451–4.
25. Weill D, Benden C, Corris PA, et al. A consensus document for the selection of lung transplant candidates: 2014–an update from the Pulmonary Transplantation Council of the International Society for Heart and Lung Transplantation. J Heart Lung Transplant 2015;34(1):1–15.
26. Shihata M, Mullen JC. Bilateral diaphragmatic plication in the setting of bilateral sequential lung transplantation. Ann Thorac Surg 2007;83(3):1201–3.
27. Raghu G, Collard HR, Egan JJ, et al. An official ATS/ERS/JRS/ALAT statement: idiopathic pulmonary fibrosis: evidence-based guidelines for diagnosis and management. Am J Respir Crit Care Med 2011;183(6):788–824.
28. Ryu JH, Moua T, Daniels CE, et al. Idiopathic pulmonary fibrosis: evolving concepts. Mayo Clin Proc 2014;89(8):1130–42.
29. Mooney JJ, Elicker BM, Urbania TH, et al. Radiographic fibrosis score predicts survival in hypersensitivity pneumonitis. Chest 2013;144(2):586–92.
30. Baughman RP, Culver DA, Judson MA. A concise review of pulmonary sarcoidosis. Am J Respir Crit Care Med 2011;183(5):573–81.
31. Trisolini R, Anevlavis S, Tinelli C, et al. CT pattern of lymphadenopathy in untreated patients undergoing

bronchoscopy for suspected sarcoidosis. Respir Med 2013;107(6):897–903.

32. Koo HJ, Chae EJ, Kim JE, et al. Presence of macronodules in thoracic sarcoidosis: prevalence and computed tomographic findings. Clin Radiol 2015; 70(8):815–21.

33. Bonifazi M, Bravi F, Gasparini S, et al. Sarcoidosis and cancer risk: systematic review and meta-analysis of observational studies. Chest 2015; 147(3):778–91.

34. de Perrot M, Chernenko S, Waddell TK, et al. Role of lung transplantation in the treatment of bronchogenic carcinomas for patients with end-stage pulmonary disease. J Clin Oncol 2004;22(21):4351–6.

35. Strollo DC, Dacic S, Ocak I, et al. Malignancies incidentally detected at lung transplantation: radiologic and pathologic features. AJR Am J Roentgenol 2013;201(1):108–16.

36. Minai OA, Shah S, Mazzone P, et al. Bronchogenic carcinoma after lung transplantation: characteristics and outcomes. J Thorac Oncol 2008;3(12):1404–9.

37. Raviv Y, Shitrit D, Amital A, et al. Lung cancer in lung transplant recipients: experience of a tertiary hospital and literature review. Lung Cancer 2011;74(2): 280–3.

38. Abrahams NA, Meziane M, Ramalingam P, et al. Incidence of primary neoplasms in explanted lungs: long-term follow-up from 214 lung transplant patients. Transplant Proc 2004;36(9):2808–11.

39. Olland AB, Falcoz PE, Santelmo N, et al. Primary lung cancer in lung transplant recipients. Ann Thorac Surg 2014;98(1):362–71.

40. MacMahon H, Austin JH, Gamsu G, et al. Guidelines for management of small pulmonary nodules detected on CT scans: a statement from the Fleischner Society. Radiology 2005;237(2):395–400.

41. Naidich DP, Bankier AA, MacMahon H, et al. Recommendations for the management of subsolid pulmonary nodules detected at CT: a statement from the Fleischner Society. Radiology 2013; 266(1):304–17.

42. Espinosa D, Baamonde C, Illana J, et al. Lung cancer in patients with lung transplants. Transplant Proc 2012;44(7):2118–9.

43. Schaffer JM, Singh SK, Reitz BA, et al. Single- vs double-lung transplantation in patients with chronic obstructive pulmonary disease and idiopathic pulmonary fibrosis since the implementation of lung allocation based on medical need. JAMA 2015; 313(9):936–48.

44. Rolla M, Anile M, Venuta F, et al. Lung transplantation for cystic fibrosis after thoracic surgical procedures. Transplant Proc 2011;43(4):1162–3.

45. Shigemura N, Bhama J, Gries CJ, et al. Lung transplantation in patients with prior cardiothoracic surgical procedures. Am J Transplant 2012;12(5): 1249–55.

46. Shigemura N, Gilbert S, Bhama JK, et al. Lung transplantation after lung volume reduction surgery. Transplantation 2013;96(4):421–5.

47. Backhus L, Sargent J, Cheng A, et al. Outcomes in lung transplantation after previous lung volume reduction surgery in a contemporary cohort. J Thorac Cardiovasc Surg 2014;147(5):1678–83.e1.

48. Almoosa KF, Ryu JH, Mendez J, et al. Management of pneumothorax in lymphangioleiomyomatosis: effects on recurrence and lung transplantation complications. Chest 2006;129(5):1274–81.

49. Curtis HJ, Bourke SJ, Dark JH, et al. Lung transplantation outcome in cystic fibrosis patients with previous pneumothorax. J Heart Lung Transplant 2005; 24(7):865–9.

50. Corris PA. Lung transplantation for cystic fibrosis and bronchiectasis. Semin Respir Crit Care Med 2013;34(3):297–304.

51. Jougon J, Dromer C, Mac Bride T, et al. Synchronous left lung transplantation and right pneumonectomy for end-stage bronchiectasis through clamshell approach. Specific problems. Eur J Cardiothorac Surg 2002;22(5):833–5.

52. Gottlieb J. Lung transplantation for interstitial lung diseases and pulmonary hypertension. Semin Respir Crit Care Med 2013;34(3):281–7.

53. Shino MY, Lynch Iii JP, Fishbein MC, et al. Sarcoidosis-associated pulmonary hypertension and lung transplantation for sarcoidosis. Semin Respir Crit Care Med 2014;35(3):362–71.

54. Handa T, Nagai S, Miki S, et al. Incidence of pulmonary hypertension and its clinical relevance in patients with sarcoidosis. Chest 2006;129(5): 1246–52.

55. Huang YS, Hsu HH, Chen JY, et al. Quantitative computed tomography of pulmonary emphysema and ventricular function in chronic obstructive pulmonary disease patients with pulmonary hypertension. Korean J Radiol 2014;15(6):871–7.

56. Khasati NH, MacHaal A, Thekkudan J, et al. An aberrant donor pulmonary vein during lung transplant: a surgical challenge. Ann Thorac Surg 2005; 79(1):330–1.

57. Macchiarini P, Chapelier A, Vouhe P, et al. Double lung transplantation in situs inversus with Kartagener's syndrome. Paris-Sud University Lung Transplant Group. J Thorac Cardiovasc Surg 1994; 108(1):86–91.

58. Duong PA, Ferson PF, Fuhrman CR, et al. 3D-multidetector CT angiography in the evaluation of potential donors for living donor lung transplantation. J Thorac Imaging 2005;20(1):17–23.

59. Frost AE. Donor criteria and evaluation. Clin Chest Med 1997;18(2):231–7.

60. Sato M, Gutierrez C, Kaneda H, et al. The effect of gender combinations on outcome in human lung transplantation: the International Society of Heart

and Lung Transplantation Registry experience. J Heart Lung Transplant 2006;25(6):634–7.

61. Eberlein M, Reed RM, Bolukbas S, et al. Lung size mismatch and survival after single and bilateral lung transplantation. Ann Thorac Surg 2013;96(2): 457–63.

62. Backhus LM, Sievers EM, Schenkel FA, et al. Pleural space problems after living lobar transplantation. J Heart Lung Transplant 2005;24(12):2086–90.

63. Massard G, Badier M, Guillot C, et al. Lung size matching for double lung transplantation based on the submammary thoracic perimeter. Accuracy and functional results. The Joint Marseille-Montreal Lung Transplant Program. J Thorac Cardiovasc Surg 1993;105(1):9–14.

64. Park SJ, Houck J, Pifarre R, et al. Optimal size matching in single lung transplantation. J Heart Lung Transplant 1995;14(4):671–5.

65. Christie JD, Edwards LB, Kucheryavaya AY, et al. The Registry of the International Society for Heart and Lung Transplantation: twenty-eighth Adult Lung and Heart-Lung Transplant Report–2011. J Heart Lung Transplant 2011;30(10):1104–22.

66. Eberlein M, Arnaoutakis GJ, Yarmus L, et al. The effect of lung size mismatch on complications and resource utilization after bilateral lung transplantation. J Heart Lung Transplant 2012;31(5):492–500.

Imaging the Complications of Lung Transplantation

Clinton Jokerst, MD[a],*, Arlene Sirajuddin, MD[b],
Tan-Lucien H. Mohammed, MD[c]

KEYWORDS

- Lung transplant • Computed tomography • Anastomotic complications • Pleural complications
- Rejection • Infection

KEY POINTS

- Radiography and computed tomography (CT) are considered workhorse imaging modalities as they are widely available and can detect and characterize most posttransplant complications.
- Within reason, the increased radiation exposure related to CT should be less of a concern in lung transplant patients given their limited long-term survival.
- Anastomotic complications are important but are becoming less common because of improvements in graft preservation, surgical technique, and immunosuppression.
- Grouping complications by their predominant imaging finding and along a timeline including the early, intermediate, and late posttransplant periods can help when generating a differential diagnosis.

INTRODUCTION

With advances in surgical technique and immuno-suppressive drug regimens, lung transplantation has become the sole treatment option for patients with a variety of end-stage lung disease. The International Society for Heart and Lung Transplantation (ISHLT) reports that through 2013 nearly 50,000 lung transplants have been performed worldwide.[1] However, long-term survival remains disappointing with only a 5.3-year median survival after transplant, primarily due to complications.[2] Detecting and treating complications are crucial to improving patient outcomes. The goal of this article is to explore the role of imaging in the diagnosis of lung transplant complications.

IMAGING MODALITIES AND TECHNIQUES

A variety of imaging modalities are available for evaluating lung transplant complications, each having its own unique strengths and weaknesses, which are covered in **Table 1**. Radiography and computed tomography serve (CT) as the workhorse modalities. Although these modalities use ionizing radiation, the risks of radiation-induced malignancy are minimal in this population with limited long-term survival.[3]

SURGICAL TECHNIQUE

Single lung transplant (SLT) is performed through a lateral thoracotomy. The lung to be removed is deflated and mobilized; the hilar structures are transected; the donor lung replaces the lung. The graft is implanted with 3 anastomoses, which are performed in their posterior-to-anterior anatomic sequence: bronchus, pulmonary artery, and pulmonary veins-left atrium. The surgical technique used for double lung transplants (DLTs) is the bilateral sequential operation, which is done through a

Disclosure: The authors of this article do not have any relevant financial disclosures.
[a] Department of Radiology, Mayo Clinic Arizona, 13400 E. Shea Blvd, Scottsdale, AZ 85259, USA; [b] Department of Medical Imaging, University of Arizona, College of Medicine, 1401 E University Blvd, Tucson, AZ 85721, USA; [c] Department of Radiology, University of Florida Gainesville, College of Medicine, P.O. Box 100215, Gainesville, FL 32610, USA
* Corresponding author.
E-mail address: clintjokerst@gmail.com

Radiol Clin N Am 54 (2016) 355–373
http://dx.doi.org/10.1016/j.rcl.2015.09.014
0033-8389/16/$ – see front matter © 2016 Elsevier Inc. All rights reserved.

Table 1
Imaging modalities: strengths and weaknesses

Imaging Modality	Indications	Strengths	Weaknesses
Chest radiography	• Evaluation of lines/ tubes • Evaluation of effusion, pneumothorax • Limited evaluation of interstitial and airspace disease	• Inexpensive • Quick • Can be done portably	• Subtle findings of infection and rejection not well evaluated • Only secondary signs of vascular complications visible
CT and CT angiography	• Evaluation of lung parenchyma, interstitium, airways, and pleura • Evaluation of vessels with addition of intravenous contrast	• Excellent resolution • Short examination time • Exhalation images can evaluate air trapping, bronchomalacia • Direct evaluation of vascular structures	• Expensive (relative to CXR) • Cannot be performed portably
MR imaging and MR angiography	• Evaluation of vascular complications • Evaluation of fluid collections	• No radiation • Superior tissue characterization	• Expensive • Long examination times • Inability to image patients with claustrophobia and certain implantable devices
Ventilation/perfusion scintigraphy	• Evaluation of quantitative lung function • Evaluation for pulmonary embolism	• Can obtain split pulmonary functional analysis	• Time consuming • Interpretation can be difficult, especially in the early posttransplant period
PET CT	• Diagnosis and staging PTLD and other malignancies	• Helpful in staging and monitoring response to treatment	• Expensive • Limited availability • Long examination times
Ultrasound	• Evaluation of pleural fluid, fluid collections	• Inexpensive • Can be done portably	• Has a limited role, aside from evaluating pleural fluid

Abbreviations: CT, computed tomography; MR, magnetic resonance; PTLD, posttransplant lymphoproliferative disorder.

clamshell incision with transverse sternotomy; it otherwise uses the same technique as SLT, just applied to both lungs sequentially.[4,5]

The bronchial anastomosis is most prone to complications due to disruption of bronchial arterial blood supply. A variety of modifications have been performed in an attempt to reduce complications. One of the more common is the telescoping anastomosis.[6] With improving surgical techniques and immunosuppression, many surgeons now favor the end-to-end anastomosis with a tissue wrap.[7] Telescoping anastomosis is still used at some centers, especially when there is size discrepancy between the native bronchus and the allograft bronchus.[6]

RELEVANT ANATOMY

Most serious posttransplant complications occur within the graft.[2] Knowledge of relevant pulmonary

anatomy helps the radiologist understand the imaging findings. The authors break pulmonary anatomy down into 3 compartments: airways, airspaces, and interstitium.

Airways

Airways within the graft constitute the conducting zone, which conveys gas to and from the airspaces. They are made up of bronchi, bronchioles, and terminal bronchioles.[8] Common findings directly visible on imaging include bronchiectasis and bronchial wall thickening. Bronchiolar disease can be inferred based on the presence of air trapping.

Airspaces

Airspaces make up the respiratory zone where gas exchange takes place. They contain respiratory bronchioles, alveolar ducts, and alveoli. Airspace disease can manifest either as ground-glass attenuation or consolidation (see **Table 4**). Ground-glass attenuation refers to increased opacity on chest x-ray (CXR) and CT in which the underlying vessels are still visible because there is still some air within the alveoli. Consolidation refers to homogenously increased opacity on radiographs and CT, which obscures the underlying vessels.[9]

Interstitium

Interstitium refers to the supportive connective tissues within the lung. Interstitial anatomy is intertwined with that of the secondary pulmonary lobule (SPL). Pulmonary interstitium can be found in the middle of the SPL along the centrilobular structures, in the subpleural regions and interlobular septa at the periphery of the SPL, and in the intralobular septae, which span the axial interstitium and peripheral interstitium.[8]

IMAGING FINDINGS OF POSTTRANSPLANT COMPLICATIONS

Complications can be grouped by their predominant imaging findings, although there is overlap. Timing is also an important consideration. When possible, the authors have grouped complications by their predominant imaging finding or anatomic compartment and subdivided chronologically into the early, intermediate, and late posttransplant periods.

VASCULAR AND ANASTOMOTIC COMPLICATIONS

Anastomotic complications can present at any time in the posttransplant period, although dehiscence and thrombosis are more common early on, whereas stenosis has a delayed presentation (**Table 2**). Anastomotic complications have become less frequent with improved graft preservation, advances in surgical technique, and improved immunosuppression.

Early Posttransplant Period (First Week)

1. Pulmonary vein thrombosis
2. Pulmonary thromboembolism (PE)

Pulmonary vein thrombosis

Pulmonary vein thrombosis is rarely seen, although one prospective series of transplant patients evaluated with transesophageal echocardiography demonstrated an incidence of approximately 15%.[10] The most common complications are systemic embolic phenomena and graft failure.[11,12] Secondary findings seen on CXR and cross-sectional imaging consist of interstitial edema, infarcts, or both. Contrast-enhanced CT or MR imaging will show a filling defect in the affected vein possibly extending into the left atrium.[13]

Pulmonary thromboembolism

PE can occur at any time after lung transplantation but is most common in the early and intermediate posttransplant periods. Postoperative immobility and hypercoagulability are important risk factor for deep vein thrombosis (DVT) and PE. PE in the setting of lung transplantation requires special attention because these patients have a higher mortality, likely related to inadequate collateral bronchial circulation occurring after lung transplantation.[14]

Secondary findings of infarction (Hampton hump) and unilateral pulmonary oligemia (Westermark sign) can occasionally be seen on CXR.[15] A centralized pulmonary artery filling defect, usually near a branch point, with a rim of surrounding contrast is the classic finding of acute PE on CT (**Fig. 1A**).[16] Magnetic resonance angiography (MRA) has a growing role in the diagnosis of PE as well, although it is less sensitive for smaller emboli.[17] The classic finding of PE on a ventilation-perfusion (V/Q) scan is multiple perfusion defects with no corresponding ventilation defects. Mortality is high in transplant patients who develop PE, so DVT prophylaxis is extremely important.

Intermediate Posttransplant Period (>1 Week, <2 Months)

1. Bronchial dehiscence
2. Pulmonary artery stenosis

Bronchial dehiscence

Bronchial dehiscence is the most common early airway complication affecting approximately 2%

Table 2 Surgical complications		
Early Posttransplant (First Week)	**Intermediate Posttransplant (>1 wk, <2 mo)**	**Late Posttransplant (>2 mo)**
• Pulmonary vein thrombosis • Pulmonary thromboembolism • Phrenic nerve paralysis	• Bronchial dehiscence • Pulmonary artery stenosis	• Bronchial stenosis • Bronchomalacia

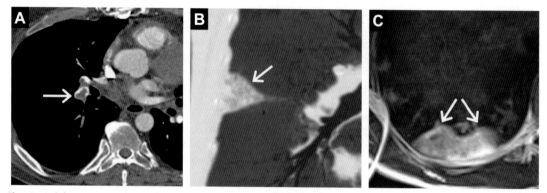

Fig. 1. Axial contrast-enhanced CT (CECT) image (*A*) demonstrating a filling defect with surrounding rim of contrast in the right lower lobe pulmonary artery (*arrow*) in a patient with a recent right-sided SLT. Coronal CT reconstruction (*B*) from a different patient with pulmonary emboli demonstrating a pulmonary infarct (*arrow*). Note the peripheral wedge-shaped appearance with internal bubbly lucencies. Axial T2-weighted MR image (*C*) from a different patient with a pulmonary infarct (*arrows*) with increased T2 signal, a classic finding.

of transplants and usually occurring 1 to 4 weeks after transplant.[7,18] Dehiscence is likely multifactorial, with ischemia related to disruption of the bronchial arterial supply being the most important contributor.[19]

Secondary signs of dehiscence, such as pneumothorax and pneumomediastinum, may be apparent on CXR (**Fig. 2**A); however, CT is more sensitive for diagnosing airway complications.[20] CT findings of bronchial dehiscence include extraluminal air, irregularity of the airway, and a defect in the bronchial wall (see **Fig. 2**B).[21] Bronchoscopy may be indicated in patients with suspected dehiscence and negative CT. Dehiscence is treated with stenting or anastomotic revision.[19]

Pulmonary artery stenosis
Pulmonary artery stenosis has been reported as both an early and late complication of lung transplantation.[22] Stenosis usually presents with shortness of breath and sometimes with pulmonary hypertension and right heart failure. Common causes of narrowing include excessive length of vascular pedicle, short allograft artery length, and presence of restrictive suture and clot.[23] Severe pulmonary artery stenosis can lead to pulmonary infarction and graft failure.

Contrast-enhanced CT and MRA will demonstrate a narrowing at the anastomotic site. V/Q scanning will show decreased perfusion to the affected lung with relatively preserved ventilation. Treatment includes angioplasty and stenting.[24]

Late Posttransplant Period (>2 Months)

1. Bronchial stenosis
2. Bronchomalacia

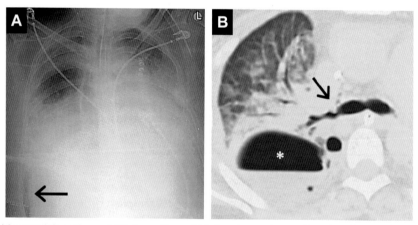

Fig. 2. Portable CXR (*A*) performed 20 days after a DLT showing a deep sulcus sign (*arrow*) from a right-sided pneumothorax. Axial image from a follow-up CT (*B*) demonstrates irregularity of the right bronchial anastomosis with adjacent extraluminal gas (*arrow*) and a loculated hydropneumothorax in the right posterior costophrenic angle (*asterisk*). Bronchial dehiscence was confirmed with bronchoscopy.

Bronchial strictures

Bronchial strictures complicate 10% to 15% of lung transplants and usually occur months after surgery.[19,25] The airflow limitations caused by strictures can be difficult to distinguish from those caused by obliterative bronchiolitis (OB) related to chronic rejection.[26] There are reports of nonanastomotic bronchial stenosis involving the bronchus intermedius, referred to as the vanishing bronchus intermedius syndrome (VBIS). VBIS is seen as early as 6 months after transplant and is associated with high morbidity and mortality.[27]

Although anastomotic strictures can be seen on CXR, CT is the study of choice (**Fig. 3**A), and multiplanar reformations and virtual bronchoscopy are excellent for demonstrating this complication.[28] Fiberoptic bronchoscopy is still the reference standard for diagnosis (see **Fig. 3**B) and can also be therapeutic via bronchoscopic debridement, dilation, and stent placement.[19]

Bronchomalacia

Bronchomalacia is a dynamic narrowing of the airway that increases during exhalation, whereas bronchial stenosis is a fixed narrowing of the airway. Both focal (usually peri-anastomotic) and diffuse forms of bronchomalacia can be seen in the posttransplant setting.[6] The latter may present with a patchy distribution of air trapping, which can mimic that seen in OB.

Paired end-inspiratory and dynamic-expiratory CT images (see **Fig. 3**C, D) are compared to identify if there is a significant reduction in bronchial cross-sectional area. A 50% loss of area was the traditional cutoff for diagnosing bronchomalacia; however, more recent data demonstrate that many normal volunteers exceed this cutoff. A higher cutoff should be used in conjunction with symptoms to reduce the number of false-positive examinations.[29] Air trapping is often seen with bronchomalacia, which can mimic OB (see **Fig. 3**D). When severe, it can be treated with stenting.[19]

PLEURAL COMPLICATIONS

Pleural complications are common affecting 22% to 34% of patients following lung transplantation (**Table 3**).[30,31] Most early forms of pleural complication can be treated conservatively; thoracostomy tubes are placed during transplantation to help mitigate these complications.

Early Posttransplant Period (First Week)

1. Pleural effusion
2. Pneumothorax
3. Hemothorax

Pleural effusions

Pleural effusions are common following lung transplantation. There are several mechanisms thought to contribute, including increased vascular permeability related to graft ischemia, denervation, reperfusion injury, disruption of graft lymphatics, and acute rejection.[30] Effusions are easily evaluated with CXR (**Fig. 4**A). CT, MR imaging, or ultrasonography (US) can be helpful to demonstrate loculations, signs of infection, and to guide thoracentesis or thoracostomy tube placement.

Pneumothorax

Pneumothorax is common in the posttransplant setting. Most pneumothoraxes spontaneously resolve within a few days; however, 10% of patients develop an air leak that lasts more than 2 weeks. These leaks are usually successfully

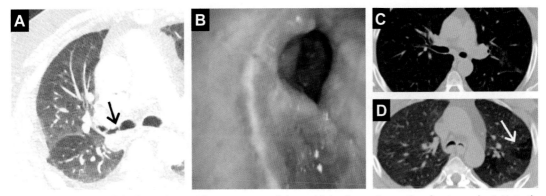

Fig. 3. Axial CT image (*A*) of a patient with an anastomotic bronchial stricture 2 months after transplant. Note the narrowing and irregularity of the bronchus (*arrow*) on CT. An image from subsequent bronchoscopy (*B*) demonstrates the stricture. Paired inspiratory (*C*) and dynamic expiratory (*D*) CT images from a patient with bronchomalacia demonstrate airway collapse and air trapping (*arrow*) on the expiratory phase. (*Courtesy of* [*A, B*] Jeffery Kanney, MD, Madison, WI.)

Table 3
Pleural complications

Early Posttransplant (First Week)	Intermediate Posttransplant (>1 wk, <2 mo)	Late Posttransplant (>2 mo)
• Pleural effusion • Pneumothorax • Hemothorax	• Chylothorax • Empyema	• Pleural thickening/scarring • Rounded atelectasis • Empyema

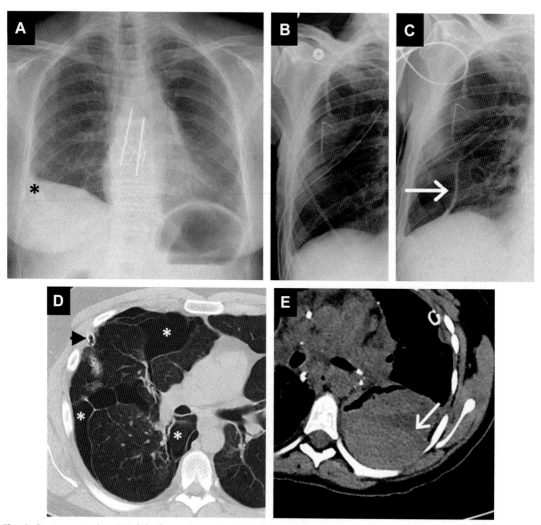

Fig. 4. Posteroanterior CXR (*A*) of a patient after DLT showing the classic appearance of a subpulmonic effusion with loss of the normal contour and lateral peaking of the right hemidiaphragm (*asterisk*). Note the transverse sternotomy transfixed with pins and cerclage wires. Frontal portable CXRs obtained 1 day apart (*B, C*) showing interval development of a pneumothorax (*arrow*) despite presence of a thoracostomy tube. Follow-up CT (*D*) shows pneumothoraxes (*asterisks*), which do not communicate with the thoracostomy tube (*arrowhead*). Axial CT image (*E*) shows layering high-density material (*arrow*) consistent with a hemothorax in another transplant patient.

treated with prolonged thoracostomy tube placement.[31]

Pneumothoraxes can be followed with serial CXRs. The upright technique is more sensitive than supine; the classic findings on an upright CXR are a thin pleural line that parallels the chest wall with no pulmonary markings beyond this line (see **Fig. 4**B, C). On supine radiographs, the deep sulcus sign can be helpful in identifying a pneumothorax (see **Fig. 2**A).[32] Rarely, cross-sectional imaging may be helpful (see **Fig. 4**D) to evaluate potential causes of persistent pneumothorax, such as bronchial dehiscence or bronchopleural fistula.

Hemothorax

Hemothorax complicates up to 15% of transplants in a recent series that found that patients with sarcoidosis, retransplantation, and dense pleural adhesions were at higher risk.[33] CXR findings of hemothorax are often indistinguishable from those of effusion. On CT, acute hemothorax will have increased attenuation, 35 to 70 Hounsfield units (see **Fig. 4**E).[34] US is also a sensitive and specific modality for detection of hemothorax.[35] Hemothoraxes require large thoracostomy tubes for effective drainage.

Intermediate Posttransplant Period (>1 Week, <2 Months)

1. Chylothorax
2. Empyema

Chylothorax

Chylothorax is usually caused by damage to the thoracic duct and is more common in technically difficult surgical cases with pleural adhesions. It is also common in patients who undergo transplant for lymphangioleiomyomatosis.[36] Chylothorax should be suspected in transplant patients with a pleural effusion that continues to increase postoperatively. From an imaging standpoint, a chylous effusion is indistinguishable from other causes of effusion. Pleural fluid analysis will yield elevated triglycerides, lymphocytes, and chylomicrons.

Empyema

Empyema complicates 4% to 7% of transplants and is the only pleural complication associated with increased mortality. Early recognition and treatment is critical.[37] Empyema should be suspected when a new effusion develops within 4 weeks of transplant, especially if the effusion appears loculated. Pleural loculations should be suspected when there is fluid that appears trapped in a non–gravity-dependent configuration.

On CXR, empyemas tend to form obtuse angles with the chest wall and, because of their lenticular shape, are much larger in one projection compared with the orthogonal projection.[38] Occasionally there will be locules of gas suggesting gas-forming organisms; gas can also be introduced via thoracentesis. The pleura will appear thickened and enhancing on contrast-enhanced CT and MR imaging. Pleural enhancement can be seen dividing into parietal and visceral layers at the margin of the empyema resulting in the split pleura sign (**Fig. 5**A, B).[38] There can be edema in the extrapleural fat. MR imaging and US are useful modalities for evaluating empyema. MR imaging is good for showing pleural enhancement and extrapleural edema (see **Fig. 5**B, C), and both MR

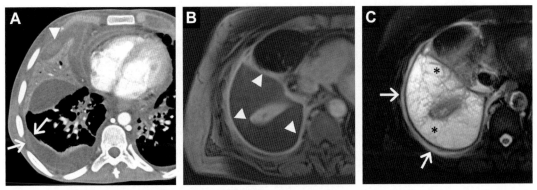

Fig. 5. Axial CECT image (*A*) from a patient who developed a hemothorax following transplant that became infected. Note the high-density material within the pleural space (*arrowhead*) consistent with blood products and the enhancing pleura resulting in a split pleura sign (*arrows*). Contrast-enhanced T1-weighted (*B*) and precontrast fat-suppressed T2-weighted (*C*) axial images from MR imaging in a different patient with empyema. Note the pleural enhancement (*B, arrowheads*), the subpleural edema (*C, arrows*), and the loculations within the pleural fluid (*C, asterisks*).

imaging and US can demonstrate septations and debris within the fluid.

Late Posttransplant Period (>2 Months)

1. Pleural scarring
2. Rounded atelectasis

Pleural scarring and rounded atelectasis

Pleural scarring and rounded atelectasis are seen in the late posttransplant period. A study demonstrated pleural fibrosis in animals that received heart-lung allografts but not in animals that received autografts, suggesting pleural scarring is related to chronic rejection.[39] Pleural thickening and blunting of the costophrenic angles are seen on CXR (**Fig. 6**A). On CT there will be pleural thickening with adjacent linear pulmonary scarring and atelectasis. Round atelectasis can be distinguished from malignancy by presence of the comet-tail sign, pulling of bronchovascular bundles into the atelectasis (see **Fig. 6**B).[40]

COMPLICATIONS MANIFESTING WITH AIRSPACE DISEASE

Airspace disease can manifest with ground-glass attenuation, consolidation, or both (**Table 4**). On imaging, airspace disease usually has a patchy cloudlike appearance where fluid fills the alveoli to a varying extent.

Early Posttransplant Period (First Week)

1. Hyperacute rejection
2. Graft size mismatch
3. Primary graft dysfunction (PGD)
4. Lobar torsion

Hyperacute rejection

Hyperacute rejection is rare and occurs when preformed antibodies to the donor graft present. Edema and graft failure occur within a few hours after transplant. Radiographs show diffuse consolidation throughout the allografts. Successful treatment with plasmapheresis and antithymocyte globulin has been described; however, death remains common.[41]

Graft size mismatch

Graft size mismatch occurs when the donor lung is placed into a hemithorax in which there is a size difference of greater than 25%. This mismatch results in areas of atelectasis that manifest as linear areas of consolidation on CXR and CT.[42]

Primary graft dysfunction

PGD is also known as reimplantation edema and ischemia/reperfusion injury. The ISHLT has diagnostic criteria and a grading system for PGD. The most important diagnostic criterion is the ratio of Pao_2 to the inspired oxygen concentration.[43–46] It has been postulated that PGD occurs from ischemia of the allograft with subsequent reperfusion. Decreased lymphatic clearance secondary to anastomotic disruption of lymphatics and lung denervation also likely contributes to PGD.[44,45,47]

Radiographs and CT show consolidation and/or interstitial opacities in a perihilar and lower lung–predominant distribution that appear in the first 24 hours and usually clear in approximately 5 to 10 days (**Fig. 7**).[48] Histopathology shows acute lung injury and diffuse alveolar damage.[49] PGD increases the risk of subsequent bronchiolitis obliterans syndrome (BOS).[50]

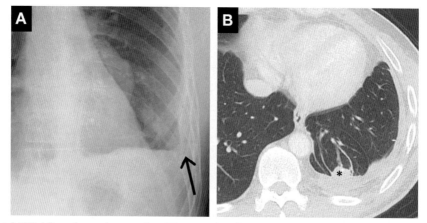

Fig. 6. Frontal CXR (*A*) performed years after SLT. Note the pleural thickening and blunting of the costophrenic angle (*arrow*). A corresponding axial image from a CT (*B*) demonstrates a nodule (*asterisk*) adjacent to some plural thickening/scarring. Note the volume loss and swirling of adjacent vessels into the nodule, the comet-tail sign.

Table 4
Differential diagnoses of imaging findings based on time from transplant

Imaging Finding	Early Posttransplant (First Week)	Intermediate Posttransplant (>1 wk, <2 mo)	Late Posttransplant (>2 mo)
Consolidation	• Hyperacute rejection • Graft size mismatch • Primary graft dysfunction • Vascular anastomotic occlusion • Lobar torsion	• Acute rejection • Infection (bacterial) • Pulmonary infarction • Acute fibrinous and organizing pneumonia	• Infection (viral, fungal, mycobacterial) • Pulmonary infarction • Acute fibrinous and organizing pneumonia
Interstitial disease	• Pulmonary edema • Primary graft dysfunction • Pulmonary vein thrombosis/stenosis	• Acute rejection	• Restrictive allograft syndrome
Air trapping	—	—	• OB • Bronchial stenosis • Bronchomalacia
Nodules	—	• Infection • Biopsy changes	• PTLD • Metastatic disease • Rounded atelectasis • Recurrent sarcoidosis

Abbreviation: PTLD, posttransplant lymphoproliferative disorder.

Lobar torsion

Lobar torsion is rare and results in ischemia and infarction of the affected lobe. Radiography may show abnormal opacity of the hilum and increased opacity of the involved lobe. Contrast-enhanced CT will show tapering of the pulmonary artery and adjacent bronchus to the involved lobe with increased soft tissue density at the hilum. The torsed lobe may show areas of ground-glass opacity, consolidation, and interlobular septal thickening.[51]

Intermediate Posttransplant Period (>1 Week, <2 Months)

1. Acute rejection
2. Infection (primarily bacterial)
3. Pulmonary infarction
4. Acute fibrinous and organizing pneumonia

Acute rejection

Acute rejection is common because lung transplants are often HLA-mismatched; it complicates

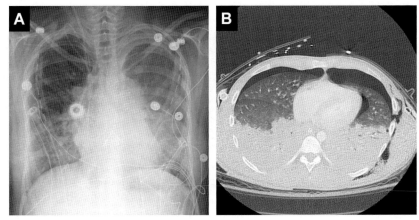

Fig. 7. DLT patient with primary graft dysfunction. CXR (*A*) performed the day after the operation showing perihilar and bibasilar interstitial and airspace disease. A corresponding axial image from a CT (*B*) performed the next day demonstrates dependent consolidation and bilateral pneumothoraces.

50% to 60% of lung transplants.[52] Acute rejection usually occurs after 5 to 10 days and presents with fever, hypoxemia, and decrease of forced expiratory volume in the first second of expiration (FEV_1) of at least 10%.[53] Diagnosis is made with transbronchial biopsy, which will show perivascular and interstitial lymphocytic infiltrate.[54]

Radiographs usually show a combination of airspace disease and interlobular septal thickening as well as pleural effusions. CT will show ill-defined centrilobular ground-glass nodules, interlobular septal thickening, scattered to diffuse ground-glass opacity, and areas of consolidation (Fig. 8). Interlobular septal thickening may be the earliest sign on acute rejection; however, ground-glass opacity is nearly always also present. Acute rejection responds rapidly to steroid therapy.[55]

Infection
Infection risk is increased in the lung allograft because of immunosuppression, exposure of the transplant to the environment, absent cough reflex from denervation, and impaired clearance of secretions from bronchial transection.[56] In the intermediate transplant period, infection is often bacterial; common pathogens include *Enterobacter*, *Staphylococcus aureus*, and *Pseudomonas aeruginosa* (Fig. 9A, B). Opportunistic infections, such as *Aspergillus* and *Candida*, are less common but may involve the bronchial anastomosis during this time period. Radiography and CT can show areas of ground-glass opacity, consolidation with air bronchograms, and centrilobular, tree-in-bud nodules (see Fig. 9C, D).[57]

Pulmonary infarction
Pulmonary infarction from pulmonary embolism can occur at any time after transplant. Pulmonary infarcts have a classic appearance on CT with peripheral, wedge-shaped consolidation often with central ground-glass opacity and absent air bronchograms (see Fig. 1B). On MR imaging, pulmonary infarcts typically demonstrate increased T1 and T2 signal (see Fig. 1C).[58] Pulmonary infarcts are often associated with pleural effusions.

Acute fibrinous and organizing pneumonia
Acute fibrinous and organizing pneumonia (AFOP) is a pattern of lung injury that is associated with both acute and chronic rejection. It manifests on chest radiography and CT as nonspecific patchy or diffuse consolidation and ground-glass opacity (Fig. 10). On histopathology, the dominant finding is balls of fibrin within the alveolar spaces. Areas of fibroblastic Masson bodies or fibroblasts surrounding the balls of fibrin are also present, consistent with areas of organizing pneumonia. Tissue sampling is necessary for definitive diagnosis. Corticosteroids are standard therapy, and prognosis is variable.[59]

Late Posttransplant Period (>2 Months)

1. Infection (primarily opportunistic)
2. Pulmonary infarction
3. AFOP

Infection
Infection in the late posttransplant period is commonly secondary to opportunistic organisms, including fungal, viral, and mycobacterial infections. Infection in the late-transplant period complicates approximately 60% of lung transplant recipients.[57]

Cytomegalovirus (CMV) infection is common and can occur as early as 1 month after transplant but is more common months to years after transplant. CMV infection may occur secondary to reactivation of latent virus in the recipient, environmental exposure to the virus, or from

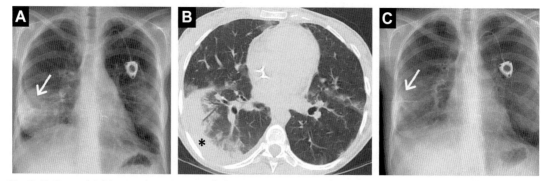

Fig. 8. Patient with biopsy-proven acute cellular rejection. Initial CXR (*A*) demonstrates peripheral consolidation in the right lower lobe (*arrow*). Subsequent CT (*B*) demonstrates patchy airspace disease (*asterisk*). A CXR obtained 2 weeks later (*C*), after escalation of immunosuppression, demonstrates improvement in the consolidation (*arrow*).

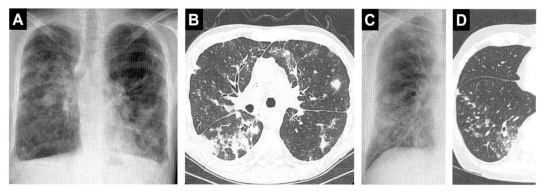

Fig. 9. CXR (*A*) taken during the intermediate posttransplant period demonstrating patchy nodular airspace disease. Corresponding axial CT (*B*) demonstrates widespread foci of ground glass and nodular consolidation. Cultures grew pseudomonas; bacterial organisms are the most common cause of pneumonia in the intermediate posttransplant period. CXR (*C*) and CT (*D*) from a different patient with tree-in-bud nodules and ground glass in the right lung base. Aspiration was suspected, but Mycobacterium avium intracellulare was isolated. (*Courtesy of* Jeffery Kanney, MD, Madison, WI.)

transmission from a CMV-infected allograft. In cases whereby transfer of a CMV seropositive allograft to a seronegative recipient must be performed, the recipient is pretreated with ganciclovir and CMV immunoglobulin before the transplant.[60] Chest radiography may show interstitial and nodular opacities. The classic CT finding is ground-glass opacity (**Fig. 11**A, B). Small centrilobular nodules, pleural effusion, or consolidation can also be present.[61] Nevertheless, CMV typically cannot be distinguished from other infections or inflammatory conditions by imaging alone.

Other viruses that cause infection in posttransplant patients include respiratory syncytial virus, influenza, parainfluenza, and herpes simplex virus.[62,63] Fungal infections include *Aspergillus* and *Candida* infections. Chest radiology and CT usually show nodules (see **Fig. 11**C, D); however, areas of patchy ground-glass opacity and consolidation may be present. A peripheral rim of ground-glass opacity (CT halo sign) surrounding nodular consolidation is highly suggestive of angioinvasive infection, particularly aspergillosis (see **Fig. 11**E).[64] Less common infections in the

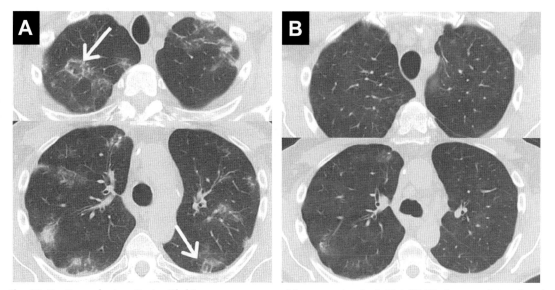

Fig. 10. Posttransplant patient with biopsy-proven organizing pneumonia. Initial CT (*A*) shows peripheral and peri-bronchovascular foci of ground glass, some with areas of central clearing, the atoll sign (*arrows*). A follow-up CT (*B*) performed 5 weeks later, after a course of steroid therapy demonstrates improvement.

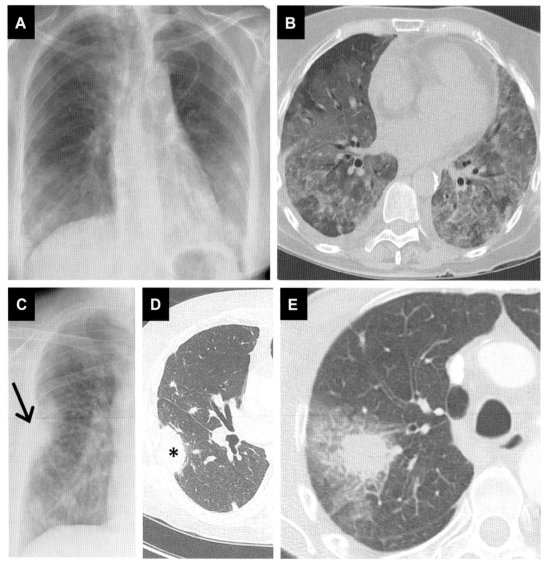

Fig. 11. CXR (*A*) from a patient with CMV pneumonia who developed dyspnea and cough 2 months after transplant. Airspace disease, predominantly ground glass, is subtle given how obvious the findings are on CT (*B*). The CT also demonstrates interstitial involvement, but the main finding is ground glass. CXR (*C*) and CT (*D*) images from a different transplant patient with a peripheral right upper lobe mass (*arrow, asterisk*). Finding suspicious for posttransplant lymphoproliferative disease but turned out to be histoplasmosis. Axial CT (*E*) from a different transplant patient with angioinvasive aspergillus. Note the nodular consolidation with a prominent ground-glass halo. (*Courtesy of* [*C, D*] Jeffery Kanney, MD, Madison, WI.)

late-transplant period include *Mycobacteria* and *Nocardia*.[65]

COMPLICATIONS MANIFESTING WITH INTERSTITIAL DISEASE

Airspace disease has a fluffy, cloudlike appearance on imaging, whereas interstitial disease consists of lines. These lines can be 1 to 2 cm long in the case of interlobular septal involvement, which may be smooth or lobular depending on the

disease process.[9] Interstitial disease can also present with reticulation, a meshlike network of subcentimeter lines; reticulation in conjunction with nodules results in a reticulonodular pattern (see Table 4).

Early Posttransplant Period (First Week)

1. Pulmonary edema
2. Primary graft dysfunction
3. Pulmonary vein stenosis/thrombosis

Pulmonary edema

Pulmonary edema from fluid overload postoperatively may be present and can present as septal thickening, consolidation, or both on radiographs. The classic finding on CXR is the Kerley-B line, peripheral 1 to 2 cm horizontal lines perpendicular to the pleura. CT shows smooth interlobular septal thickening (**Fig. 12A**).

Pulmonary vein stenosis

Pulmonary vein stenosis can manifest with interlobular septal thickening involving the affected lobe. Occlusion of the pulmonary vein can result in superimposed airspace disease representing hemorrhage in the affected lobe.[66]

Intermediate Posttransplant Period (>1 Week, <2 Months)

1. Acute rejection
2. Infection (**Fig. 12B**)

Late Posttransplant Period (>2 Months)

1. Restrictive allograft syndrome (RAS)

Restrictive allograft syndrome

RAS, often referred to as upper lobe fibrosis, is a recently described form of chronic lung allograft dysfunction (CLAD).[67] CLAD is defined as an irreversible decline in FEV_1 to less than 80% of patients' baseline on spirometry.[67] RAS is defined as CLAD found in conjunction with restrictive changes, defined as an irreversible decline in total lung capacity to less than 90% of patients' baseline.[67] Recently, pleuroparenchymal fibroelastosis has been identified as the underlying histopathologic finding in RAS.[68]

RAS eventually affects approximately 10% of transplant patients, and survival is significantly worse when compared with patients with the other major form of CLAD, OB.[67] Both radiographs and CT will show findings of fibrosis, including reticulation, traction bronchiectasis, and volume loss with architectural distortion and pleural scarring with an upper-lung predilection (**Fig. 13**).[67,69]

COMPLICATIONS MANIFESTING WITH AIR TRAPPING

Air trapping commonly manifests as mosaic attenuation whereby the lung parenchyma appears as a patchwork of regions of differing attenuation on CT.[9] If air trapping is suspected, it can be confirmed using expiratory CT, which will show persistence of low attenuation in areas with air trapping (see **Table 4**).

Late Posttransplant Period (>2 Months)

1. OB/BOS
2. Bronchial stenosis
3. Bronchomalacia

Obliterative bronchiolitis

OB is the classic cause of CLAD and is the principal factor limiting long-term survival. It affects more than half of patients surviving to 5 years post-transplant.[70] The histopathologic manifestations are those of constrictive bronchiolitis (CB), whereby the bronchioles are narrowed and eventually obliterated by chronic inflammation and fibrosis. Risk factors include recurrent episodes of acute rejection, infection, and gastroesophageal reflux. Patients generally present with a

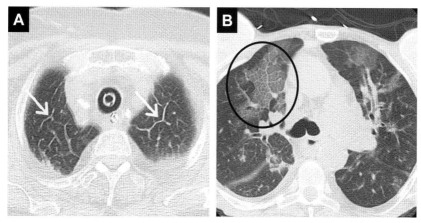

Fig. 12. Axial CT (*A*) demonstrating smooth septal line thickening typical of cardiogenic edema (*arrows*). Volume overload is common in the immediate posttransplant period. CT from a different posttransplant patient (*B*) with patchy ground glass and superimposed interlobular and intralobular thickening consistent with crazy paving (*circle*). Sputum cultures were positive for strep pneumonia.

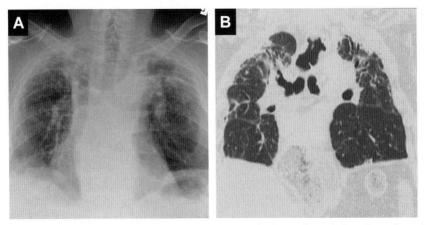

Fig. 13. CXR (*A*) and coronal CT reconstruction (*B*) demonstrating findings of restrictive allograft syndrome. There is upper lobe reticulation, bronchiectasis, and volume loss with architectural distortion. (*Courtesy of [A, B]* Jeffery Kanney, MD, Madison, WI.)

cough, worsening dyspnea, and progressive airflow obstruction.[71]

Demonstration of CB within a path specimen is the gold standard for diagnosis; however, pulmonary involvement is patchy and yield of transbronchial biopsy is low.[72] Surgical biopsy has a higher yield but is expensive and invasive.[73] Because OB is difficult to document pathologically, the ISHLT Working Group has adopted the term *BOS* to describe and chronic allograft rejection *in the absence of histologic confirmation.*[74] *BOS is diagnosed and graded with spirometry with updated criteria being published in 2002.*[75]

The imaging findings of OB can be subtle and are most apparent on CT. Findings include mosaic attenuation, mild bronchiectasis, bronchial wall thickening, and expiratory air trapping (**Fig. 14**).[76] Spirometry has proven to be more sensitive than CT for BOS.[77] CT is more useful as an adjunct, allowing distinction of OB from other causes of airflow obstruction.[73] Treatment consists of escalating immunosuppression.

COMPLICATIONS MANIFESTING WITH NODULES

Nodules are defined as solid, rounded lesions measuring up to 30 mm. Micronodules are defined as nodules smaller than 3 mm and can occur in a variety of patterns, including centrilobular, perilymphatic, and random (see **Table 4**).[78]

Intermediate Posttransplant Period (>1 Week, <2 Months)

1. Infection
2. Effects from biopsy

Transbronchial biopsy

Transbronchial biopsy is most often used to aid in the diagnosis of acute and chronic rejection,

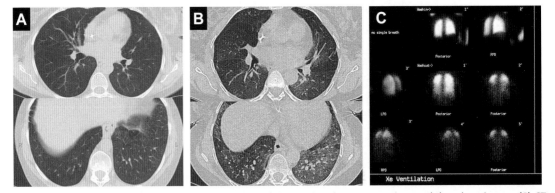

Fig. 14. A 56-year-old woman after DLT 7 years ago with increasing dyspnea. Inspiratory (*A*) and expiratory (*B*) CT images demonstrate widespread air trapping (*asterisk*) consistent with CB related to chronic rejection. Xenon ventilation images from a V/Q scan (*C*) demonstrate delayed washout of tracer consistent with air trapping.

infection, and recurrence of primary disease.[79] One of the most common postbiopsy findings are small focal nodular opacities that are usually located within 2 cm of the pleura and correspond to biopsy sites.[80] On CT these nodules may be solid or cavitary and are often surrounded by a halo of ground-glass opacity representing hemorrhage.

Late Posttransplant Period (>2 Months)

1. Posttransplant lymphoproliferative disorder (PTLD)
2. Metastases
3. Rounded atelectasis
4. Recurrent sarcoidosis

Posttransplant lymphoproliferative disorder

PTLD represents a heterogeneous group of abnormal B-cell proliferative responses. Most cases are associated with Epstein-Barr virus (EBV) infection of B cells, either from reactivation of the virus within an EBV-positive recipient or from primary infection. Primary infection can occur when an EBV-naïve recipient receives a graft from an EBV-positive donor. PTLD occurs in approximately 5% of lung transplant recipients.[81] Most cases of PTLD occur within the first year after transplant.[82] The initial treatment of PTLD involves reduction in immunosuppression, which increases the risk of developing rejection.

The most common imaging manifestations of PTLD are pulmonary nodules and masses

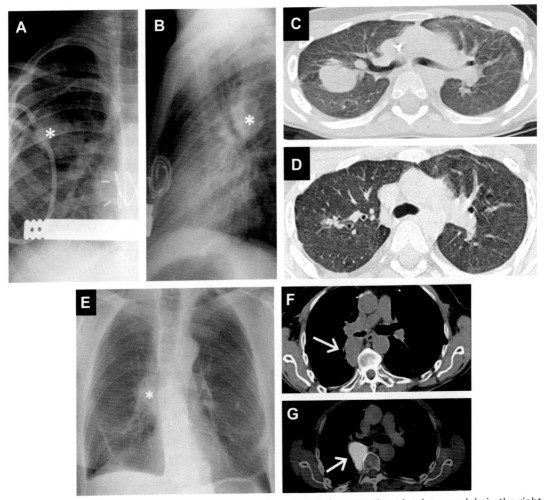

Fig. 15. Frontal (*A*) and lateral (*B*) CXR of a 6-year-old 3 months after DLT. There is a large nodule in the right upper lobe (*asterisk*). Biopsy yielded PTLD. CT performed before (*C*) and after (*D*) therapy demonstrates a favorable response. (*E*) CXR from a different patient with PTLD 15 months after DLT demonstrates a nodule superimposed on the right hilum (*asterisk*). CT (*F*) and PET-CT (*G*) confirm the finding (*arrow*). PET-CT is useful for diagnosis and staging of PTLD.

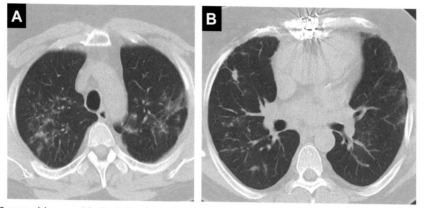

Fig. 16. A 46-year-old man with declining lung function years after DLT for sarcoidosis. CT images (*A, B*) demonstrate scattered upper-lung predominant nodules with a perilymphatic distribution. Transbronchial biopsy demonstrated recurrent sarcoidosis.

(**Fig. 15**), which can be associated with lymphadenopathy and pleural effusions.[83] Although most of these findings are recognizable on CXR, CT best characterizes these findings (see **Fig. 15F**). PET-CT allows for more accurate initial staging of PTLD and can also be used to monitor response to therapy (see **Fig. 15G**).[84]

Metastatic disease

Metastatic disease is seen with increased frequency in transplant patients. Immunosuppression increases the risk of developing malignancies, especially skin cancer. There is a 65- to 100-fold greater risk of nonmelanoma skin cancer, particularly squamous cell carcinoma.[85,86] These neoplasms are more aggressive, difficult to treat, and have higher rates of metastases.[87] Lung metastases usually manifest as multiple nodules of varying sizes. CT is the modality of choice for diagnosis and evaluation of pulmonary metastases.

Recurrent sarcoidosis

Recurrent sarcoidosis is the most commonly reported disease to recur in lung transplant patients. Recurrence can occur in the intermediate or late posttransplant periods, and the rate of recurrence is 35%.[88] The classic findings in sarcoidosis are mediastinal and hilar lymphadenopathy and perilymphatic lung nodules (**Fig. 16**).

SUMMARY

Imaging plays a key role in detection and management of complications following lung transplantation. Knowing the strengths and weaknesses of the various imaging modalities available allows one to tailor the study to answer the relevant clinical question. CXR and CT serve as workhorse modalities with other modalities filling niche roles. An understanding of underlying anatomy and surgical technique helps to accurately describe imaging findings. The predominant imaging findings, in conjunction with timing of presentation, can be used to narrow the differential diagnosis when faced with potential complications following transplantation.

REFERENCES

1. Yusen RD, Edwards LB, Kucheryavaya AY, et al. The registry of the International Society for Heart and Lung Transplantation: thirty-first adult lung and heart-lung transplant report–2014; focus theme: re-transplantation. J Heart Lung Transplant 2014;33: 1009.
2. Christie JD, Edwards LB, Kucheryavaya AY, et al. The Registry of the International Society for Heart and Lung Transplantation: twenty-seventh official adult lung and heart-lung transplant report–2010. J Heart Lung Transplant 2010;29:1104–18.
3. Rosengarten D, Raviv Y, Rusanov V, et al. Radiation exposure and attributed cancer risk following lung transplantation. Clin Transplant 2014;28(3):324–9.
4. Pasque MK, Cooper JD, Kaiser LR, et al. Improved technique for bilateral lung transplantation: rationale and initial clinical experience. Ann Thorac Surg 1990;49:785.
5. Egan TM, Detterbeck FC. Technique and results of double lung transplantation. Chest Surg Clin N Am 1993;3:89.
6. Santacruz JF, Mehta AC. Airway complications and management after lung transplantation. Proc Am Thorac Soc 2009;6(1):79–93.
7. Date H, Trulock EP, Arcidi JM, et al. Improved airway healing after lung transplantation: an analysis of 348 bronchial anastomoses. J Thorac Cardiovasc Surg 1995;110:1424–33.

8. Karthikeyan D. High resolution computed tomography of the lungs: a practical guide. New Delhi (India): Jaypee Brothers Medical Publishing; 2013.

9. Hansell DM, Bankier AA, MacMahon H, et al. Fleischner Society: glossary of terms for thoracic imaging. Radiology 2008;246(3):697–722.

10. Schulman LL, Anandarangam T, Leibowitz DW. Four-year prospective study of pulmonary venous thrombosis after lung transplantation. J Am Soc Echocardiogr 2001;14(8):806–12.

11. Sarsam MA, Yonan NA, Beton D, et al. Early pulmonary vein thrombosis after single lung transplantation. J Heart Lung Transplant 1993;12:17–9.

12. Uhlmann EJ, Dunitz JM, Fiol ME. Pulmonary vein thrombosis after lung transplantation presenting as stroke. J Heart Lung Transplant 2009;28(2):209–10.

13. Selvidge SDD, Gavant ML. Idiopathic pulmonary vein thrombosis: detection by CT and MR imaging. Am J Roentgenol 1999;172(6):1639–41.

14. Krivokuca I, van de Graaf EA, van Kessel DA, et al. Pulmonary embolism and pulmonary infarction after lung transplantation. Clin Appl Thromb Hemost 2011;17(4):421–514.

15. Worsley DF, Alavi A, Aronchick JM, et al. Chest radiographic findings in patients with acute pulmonary embolism: observations from the PIOPED Study. Radiology 1993;189(1):133–6.

16. Wittram C, Maher MM, Yoo AJ, et al. CT angiography of pulmonary embolism: diagnostic criteria and causes of misdiagnosis. Radiographics 2004;24(5):1219–38.

17. Revel MP, Sanchez O, Couchon S, et al. Diagnostic accuracy of magnetic resonance imaging for an acute pulmonary embolism: results of the 'IRM-EP' study. J Thromb Haemost 2012;10(5):743–50.

18. de Perrot M, Chaparro C, McRae K, et al. Twenty-year experience of lung transplantation at a single center: influence of recipient diagnosis on long-term survival. J Thorac Cardiovasc Surg 2004;127:1493–501.

19. Kshettry VR, Kroshus TJ, Hertz MI, et al. Early and late airway complications: incidence and management. Ann Thorac Surg 1997;63:1576–83.

20. Herman SJ, Weisbrod GL, Weisbrod L, et al. Chest radiographic findings after bilateral lung transplantation. Am J Roentgenol 1989;153:1181–5.

21. Semenkovich JW, Glazer HS, Anderson DC, et al. Bronchial dehiscence in lung transplantation: CT evaluation. Radiology 1995;194:205–8.

22. Lumsden AB, Anaya-Ayala JE, Birnbaum I, et al. Robot-assisted stenting of a high-grade anastomotic pulmonary artery stenosis following single lung transplantation. J Endovasc Ther 2010;17:612–6.

23. Madan R, Chansakul T, Goldberg HJ. Imaging in lung transplants: checklist for the radiologist. Indian J Radiol Imaging 2014;24(4):318–26.

24. Banerjee SK, Santhanakrishnan K, Shapiro L, et al. Successful stenting of anastomotic stenosis of the left pulmonary artery after single lung transplantation. Eur Respir Rev 2011;20:59.

25. Shennib H, Massard G. Airway complications in lung transplantation. Ann Thorac Surg 1994;57:506–11.

26. Ross DJ, Belman MJ, Mohsenlfar Z, et al. Obstructive flow-volume loop contours after single lung transplantation. J Heart Lung Transplant 1994;13:508–13.

27. Shah SS, Karnak D, Minai O, et al. Symptomatic narrowing or atresia of bronchus intermedius following lung transplantation vanishing bronchus intermedius syndrome (VBIS). Chest 2006;130:236S.

28. McAdams HP, Palmer SM, Erasmus JJ, et al. Bronchial anastomotic complications in lung transplant recipients: virtual bronchoscopy for noninvasive assessment. Radiology 1998;209(3):689–95.

29. Litmanovich D, O'Donnell CR, Bankier AA, et al. Bronchial collapsibility at forced expiration in healthy volunteers: assessment with multidetector CT. Radiology 2010;257(2):560–7.

30. Ferrer J, Roldan J, Roman A, et al. Acute and chronic pleural complications in lung transplantation. J Heart Lung Transplant 2003;22:1217–25.

31. Herridge MS, de Hoyos AL, Chaparro C, et al. Pleural complications in lung transplant recipients. J Thorac Cardiovasc Surg 1995;110:22–6.

32. Tocino IM, Miller MH, Fairfax WR. Distribution of pneumothorax in the supine and semirecumbent critically ill adult. Am J Roentgenol 1985;144(5):901–5.

33. Hong A, Khandhar S, Brown AW, et al. Hemothorax after lung transplantation. [abstract]. In: A44. Lung transplantation outcomes and complications. San Diego (CA): 2014. p. A1593.

34. Kaewlai R, Avery LL, Asrani AV, et al. Multidetector CT of blunt thoracic trauma. Radiographics 2008;28(6):1555–70.

35. Brooks A, Davies B, Smethhurst M, et al. Emergency ultrasound in the acute assessment of haemothorax. Emerg Med J 2005;21(1):44–6.

36. Fremont RD, Milstone AP, Light RW, et al. Chylothoraces after lung transplantation for lymphangioleiomyomatosis: review of the literature and utilization of a pleurovenous shunt. J Heart Lung Transplant 2007;26:953.

37. Wahidi MM, Willner DA, Snyder LD, et al. Diagnosis and outcome of early pleural space infection following lung transplantation. Chest 2009;135:484.

38. Stark DD, Federle MP, Goodman PC, et al. Differentiating lung abscess and empyema: radiography and computed tomography. Am J Roentgenol 1983;141(1):163–7.

39. Haverich A, Dawkins KD, Baldwin JC, et al. Long-term cardiac and pulmonary histology in primates

following combined heart and lung transplantation. Transplantation 1985;39:356.

40. Partap VA. The comet tail sign. Radiology 1999; 213(2):553–4.

41. Bittner HB, Dunitz J, Hertz M, et al. Hyperacute rejection in single lung transplantation –case report of successful management by means of plasmapheresis and antithymocyte globulin treatment. Transplantation 2001;71(5):649–51.

42. Frost AE. Donor criteria and evaluation. Clin Chest Med 1997;18(2):231–7.

43. Christie JD, Carby M, Bag R, et al. Report of the ISHLT Working Group on primary lung graft dysfunction part II: definition. A consensus statement of the International Society for Heart and Lung Transplantation. J Heart Lung Transplant 2005;24(10):1454–9.

44. de Perrot M, Bonser RS, Dark J, et al. Report of the ISHLT Working Group on primary lung graft dysfunction part III: donor-related risk factors and markers. J Heart Lung Transplant 2005;24(10):1460–7.

45. Barr ML, Kawut SM, Whelan TP, et al. Report of the ISHLT Working Group on Primary lung graft dysfunction part IV: recipient-related risk factors and markers. J Heart Lung Transplant 2005;24(10): 1468–82.

46. Prekker ME, Nath DS, Walker AR, et al. Validation of the proposed International Society for Heart and Lung Transplantation grading system for primary graft dysfunction after lung transplantation. J Heart Lung Transplant 2006;25(4):371–8.

47. Carter YM, Davis RD. Primary graft dysfunction in lung transplantation. Semin Respir Crit Care Med 2006;27(5):501–7.

48. Anderson DC, Glazer HS, Semenkovich JW, et al. Lung transplant edema: chest radiography after lung transplantation-the first 10 days. Radiology 1995;195(1):275–81.

49. Paradis IL, Duncan SR, Dauber JH, et al. Distinguishing between infection, rejection, and the adult respiratory distress syndrome after human lung transplantation. J Heart Lung Transplant 1992;11(4 Pt 2):S232–6.

50. Daud SA, Yusen RD, Meyers BF. Impact of immediate primary lung allograft dysfunction on bronchiolitis obliterans syndrome. Am J Respir Crit Care Med 2007;175(5):507–13.

51. Grazia TJ, Hodges TN, Cleveland JC Jr, et al. Lobar torsion complicating bilateral lung transplantation. J Heart Lung Transplant 2003;22(1):102–6.

52. Knoop C, Estenne M. Acute and chronic rejection after lung transplantation. Semin Respir Crit Care Med 2006;27(5):521–33.

53. Kirby TJ, Mehta A, Rice TW, et al. Diagnosis and management of acute and chronic lung rejection. Semin Thorac Cardiovasc Surg 1992;4(2):126–31.

54. Stewart S, Fishbein MC, Snell GI, et al. Revision of the 1996 working formulation for the standardization

55. Bergin CJ, Castellino RA, Blank N, et al. Acute lung rejection after heart-lung transplantation: correlation of findings on chest radiographs with lung biopsy results. Am J Roentgenol 1990;155(1):23–7.

56. Herve P, Silbert D, Cerrina J, et al. Impairment of bronchial mucociliary clearance in long-term survivors of heart/lung and double-lung transplantation. The Paris-Sud Lung Transplant Group. Chest 1993; 103(1):59–63.

57. Dauber JH, Paradis IL, Dummer JS. Infectious complications in pulmonary allograft recipients. Clin Chest Med 1990;11(2):291–308.

58. Kessler R, Fraisse P, Krause D, et al. Magnetic resonance imaging in the diagnosis of pulmonary infarction. Chest 1991;99(2):298–300.

59. Alici IO, Yekeler E, Yazicioglu A, et al. A case of acute fibrinous and organizing pneumonia during early postoperative period after lung transplantation. Transplant Proc 2014;47(3):836–40.

60. Valantine HA, Luikart H, Doyle R, et al. Impact of cytomegalovirus hyperimmune globulin on outcome after cardiothoracic transplantation: a comparative study of combined prophylaxis with CMV hyperimmune globulin plus ganciclovir versus ganciclovir alone. Transplantation 2001;72(10):1647–52.

61. Kang EY, Patz EF Jr, Muller NL. Cytomegalovirus pneumonia in transplant patients: CT findings. J Comput Assist Tomogr 1996;20(2):295–9.

62. Garantziotis S, Howell DN, McAdams HP, et al. Influenza pneumonia in lung transplant recipients: clinical features and association with bronchiolitis obliterans syndrome. Chest 2001;119(4):1277–80.

63. Ko JP, Shepard JA, Sproule MW, et al. CT manifestations of respiratory syncytial virus infection in lung transplant recipients. J Comput Assist Tomogr 2000;24(2):235–41.

64. Schulman LL, Htun T, Staniloae C, et al. Pulmonary nodules and masses after lung and heart-transplantation. J Thorac Imaging 2000;15(3):173–9.

65. Avery RK. Infections after lung transplantation. Semin Respir Crit Care Med 2006;27(5):544–51.

66. Shoji T, Hanaoka N, Wada H, et al. Balloon angioplasty for pulmonary artery stenosis after lung transplantation. Eur J Cardiothorac Surg 2008; 34(3):693–4.

67. Sato M, Waddell TK, Wagnetz U, et al. Restrictive allograft syndrome (RAS): a novel form of chronic lung allograft dysfunction. J Heart Lung Transplant 2011;30(7):735–42.

68. Ofek E, Sato M, Saito T, et al. Restrictive allograft syndrome post lung transplantation is characterized by pleuroparenchymal fibroelastosis. Mod Pathol 2013;26(3):350–6.

69. Konen E, Weisbrod GL, Pahkale S, et al. Fibrosis of the upper lobes: a newly identified late-onset

of nomenclature in the diagnosis of lung rejection. J Heart Lung Transplant 2007;26(12):1229–42.

complication after lung transplantation? Am J Roentgenol 2003;181(6):1539–43.

70. Christie JD, Edwards LB, Aurora P, et al. Registry of the International Society for Heart and Lung Transplantation: twenty-fifth official adult lung and heart/lung transplantation report-2008. J Heart Lung Transplant 2008;279:957–69.

71. Nicod LP. Mechanisms of airway obliteration after lung transplantation. Proc Am Thorac Soc 2006;3: 444–9.

72. Kramer MR, Stoehr C, Whang JL, et al. The diagnosis of obliterative bronchiolitis after heart-lung and lung transplantation: low yield of transbronchial lung biopsy. J Heart Lung Transplant 1993; 12:675–81.

73. Belperio JA, Lake K, Tazelaar H, et al. Bronchiolitis obliterans syndrome complicating lung or heart-lung transplantation. Semin Respir Crit Care Med 2003;24(5):499–530.

74. Cooper JD, Billingham M, Egan T, et al. A working formulation for the standardization of nomenclature and for clinical staging of chronic dysfunction in lung allografts. International Society for Heart and Lung Transplantation. J Heart Lung Transplant 1993;12:713–6.

75. Estenne M, Maurer JR, Boehler A, et al. Bronchiolitis obliterans syndrome 2001: an update of the diagnostic criteria. J Heart Lung Transplant 2002;21: 297–310.

76. Morrish WF, Herman SJ, Weisbrod GL, et al. Bronchiolitis obliterans after lung transplantation: findings at chest radiography and high-resolution CT. The Toronto Lung Transplant Group. Radiology 1991;179:487–90.

77. Konen E, Gutierrez C, Chaparro C, et al. Bronchiolitis obliterans syndrome in lung transplant recipients: can thin-section CT findings predict disease before its clinical appearance? Radiology 2004;231(2): 467–73.

78. Brauner MW, Lenoir S, Grenier P, et al. Pulmonary sarcoidosis: CT assessment of lesion reversibility. Radiology 1992;182:349–54.

79. Collins J, Muller NL, Kazerooni EA, et al. CT findings of pneumonia after lung transplantation. Am J Roentgenol 2000;175:811–8.

80. Kazerooni EA, Cascade PN, Gross BH. Transplanted lungs: nodules following transbronchial biopsy. Radiology 1995;194:209–12.

81. Kotloff RM, Ahya VN. Medical complications of lung transplantation. Eur Respir J 2004;23:334.

82. Garg K, Zamora MR, Tuder R, et al. Lung transplantation: indications, donor and recipient selection, and imaging of complications. RadioGraphics 1996;16:355–67.

83. Reams BD, McAdams HP, Howell DN, et al. Posttransplant lymphoproliferative disorder: incidence, presentation and response to treatment in lung transplant recipients. Chest 2003;124:1242–9.

84. Zahiri H, Bierman P, Holdeman KP, et al. The role of FDG-PET/CT scans in early detection, staging, and management of posttransplant lymphoproliferative disease. Radiological Society of North America 2010 Scientific Assembly and Annual Meeting. Chicago (IL), November 28-December 3, 2010.

85. Jensen P, Møller B, Hansen S. Skin cancer in kidney and heart transplant recipients and different long-term immunosuppressive therapy regimens. J Am Acad Dermatol 1999;40:177–86.

86. Lindelöf B, Sigurgeirsson B, Gäbel H, et al. Incidence of skin cancer in 5,356 patients following organ transplantation. Br J Dermatol 2000;143:513–9.

87. Kanitakis J, Euvrard S, Claudy A. Skin cancers in organ transplant recipients. J Am Acad Dermatol 2006;54:1115.

88. Collins J, Hartman MJ, Warner TF, et al. Frequency and CT findings of recurrent disease after lung transplantation. Radiology 2001;219:503–9.

Current Indications, Techniques, and Imaging Findings of Stem Cell Treatment and Bone Marrow Transplant

Tarun Pandey, MD, FRCR (U.K)[a],*, Stephen Thomas, MD[b],
Matthew T. Heller, MD, FSAR[c]

KEYWORDS

- Hematopoietic stem cell transplant imaging (HSCT) • Bone marrow transplant imaging
- Computed tomography

KEY POINTS

- The goal of immunoablative therapy followed by hematopoietic stem cell transplant (HSCT) is to allow outgrowth of a nonautogressive immune system from reinfused hematopoietic stem cells.
- Complications of HSCT can manifest in almost all organ systems and follow a predictable temporal sequence that mirrors the periods of immunosuppression and recovery after transplantation.
- During the preengraftment phase (phase I), neutropenia is common and mucositis, acute graft-versus-host disease (GVHD), and complications associated with lines and tubes are most frequently encountered.
- The early posttransplant phase (phase II) is characterized by impaired cellular immunity; acute GVHD is encountered commonly.
- The late posttransplantation phase (phase III) consists of impairment in both humoral and cellular immunity, with chronic GVHD being most common.

INTRODUCTION

Stem cell therapy has made rapid strides in recent years and has generated considerable interest among scientific communities, clinicians, and the general public. Much of the attention emanates from the great promise offered by this technique, most notably with regard to the application of stem cell therapy for diseases that are currently difficult to treat or incurable, such as Parkinson disease or diabetes mellitus. Traditionally viewed as a core research area, the study of stem cells and cell-based therapies is no longer limited to basic researchers and scientists and is rapidly getting into the paradigm of clinical care.

For radiologists, it is particularly advantageous to be involved actively in the bench to bedside development of these therapies. Stem cell imaging encompasses a wide spectrum, including molecular imaging, and diagnostic and interventional radiology. Molecular imaging offers diverse imaging applications, including imaging, tracking, and monitoring of stem cells and in the assessment of engraftment efficiency. In addition, diagnostic radiologists play an important role in the imaging of transplant diseases and complications associated with stem cell transplantation. The interventional radiologist can also be highly valuable in targeted stem cell delivery by means of different

[a] Department of Radiology, University of Arkansas for Medical Sciences, Slot #556 West Markham Street, Little Rock, AR 72205, USA; [b] Department of Radiology, University of Chicago, 5841 South Maryland Avenue, MC 2026, Chicago, IL 60611, USA; [c] Radiology Residency Program, Division of Abdominal Imaging, University of Pittsburgh Medical Center, 200 Lothrop Street, Suite 201 East, Wing PUH, Pittsburgh, PA 15213, USA
* Corresponding author.
E-mail address: TPandey@uams.edu

Radiol Clin N Am 54 (2016) 375–396
http://dx.doi.org/10.1016/j.rcl.2015.09.015
0033-8389/16/$ – see front matter © 2016 Elsevier Inc. All rights reserved.

routes (percutaneous, selective intravenous, or intraarterial).

The current review presents a simplified overview of stem cell applications and techniques with focus on hematopoietic stem cell transplant imaging.

Stem Cell Biology and Differentiation

Stem cells are undifferentiated biological cells that can differentiate into specialized cells and can undergo mitosis to produce more stem cells. Regardless of their source, all stem cells have 3 general properties: they are capable of dividing and renewing themselves for long periods (long-term self-renewal); they are unspecialized, that is, they lack tissue specific structure and function (plasticity); and they can give rise to specialized cell types (differentiation).[1,2] Stem cells are distinguished on the basis of their plasticity. Not all stem cells have the same degree of plasticity, or developmental versatility. Some stem cells are more committed to becoming any particular type of cell than others. The categories into which the various stem cells fall include the totipotent stem cell, the pluripotent stem cell, multipotent stem cell, and the adult stem cell (a certain type of multipotent stem cell). These properties of stem cells are described in **Table 1**.

Embryonic stem cells are examples of totipotent stem cells, allowing them to give rise to any mature cell type. This property implies that an entire organism can be constructed from these embryonic stem cells. Adult stem cells are examples of pluripotent stem cells, very similar to totipotent stem cells in that they can give rise to all tissue types. But, unlike totipotent stem cells, they cannot give rise to an entire organism. Multipotent cells can differentiate into a number of cell types; however, these are a closely related family of cells. Oligopotent cells are further limited to differentiate into only a few cell types (eg, lymphoid or myeloid cells), whereas unipotent cells can only produce 1 cell line. It is important to note that the property of self-renewal in stem cells is unlimited. This differentiates them from other non–stem cells like progenitor cells that have a limited capacity of self-renewal. **Fig. 1** presents a simplified representation of the stem cells and their lineages in the body.

CLINICAL APPLICATIONS OF STEM CELLS

Stem cells can be used for a variety of applications. Some of the uses are summarized herein.

Understanding the Genetic and Molecular Controls of Cell Division and Differentiation

The control of cell division and differentiation depends on an orderly control of the genes. Understanding how undifferentiated stem cells become differentiated to form tissues and organs is central to the study of abnormal cell division in conditions like cancer and birth defects. The information gained from the study of the genetic and molecular mechanisms underlying cell division and differentiation may help to better understand the molecular basis of these diseases and can suggest novel therapeutic approaches.

Table 1
Stem cells and their properties

Stem Cell Types Properties	Totipotent/Omnipotent	Pluripotent	Multipotent
Plasticity	*Maximum:* The cells can give rise to any and all cells; possible to regenerate the entire organism.	*Intermediate:* Can give rise to all tissue types; however, they cannot give rise to an entire organism.	*Limited:* They give rise to a limited range of cells within a tissue type.
Long-term cell renewal	Unlimited capacity of self-renewal	Unlimited capacity of self-renewal	Unlimited capacity of self-renewal
Differentiation	Completely undifferentiated and remain noncommitted. Can differentiate into any unrelated cell type	Undifferentiated to start with but become committed after some time to differentiate into different cell types of their tissue of origin.	Most differentiated among stem cells. Differentiate into a number of cell types that are closely related family of cells.
Example	Embryonic stem cells	Adult stem cell	Hematopoietic stem cells

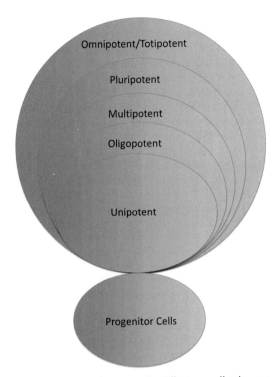

Fig. 1. Lineage of stem cells. All stem cells share a common property of long-term self-renewal unlike non–stem cells, like progenitor cells, that have a limited capacity for self-renewal.

Drug Testing

The safety and efficacy of new drugs can be tested on differentiated cells generated from human pluripotent cell lines. Similarly, cancer cell lines are used to screen potential antitumor drugs. Pluripotent cell lines can generate a number of differentiated cell types, allowing a variety of cell substrate for drug testing.

Cell-based Therapy

Approximately 128 million people suffer from chronic, degenerative, and acute diseases, and stem cell therapies hold great promise in the treatment of many of these diseases. Advances in stem cell biology have allowed expanded the use of stem cells to treat nonmalignant diseases. These applications include treatment of autoimmune diseases, restoring or normalizing hematopoietic function, and treating inborn errors of metabolism. With stem cell–derived cells, tissues and possibly organs may become a renewable source of replacement cells and tissues to treat diseases including cancer, diabetes, macular degeneration, spinal cord injury, stroke, burns, heart disease, osteoarthritis, and rheumatoid arthritis (RA).

Hematopoietic stem cell transplantation for autoimmune diseases

The goal of immunoablative therapy followed by hematopoietic stem cell transplantation (HSCT) is aimed at resetting the patient's immune system and allow outgrowth of a nonautogressive immune system from reinfused hematopoietic stem cells allowing the immune system to shift from a highly proinflammatory disease environment to a less inflammatory one.[3,4]

Both autologous and allogeneic stem cells can been used to treat various immune mediated diseases including multiple sclerosis (MS), systemic sclerosis, systemic lupus erythematosus, and RA.[5]

Multiple sclerosis

Autologous HSCT has been used to treat patient with progressive forms of MS and refractory relapsing-remitting MS with promising outcomes.[5,6] The outcomes for treating MS are partly dependent on the conditioning regimens prior to allogeneic stem cell transplantation. The long-term progression-free survival was better in patients who received intermediate-intensity regimens conditioning 79.4% (95% CI: 69.9%–86.5%) with a median follow-up of 39 months versus high-intensity regimens 44.6% (95% CI: 26.5%–64.5%) with a median follow-up of 24 months.[7]

Systemic sclerosis

Systemic sclerosis with skin involvement and internal organ involvement is a progressive life threatening disease that has a mortality of 30% to 50% at 5 years.[8] The rationale behind HSCT is to significantly reduce the bulk of autoaggressive immune competent cells and then rescue the ablated hematopoiesis via an autologous HSCT. Clinical trials have reported significant therapeutic benefits in approximately a third of the patients and a relapse rate of 25%. Treatment related mortality ranged from 6% to 23% across different studies.[9,10]

Systemic lupus erythematosus

Systemic lupus erythematosus is a multisystem immune disorder characterized by autoantibody production against cellular components. Autologous stem cell transplantation has been used successfully to treat mild to severe systemic lupus erythematosus with an estimated 50% to 70% disease free survival at 5 years and an overall transplant-related mortality ranging from 0% to 25 %.[11]

Rheumatoid arthritis

RA is T-cell–mediated autoimmune disease characterized by synovial inflammation and articular destruction. RA has been effectively treated using biologic therapies and disease-modifying anti-rheumatic agents and is the reason why there are few studies on the use of HSCT in its treatment. In a study of refractory RA patients, Snowden and colleagues[12] reported 67% of patients achieved an American College of Rheumatology 50% improvement response after autologous HSCT.

Hematopoietic stem cell transplantation for anemia

Aplastic anemia Most causes of aplastic anemia result from immune-mediated depletion of hematopoietic stem cells. Aplastic anemia can result from inborn errors of metabolism such as Fanconi's anemia and Diamond-Blackfan anemia. Toxic exposure from radiation, chemicals, drugs, and infections can also cause aplastic anemia. Allogenic stem cell transplantation has had produced excellent results in aplastic anemia; however, its success is related to age with a decline in survival in older patients. Reported survival data from HLA identical siblings over 10 years is 83% (aged 1–10), 73% (aged 21–30), 68% (aged 31–40), and 51% in patients over 40.[13]

Thalassemia and sickle cell anemia Allogenic stem cell transplantation can be curative in patients with β-thalassemia major with disease-free survival rates as high as 86% and 80% for HLA-identical sibling cord blood transplantation and bone marrow transplantation, respectively.[14] Unrelated cord blood transplantation has also been successful in curing the disease.[15] Similarly, disease-free survival rates for sickle cell disease was 92% and 90% for sibling cord blood and bone marrow transplantation, respectively.[14]

Allogenic HSCT has also had success in treating other diseases such as severe combined immunodeficiency, Wiskott-Aldrich disease, mucopolysaccharidoses, amyloidosis, Gaucher's disease, globosidoses, and Pompeacute; disease. With improvements in ablative regimens and improved management transplant related complications, HSCT can produce durable responses in patients with wide range of nonmalignant diseases who have failed conventional therapies. Transplant-related mortality remains the significant hurdle in application.

OVERVIEW OF HEMATOPOIETIC STEM CELL TRANSPLANTATION PROCEDURE

The HSCT procedure, also called as bone marrow transplant in common parlance, is a process that involves the infusion of stem cells into the body to replace damaged or diseased bone marrow from various neoplastic or nonneoplastic conditions. The transplanted cells can be derived from the patient's own body (autologous transplant) or from a donor (allogenic transplant). Apart from replenishing the diseased or damaged marrow with new stem cells, the HSCT procedure may provide an immune boost owing to the direct tumoricidal effect of the infused stem cells. Additionally, it may act as a back up, allowing treatment of the diseased marrow with high doses of chemotherapy or radiation and subsequent restoration of the marrow after successful treatment.

There are several steps involved in an HSCT procedure.[16] A rigorous health assessment of the subject undergoing the transplant is done to ensure success of the procedure using a series of tests and procedures. A central line is placed during this period and typically left in place for subsequent infusion of stem cells, medications, and transfusions.

The harvesting of stem cell depends on the type of the HSCT procedure. For allogenic transplant stem, cells are collected from the donor blood or bone marrow. For autologous stem cell harvest, the subject's stem cell production is first increased by administration of daily injections of growth factor, after which the subject's blood is collected and circulated through a machine that separates the blood into different components, a process called apheresis.

As a final step before the HSCT procedure, the patient undergoes a conditioning process wherein pre transplant chemotherapy and/or radiation are used to destroy any existing cancer cells and to suppress the immune system. Those who cannot tolerate the conditioning regimen may receive lower doses or potentially less toxic medications, a process called reduced intensity conditioning. The patient typically receives a number of medications, red blood and platelet transfusions, and intravenous fluids to control the side effects of the conditioning regimen.

After conditioning, stem cells are simply infused through a central line. Over the course of several weeks, the stem cells home into the marrow and start producing new blood cells. During this period of engraftment, the patient is monitored closely for the success of the procedure and development of complications. A patient who has undergone HSCT may be at greater risk of infections or other complications for months to years after the transplant.

Transplantation of stem cells has been associated with a myriad of systemic complications ranging from infection, graft-versus-host disease (GVHD), and neoplasia, predominantly owing to the immunosuppression associated with stem cell transplantation. These complications follow a predictable pattern in that recipients of allo-genic transplant are at risk for developing GVHD and those receiving autologous transplant, although not at risk of GVHD, have greater chances of developing infections or relapse of the disease.

After HSCT, the risk of developing complications depends on several factors. The type of transplantation, whether allogenic or autologous plays, a vital role. The potency of the conditioning regimen is another important prognostic factor; it determines how much residual disease is present at the time of transplantation. Other factors include the patient's age and the underlying disease condition. In general, the prognosis is poorer in adults, those with autologous transplant, and in whom residual disease was present.[17]

IMAGING OF STEM CELL TRANSPLANT COMPLICATIONS

Complications can manifest in almost all organ systems of the body and follow a predictable temporal sequence that mirrors the periods of immunosuppression and recovery after transplantation. In general, there are 3 phases after transplantation: the preengraftment phase (0–30 days posttransplant), early posttransplantation phase (30–100 days posttransplant), and late posttransplant phase (>100 days posttransplant).[18] The immune defect underlying these complications also varies during each of these periods. Neutropenia is most operative during phase 1 (preengraftment) with mucositis, acute GVHD, and complications associated with lines and tubes most frequently encountered. Phase II (early posttransplantation) is characterized by impaired cellular immunity. Acute GVHD is commonly encountered. Phase III consists of impairment in both humoral and cellular immunity with chronic GVHD being most common. **Fig. 2** lists the location, relative frequency, and temporal course of complications after HSCT.

Pulmonary Diseases in Hematopoietic Stem Cell Transplantation

Pulmonary complications are the cause of significant mortality and morbidity in patients after HSCT seen in approximately 40% to 60% of patients after HSCT.[19] These occur despite the advances in HSCT, including the use of reduced intensity conditioning.[20,21] Pulmonary complications can be classified as either infectious or noninfectious and vary depending on the time course after HSCT.

Imaging plays an important role in evaluation of pulmonary infections with high-resolution computed tomography (HRCT) being the workhorse.[22] The role of imaging is 3-fold. Imaging, especially using HRCT, confirms the presence or absence of a pulmonary abnormality, because clinical abnormalities are infrequently nonspecific. Imaging patterns can be combined with time course of the illness and the differential diagnosis can be narrowed. Imaging can also help in the localization of an area for biopsy or sampling.

Before delving into the specifics of pulmonary imaging, it should be noted that the imaging

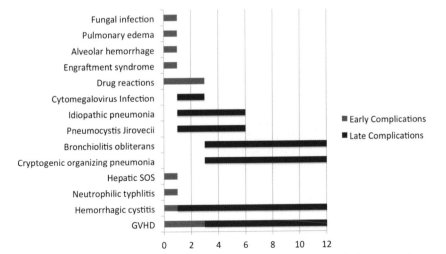

Fig. 2. Relative onset and duration of common complications after hematopoietic stem cell transplantation (HSCT). The x-axis plots the timeline since HSCT in months and is divided into early (<1 month) and late (>3 months) phases. Notice that a few complications can span both groups. GVHD, graft-versus-host disease; SOS, sinusoidal obstruction syndrome.

appearance of a particular complication remains the same regardless of its temporal occurrence and there may be an overlap in the radiologic manifestation of different complications. For example, bacterial infection, drug toxicity, and diffuse pulmonary hemorrhage may manifest as consolidation and air space opacities. Although it may not be possible to differentiate these entities on imaging, it is still useful to perform imaging to rule out other conditions like fungal infection that manifest as nodules, nodular infiltrates, or masses, and can alter therapeutic decisions. As a general rule, empiric treatment is started based on clinical suspicion.

Although HRCT is used frequently in the evaluation of pulmonary complications, information obtained from a plain chest radiograph may also be valuable in narrowing the differential diagnosis of chest complications after HRCT (**Fig. 3**). Because the differential diagnosis is based on time course of the development of these complications after transplantation, the subsequent review subgroups complications accordingly.

Preengraftment phase

Lung infections In the preengraftment phase, both infectious and noninfectious complications can occur with equal frequency. Despite prophylactic strategies and advances in diagnosis and treatment of pulmonary infections, pneumonia remains an important cause of nonrelapse mortality after HSCT.[23] Infectious complications are more common in patients undergoing allogeneic transplants owing to prolonged immunosuppressive therapy and GVHD.

Fungal infections manifest more often because most patients who are febrile receive empiric antibiotics for assumed bacterial infections, giving mostly negative cultures.[18,24] As many as 50% of all pulmonary infections in the allogenic stem cell transplant setting are fungal in origin. Invasive pulmonary aspergillosis is the most common invasive fungal infection among HSCT recipients with reported incidence of 5% to 30% in allogeneic and 1% to 5% in autologous HSCT.[25] The incidence of aspergillosis continues to decrease with the increased use of aspergillus prophylaxis. Although a number of randomized, controlled trials have shown that prophylaxis for aspergillus infection is correlated with reduced all-cause mortality, long-term mortality (>36 months) is unchanged.[26] Hence, it is important to diagnose aspergillus infection early. HRCT can show multiple nodules, masses, and air space opacities as well as the halo sign, suggestive of the diagnosis (**Fig. 4**).

Pulmonary edema In the setting of HSCT, some specific causes of pulmonary edema are secondary to drug-induced toxicity or sepsis, are related to transfusion, or are from intravenous fluid overload. The diagnosis is typically made clinically and on chest radiographs. Radiologic differential diagnosis includes various lung injury syndrome in the post HSCT setting like postengraftment syndrome (**Fig. 5**), diffuse alveolar hemorrhage (**Fig. 6**), and idiopathic pneumonia syndrome (IPS; **Table 2**).

Engraftment syndrome This is a clinical syndrome, also called periengraftment respiratory distress syndrome and is characterized by fever,

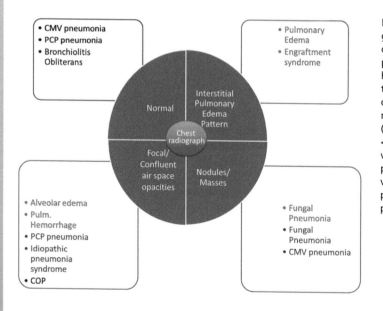

Fig. 3. A simplified pattern radiographic approach to evaluate most commonly occurring pulmonary complications on chest radiographs after hematopoietic stem cell transplantation. Within each pattern the conditions are color coded based on most likely time of occurrence (*green* = neutropenic phase, <3 weeks; *red* = early phase, 3 weeks–3 months; *blue* = late phase, >3 months). CMV, cytomegalovirus; COP, cryptogenic-organizing pneumonia; PCP, *Pneumocystis carinii* pneumonia.

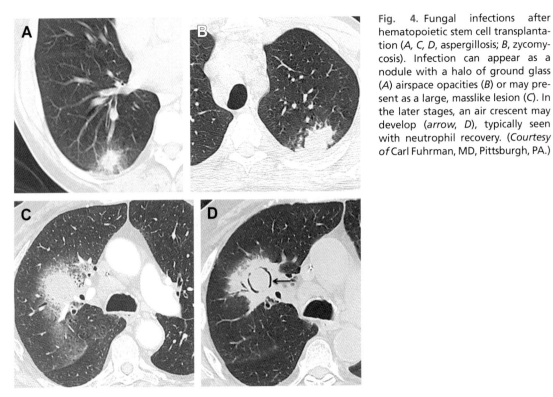

Fig. 4. Fungal infections after hematopoietic stem cell transplantation (*A, C, D*, aspergillosis; *B*, zycomycosis). Infection can appear as a nodule with a halo of ground glass (*A*) airspace opacities (*B*) or may present as a large, masslike lesion (*C*). In the later stages, an air crescent may develop (*arrow, D*), typically seen with neutrophil recovery. (*Courtesy of* Carl Fuhrman, MD, Pittsburgh, PA.)

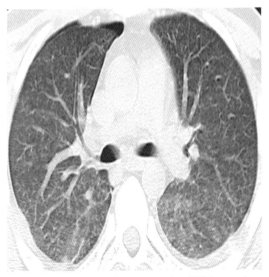

Fig. 5. Axial computed tomography (CT) image in a 32-year-old patient who presented with shortness of breath within a few hours after hematopoietic stem cell transplantation. CT shows mild bilateral interstitial thickening, similar to pulmonary edema. The clinical presentation prompted a diagnosis of engraftment syndrome. A trace right pneumothorax is incidentally noted. (*Courtesy of* Carl Fuhrman, MD, Pittsburgh, PA.)

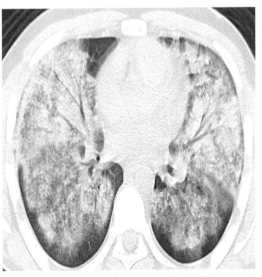

Fig. 6. Axial computed tomography (CT) image in lung window from a CT performed on a 37-year-old woman with hemoptysis, dyspnea, and oxygen desaturation. Diffuse alveolar opacities are visualized owing to alveolar hemorrhage. (*Courtesy of* Carl Fuhrman, MD, Pittsburgh, PA.)

Table 2
Summary of noninfectious acute, subacute, and chronic lung conditions in patients with hematopoietic stem cell transplantation (HSCT)

Feature	Engraftment Syndrome	Diffuse Alveolar Hemorrhage	Idiopathic Pneumonia Syndrome	Cryptogenic Organizing Pneumonia	Bronchiolitis Obliterans
Incidence and onset	Acute onset; within 96 h of engraftment (4–25 d). More common in autologous HSCT.	Acute to early onset. Occurs with equal frequency in allogeneic vs autologous HSCT.	Subacute-late (30–180 d); more common in allogenic HSCT.	<2%; Allogenic and autologous HSCT; Onset usually in the first 100 d.	0%–48%; Allogenic HSCT; late onset (1 y).
Etiology and pathogenesis	Release of proinflammatory cytokines and neutrophils influx into lungs; Use of G-CSF	Bleeding into the alveolar spaces owing to injury or inflammation of the arterioles, venules, or alveolar septal capillaries.	Interstitial pneumonitis and/or diffuse alveolar damage; associated with aggressive conditioning.	Granular plugs of bronchioles, extending into alveoli; interstitial inflammation and fibrosis.	Fibrotic plugs obliterating bronchioles with inflammation and scarring; spare alveoli and alveolar ducts.
Clinical features and diagnostic tests	Characterized by erythematous rash over 25% of body surface area.	Tachypnea and dyspnea; hemoptysis is not a feature. Progressive bloodier bloodier lavage from >3 subsegmental lobes >20% hemosiderin-laden macrophage in the absence of infection.	Needs 2 main criteria: a. Presence of wide-spread alveolar injury, and b. Absence of lower respiratory tract infection (confirmed on 2 negative BAL or lung biopsy within 2 wk).	Dyspnea, cough, fever; Restrictive; reduction in diffusing capacity; diagnosis is made on tissue biopsy.	Cough, dyspnea, wheeze; obstructive; normal diffusion capacity; diagnosis is based on clinical, radiologic and physiologic testing.
Radiologic features	Indistinguishable from noncardiogenic pulmonary edema.	Patchy alveolar infiltrates becoming more confluent with central, mid, and lower lung predominance.	Nonspecific findings like noncardiogenic pulmonary edema; bilateral air space opacities and consolidations with basilar predominance.	Patchy consolidation, ground glass opacities, nodular opacities.	Normal; hyperinflated lungs, air trapping, bronchiectasis.
Prognosis	Generally responds well to steroids; discontinue G-CSF.	Poor prognosis. Moderate response to steroids. Usually die of multiorgan failure and sepsis.	Poor prognosis; does not respond well to steroids; 70%–85% mortality.	Responds well to steroids; potentially reversible.	Poor response to therapy; progressive disease with high mortality.

Abbreviations: BAL, bronchoalveolar lavage; G-CSF, granulocytic-colony stimulating factor.

erythematous rash, and noncardiogenic pulmonary edema. It usually occurs at the time of neutrophil recovery.[27] Periengraftment respiratory distress syndrome is seen more frequently in autologous patients who underwent HSCT, with an incidence of 7% to 11%.[26] Imaging may be normal or show nonspecific findings like ground glass opacities, hilar/peribronchial air space consolidations, septal thickening, and effusions that can mimic pulmonary edema, infections, or GVHD.[28]

Treatment-related toxicity Lung injury can also result from total body irradiation or chemotherapy with lung toxicity (carmustine/methotrexate) in the immediate posttransplant period. Chemotherapy and radiation have synergistic risk of producing lung damage.[29] Both imaging and biopsy findings are nonspecific. Imaging may show a pattern similar to acute respiratory distress syndrome, hypersensitivity pneumonitis, and organizing pneumonia.[30] Biopsy may show diffuse alveolar damage, histologic equivalent of acute respiratory distress syndrome, type II alveolar epithelial cell atypia and hyperplasia, interstitial pneumonitis, and fibrosis. It is a diagnosis of exclusion.

Early posttransplant phase (days 31–100)
Among infectious complications pneumonia remains the most common, although less common compared with the preengraftment phase. Despite gradual resolution of severe neutropenia by day 100 and waning of the induction chemotherapy and radiation effects, several factors account for patient's susceptibility to infections, like T-cell dysfunction, hypogammaglobulinemia, diminished phagocyte function, acute GVHD, and use of immunosuppressants to manage the GVHD. Acute GVHD and idiopathic pneumonia are the other noninfectious complications in this period.

Overall, viral (cytomegalovirus [CMV], adenovirus) and fungal infections (*Pneumocystis jiroveci*, aspergillus) are more common than bacterial

infections.[31] Among bacterial infections, *Staphylococcus* may be seen in patients with an indwelling central line. The patients are also prone to infections with encapsulated bacteria like *Streptococcus pneumonia* and *Haemophilus influenza*.[32] Owing to effective prophylaxis, *P jiroveci* infection is rare.

Fungal pneumonia CMV pneumonia is the most important cause of viral pneumonia in the post HSCT setting, even though its occurrence has decreased with CMV monitoring and preemptive treatment. It should be noted that CMV infection not only manifests as pneumonia, but can also cause hepatitis and colitis. Most CMV infections result from reactivation of the latent virus in seropositive recipients from the peripheral blood leukocytes or as primary infection from a seropositive donor.

CMV pneumonia carries a 15% to 20% mortality rate with a high case fatality rate of 80% to 90%. Chest radiographs may be normal, but typically show patchy areas of ground glass or consolidation. HRCT may show ground-glass opacities, air space consolidations, or small (<5 mm) centrilobular nodules[33] (**Fig. 7**). Routine prophylaxis is not recommended owing to toxicity. Given the high mortality, presumptive therapy is started once clinical and/or radiologic features are seen and the presence of CMV in blood or bronchoalveolar lavage fluid is confirmed with either CMV DNA polymerase chain reaction shell assay or positive viral cultures. Other respiratory and enteric viruses (respiratory syncytial virus, respiratory syncytial virus, and adenovirus) account for the majority of non-CMV viral infections in the HSCT population. These either produce no radiologic findings or may show diffuse ground glass opacities.

Pneumocystis jiroveci **pneumonia** *Pneumocystis jiroveci* pneumonia is rare in patients who receive prophylaxis. Chest radiographs can be normal early on or show reticulonodular infiltrates that progress to air space consolidations. In cases

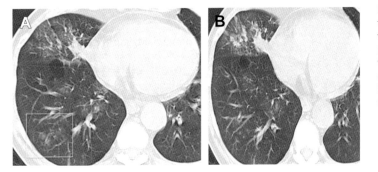

Fig. 7. (*A*, *B*) Cytomegalovirus infection after hematopoietic stem cell transplantation. Computed tomography shows a combination of centrilobular nodules (*box*), ground class opacities and consolidations in the right lung. (*Courtesy of* Carl Fuhrman, MD, Pittsburgh, PA.)

where radiographs are negative, HRCT may show the characteristic ground glass opacities and/or consolidations, either diffuse or perihilar in distribution (**Fig. 8**). Sparing of the secondary pulmonary lobules has been described on HRCT.[34] Other features include focal opacities, cavitations/pneumatoceles, or air cysts.

Idiopathic pneumonia syndrome The most recent definition of IPS by the American Thoracic Society is "an idiopathic syndrome of pneumopathy after HSCT, with evidence of widespread alveolar injury and in which an infectious etiology and cardiac dysfunction, acute renal failure or iatrogenic fluid overload have been excluded."[35,36] IPS is the most common cause of diffuse radiographic abnormalities between 30 and 180 days after transplantation.[35] The mean estimated incidence of this syndrome is 1% to 10% and is less common in the patient undergoing autologous HSCT (5.8%).[37] IPS is a group of disorders that show common pathologic findings of interstitial pneumonitis and/or diffuse alveolar damage. The etiopathogenesis, diagnostic criteria, and radiologic findings are summarized in **Table 2**. There is no optimal therapy for IPS. High–dose glucocorticoids have been tried, but overall the prognosis is poor.

Late posttransplant period (>100 days)
This period is characterized by the recovery of host cell–mediated and humoral immunity. The main complication during this phase is chronic GVHD, which is a reaction of donor T cells and natural killer cells to host antigens, treating them as foreign. Although rare in autologous HSCT, it can be seen in 40% to 80% of allogenic transplant recipients. Ironically, it needs immunosuppressive medications for both prophylaxis and treatment, halting the recovery of the host immunity. Hence, this phase continues until the stem cell recipient stops all immunosuppressive medications for GVHD, which is at approximately 18 to 36 months posttransplantation.

Infections are unusual in this period, except as a complication of chronic GVHD. Most infections are localized to exposed areas like skin and respiratory tract owing to loss of skin and mucosal barriers. Although these patients are at risk for pulmonary infections from a variety of organisms, viral infections, especially secondary to varicella zoster virus, are responsible for more than 40% of infections during this phase, bacteria are responsible for approximately 33%, and fungi cause approximately 20% of infections.[32]

Additionally, patients with GVHD are at risk for noninfectious pulmonary complications including bronchiolitis obliterans (BO), cryptogenic-organizing pneumonia (COP), posttransplant lymphoproliferative disorder (PTLD), and pulmonary venoocclusive disease.

Bronchiolitis obliterans Although mild airflow obstruction and decrements in lung function are common after HSCT, moderate-to-severe airflow obstruction indicates the presence of BO. It has a strong association with chronic GVHD.[38] BO can mimic infection and cryptogenic organizing pneumonia; however, in a setting of an allogeneic HSCT, especially with chronic GVHD, and absence of signs of infection (based on clinical symptoms, radiographs, microbiologic cultures, sputum culture, or bronchoalveolar lavage), BO should be favored. The diagnosis of BO is established on the basis of pulmonary function tests showing reduced forced expiratory volume in 1 second and HRCT findings of expiratory air trapping, mosaic attenuation, and bronchiolectasis (**Fig. 9**). The airflow obstruction is nonreversible and characterized by intraluminal fibrosis on histology. Pathologic confirmation of constrictive bronchiolitis is not required for clinical diagnosis if all above criteria are met. Because BO has an insidious presentation, including dry cough and dyspnea, recent guidelines by the American Society for Blood and Marrow Transplantation recommend pulmonary function testing at 6 months and then yearly after HSCT.[39]

Cryptogenic organizing pneumonia COP was previously known as BO organizing pneumonia

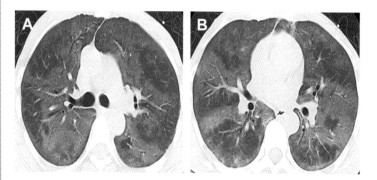

Fig. 8. (*A*, *B*) *Pneumocystis jiroveci* pneumonia. A 52-year-old man, status post hematopoietic stem cell transplantation, presented with fever. High-resolution computed tomography shows characteristic ground glass opacities in with perihilar predominance. (*Courtesy of* Carl Fuhrman, MD, Pittsburgh, PA.)

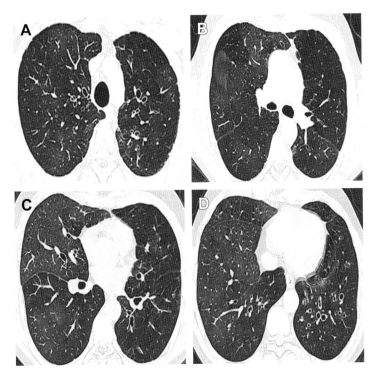

Fig. 9. (*A–D*) Bronchiolitis obliterans in a setting of hematopoietic stem cell transplantation. Computed tomography shows bronchiectasis, peribronchial thickening, air trapping, and simplification of pulmonary parenchyma owing to destruction. (*Courtesy of* Carl Fuhrman, MD, Pittsburgh, PA.)

or BOOP and it should not be confused with BO. BO is primarily an airway-isolated process with normal interstitial tissue, compared with COP, which has both small airway fibrosis and accompanying interstitial and alveolar inflammation. Additionally, COP can occur in both autologous and allogeneic patients who underwent HSCT as opposed to BO, which occurs primarily in allogeneic patients who underwent HSCT. These differences are summarized in **Table 2**. Several etiologic factors might be operative for COP in a post-HSCT setting. Apart from chronic GVHD, it may be related to lung irradiation, after CMV pneumonitis, or may be idiopathic.[40] Histologically, it is characterized by polypoid granulation tissue in the lumina of bronchioles and alveolar ducts, associated with a variable amount of interstitial and air space mononuclear cell infiltration. HRCT may show bilateral, peripheral, and basilar predominant patchy air space consolidation, randomly distributed ground glass opacities, and bronchial wall thickening with dilatation, also described as the open bronchus sign (**Fig. 10**).

Hepatic Diseases in Hematopoietic Stem Cell Transplantation

Hepatic complications afflict 80% of allogeneic HSCT patients and have an overall mortality rate of 37%. Several hepatic diseases can be encountered in the setting of HSCT. Acute GVHD of the

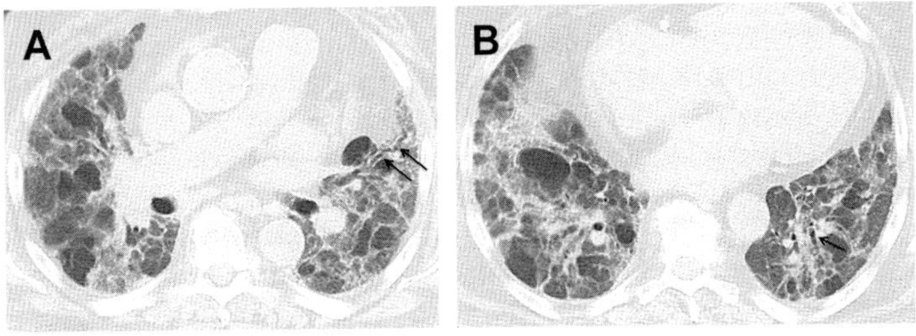

Fig. 10. (*A, B*) Transverse thin-section computed tomography scans through lower lobes in a patient with cryptogenic organizing pneumonia. There are arcadelike and polygonal opacities in lower lobes in both subpleural and central regions of the lung. These bandlike perilobular opacities resemble thickened interlobular septa. There is dilatation and distortion of airways (*arrows*) indicating presence of interstitial fibrosis (open bronchus sign). (*Courtesy of* Carl Fuhrman, MD, Pittsburgh, PA.)

liver, drug-induced hepatotoxicity, and viral hepatitis are the top 3 causes of liver disease in HSCT patients. Other notable complications include hepatic sinusoidal obstruction syndrome (SOS) and liver infections.[41] Clinical, laboratory, and radiologic findings usually suffice for diagnosing drug-induced cholestasis and infection.[42] In GVHD and VOD, however, findings may be nonspecific and liver biopsy may be required.[41]

Acute graft-versus-host disease of the liver

This is the most common hepatic complication after HSCT. Liver involvement is rarely in isolation, and is seen in approximately 50% patients with cutaneous and/or acute gastrointestinal (GI) GVHD. Hepatic involvement manifests as cholestatic jaundice or liver failure with rare progression to hepatic encephalopathy. However, these findings are nonspecific and can be seen in hepatic SOS, viral hepatitis, and drug toxicity. Imaging is also nonspecific and may show dilatation of common bile duct paralleling the serum bilirubin concentration, biliary tract enhancement, and wall thickening.[43] Given no truly reliable GVHD-specific imaging findings and the frequent coexistence of GVHD of the gut, some investigators have suggested routine abdominal computed tomography (CT) scan in search for GI GVHD. Detection of bowel wall thickening in a setting of biliary abnormalities is a strong pointer toward a diagnosis of hepatic GVHD and can also help to differentiate other hepatic conditions like VOD.[44] Similarly, clinical features like presence of a rash concurrent with the liver function abnormalities are also suggestive of the diagnosis. Liver biopsy may be required for confirming damage to the bile canaliculi (bile duct atypia and degeneration, epithelial cell dropout, lymphocytic infiltration of small bile ducts) in ambiguous cases.

Hepatic infections

The development of abnormal serum liver enzymes in conjunction with serologic evidence of active viral infection is indicative of viral hepatitis. Reactivation of latent hepatitis B virus (HBV) can occur owing to the impaired cellular immunity after HSCT. HBV vaccination is needed in patients who are negative for hepatitis B surface antigen and prophylactic antiviral therapy is required for those who are hepatitis B surface antigen positive because HBV infection can lead to that can result in fulminant hepatic failure. Unlike HBV, infection with hepatitis C virus does not result in acute or fulminant disease. However, in the long term, it is a risk factor for hepatic venoocclusive disease and GVHD. Imaging does not have much of a role to play in the diagnosis and management of viral hepatitis, other than ruling out other confounding complications like GVHD or SOS.

Liver abscess

Bacterial or fungal liver abscesses can develop after HSCT. Candidiasis is the most common fungal infection of the liver. The imaging appearance of fungal infection varies according to the stages of its evolution and presence or absence of neutropenia. During the active phase, the lesion is predominantly hypoechoic on ultrasonography (US) with or without characteristic halo, bull's eye, or wagon wheel appearance. The halo occurs owing to the host response and hence may not be seen early on making the lesions inconspicuous. MR imaging may be more sensitive in this phase owing to superior contrast resolution compared with CT and US (Fig. 11). As neutropenia improves, the host mounts a response against the infection, imparting the characteristic halo and enhancement that makes them conspicuous. The lesion becomes echogenic in the late phase. On CT and MR imaging, similar phases have been described.[44–46] In cases when the initial scan is negative and there is a strong clinical suspicion for fungal infection, repeat imaging in 2 weeks may be performed.

Hepatic venoocclusive disease

VOD represents the most common cause of liver disease during the first 20 days after HSCT, affecting 10% to 60% of HSCT patients.[47] In most cases, VOD develops within 1 week before to 3 weeks after cell transplantation and is diagnosed by the modified Seattle criteria (presence of hyperbilirubinemia, painful hepatomegaly and >2% weight gain over baseline within 20 days of HCT).[48] This was earlier called hepatic venoocclusive disease and clinically even mimics Budd–Chiari syndrome. However, it is now known to result from endothelial damage to the hepatic sinusoids causing fibrosis and occlusion of the hepatic outflow. The hepatic veins and inferior vena cava remain patent.[49] In patients with HSCT, SOS is thought to result directly from chemotherapy-induced or radiation-induced destruction of hepatic microvasculature during the conditioning phase. However, SOS is not unique to HSCT and can be induced by the ingestion of pyrrolizidine alkaloids, like herbal tea, high-dose (>30 Gy) radiation therapy to the liver, radioembolization of liver tumors, and after liver transplantation. No single factor is implicated in its causation. Preexisting liver disease, aggressive conditioning therapy, young age, and poor baseline performance status of the host are the risk factors for SOS.[50]

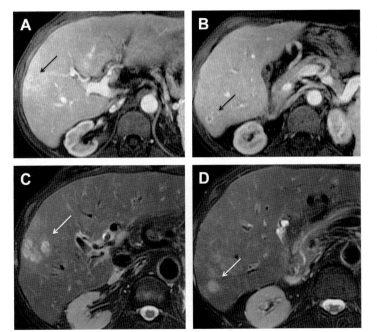

Fig. 11. Hepatic microabscesses in a 43-year-old man who presented with fever and leukocytosis after transplant. Axial post contrast T1-weighted images through the liver (*A, C*) and T2-weighted fat sat images (*B, D*) show multiple T2 hyperintense liver lesions that show ring like enhancement on post contrast images (*arrows*).

Radiologic evaluation in VOD may reveal morphologic changes, including hepatomegaly, splenomegaly, gallbladder wall thickening, increased hepatic echotexture, ascites, and periportal cuffing, as well as signs of blood flow abnormality in the hepatic arterial or portal venous systems. No grayscale US finding is strongly associated with VOD.[51] Doppler evaluation may be more useful (**Fig. 12**). A hepatic arterial resistive index of 0.75 or greater was the best indicator of VOD, occurring in 95% of VOD patients. In HSCT patients without VOD, including those with GVHD and hepatitis, the resistive index values always remained less than 0.70.[51] Other Doppler findings, including portal vein pulsatility and to-and-fro and hepatofugal flow, are considered more specific for VOD, but they typically occur very late in the disease, are seen in a minority of patients, and may represent more severe VOD; hence, they are of limited value in diagnosing early or clinically ambiguous liver disease.

However, imaging may help in the differential diagnosis. For example, the clinical findings of SOS are indistinguishable from those of acute Budd–Chiari syndrome. Doppler US, CT, or MR imaging can noninvasively show the thrombosis of hepatic veins and/or intrahepatic or suprahepatic vena cava, differentiating it from SOS where the hepatic venous outflow obstruction is at the level of the sinusoids and terminal hepatic venules. This distinction may be critical because untreated SOS is associated with significant mortality and morbidity. Unlike Budd–Chiari syndrome, anticoagulation with heparin has not proved to be beneficial. Most patients are treated symptomatically with sodium and fluid restriction along with diuretic therapy. Similarly, imaging can be useful to distinguish SOS from hepatic GVHD, another potential mimic in this setting. CT findings of periportal edema, ascites, and narrowed right hepatic vein have been shown to be associated with SOS more than GVHD.[44] It is important to note that this distinction is not entirely reliable and final diagnosis may require biopsy. **Table 3** summarizes the salient features of hepatic SOS, GVHD, and Budd–Chiari syndrome.

Bowel Diseases in Hematopoietic Stem Cell Transplantation

Several bowel complications can be seen in the post-HSCT setting like typhlitis, pseudomembranous colitis, CMV enterocolitis, and PTLD. The salient complications have been summarized in **Table 4**. GVHD is by far the most common complication.

Gastrointestinal tract graft-versus-host disease

GVHD develops in 55% of the allogenic marrow recipients.[52] The GI tract is one of the most commonly affected target sites of acute GVHD (74%); the other sites are the skin (70%) and liver (44%).[53] GVHD is classified based on clinical features and timing of presentation. The acute and chronic forms of the disease have mutually

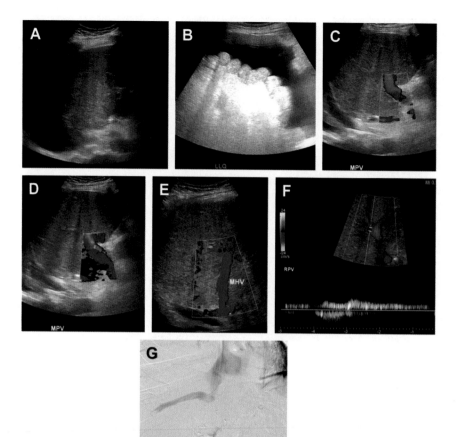

Fig. 12. Hepatic venoocclusive disease (VOD). A 39-year-old woman with a history of acute myelogenous leukemia presents with hepatic dysfunction after transplant. Gray scale shows new, subtle parenchymal heterogeneity owing to congestion at the sinusoidal level and new onset ascites (*A*, *B*). Doppler ultrasonography (US) showed bidirectional portal venous flow that varied with respiration (*C*, *D*); this was a new finding compared with recent prior US and indicated obstruction at the sinusoidal level resulting in increased pressure in the portal venous system. Also, notice patency of the middle hepatic vein (*E*), allowing differentiation from Budd–Chiari syndrome. Doppler US also shows slow portal vein (PV) flow with lack of the normal mild undulation characteristic of the PV waveform (*F*). Finally, image from venogram with catheter in the right hepatic vein (*G*); sinusoidal pressure was measured at 9 mm Hg. A transjugular liver biopsy was performed and results were consistent with hepatic VOD. LLQ, lower left quadrant; MHV, middle hepatic vein; MPV, middle portal vein; RPV, right portal vein.

exclusive features forming opposite ends of the spectrum with an intermediate form having features of both acute and chronic GVHD. Clinically, acute GVHD presents with a maculopapular rash, symptoms of GI upset like odynophagia, nausea, vomiting, diarrhea, and an increasing serum bilirubin concentration. In contrast, patients with chronic GVHD commonly demonstrate skin involvement resembling lichen planus or the cutaneous manifestations of scleroderma, namely, dry oral mucosa with ulcerations and sclerosis of the GI tract. Radiologic findings are not diagnostic of GVHD. Upper GI tract involvement is best evaluated on endoscopy and biopsy of the involved

mucosa showing mucosal erythema, denudation, and aphthous ulcers. An important caveat is that visually normal mucosa does not rule out GVHD. Hence, histologic evaluation is necessary. Lower GI involvement can also be easily established on rectal biopsy with high sensitivity.[54]

On imaging, fluid-distended bowel loops with thickened walls may be seen. Although these findings are nonspecific and may be seen with infectious enterocolitis, radiation enteritis, and drug-induced or neutropenic colitis (typhlitis; **Fig. 13**), a few differentiating features include more extensive involvement in GVHD compared with other diseases like typhlitis or pseudomembranous colitis.

Table 3
Table summarizing salient features of hepatic complications after hematopoietic stem cell transplant

Features	Sinusoidal Obstruction Syndrome	Budd–Chiari Syndrome	Acute GVHD
Risk factors/ etiology	Endothelial injury is result of conditioning regiment in stem cell transplant	Polycythemia, pregnancy, post partum, oral contraceptives, HCC	Allogenic stem cell transplant
Pathology	Endothelial damage hepatic sinusoids causing fibrosis/ occlusion of the hepatic outflow	Intraluminal or extraluminal obstruction of hepatic veins, owing to thrombus or extrinsic compression	Damage to bile canaliculi with degeneration and lymphocytic infiltration
Clinical features	Weight gain, tender hepatomegaly, increased bilirubin, ascites	Pain, jaundice, hepatomegaly, ascites, liver dysfunction	Rash Liver function abnormal, elevated bilirubin and alkaline phosphatase Associated gastrointestinal and skin findings
Imaging	Ultrasonography, ascites, hepatosplenomegaly, PV enlargement, gallbladder wall edema, abnormal Doppler parameters	Thrombus will differentiate from SOS Ascites, hepatosplenomegaly, decreased/absent hepatic vein flow	Temporary fluctuation in size of CBD correlating with changes in serum bilirubin
Treatment	Sodium/fluid restriction, diuretics; Anticoagulation of no use	Sodium/fluid restriction, diuretics; anticoagulation; severe cases can be shunted	Steroids

Abbreviations: CBD, common bile duct; GVHD, graft-versus-host disease; HCC, hepatocellular carcinoma; PV, portal vein; SOS, sinusoidal obstruction syndrome.

Also, luminal distention is more common in GVHD than wall thickening compared with the other entities. On the other hand, there is a higher incidence of pneumatosis, mesenteric stranding, and ascites with neutropenic colitis (see **Table 4**). In cases suspected to have GVHD, CT with negative oral contrast (water) should be performed as patient may not be able to tolerate oral contrast and also negative contrast is advantageous to show mucosal hyperemia and the characteristic "halo sign."

Genitourinary Diseases in Hematopoietic Stem Cell Transplantation

Acute renal injury
Acute kidney injury after HSCT typically develops 10 to 21 days after HCT. Acute kidney injury is defined as a 50% or greater reduction in the glomerular filtration rate and/or more than doubling of the serum creatinine and/or the requirement for dialysis. The incidence ranges from 23% in patients with autologous HSCT to as high as 76% in patients with myeloablative allogenic HSCT. The most common causes of acute kidney injury after HSCT are acute tubular

necrosis, toxicity from medications such as calcineurin inhibitors, and hepatic sinusoidal obstructive syndrome (SOS). Less frequent etiologies include tumor lysis syndrome, thrombotic microangiopathy, GVHD, and hemolysis associated with ABO incompatible transplants. Severe renal toxicity requiring hemodialysis rarely occurs, but mortality in bone marrow transplant recipients requiring hemodialysis is high (up to 80%).[55] Imaging findings are nonspecific.

Renal infections
Renal parenchymal infections occur early on in the posttransplant period. Fungal and/or bacterial abscess can occur. The imaging is similar to infections in non-transplant setting (**Fig. 14**).

Hemorrhagic cystitis
Hemorrhagic cystitis occurs in as many as 70% of patients after high-dose chemotherapy and stem cell transplant without any prophylaxis. The incidence is much less in patients who receive prophylaxis (5%–35%) especially, high-dose chemotherapy with ifosfamide or cyclophosphamide. Irradiation, and some viruses (such as BK polyomavirus, CMV, or adenovirus) can also

Table 4
Summary of GI complications after hematopoietic stem cell transplantation

Feature	Neutropenic Colitis	PMC	CMV Gastroenteritis	GVHD
Onset	Preengraftment period (0–30 d)	Preengraftment period (0–30 d)	Early postengraftment period (31–100 d)	Acute GVHD: Early postengraftment period (31–100 d) Chronic GVHD: late-post engraftment (>100 d)
Etiopathogenesis	Chemotherapy-related neutropenia; damaged mucosa predispose to bacterial infection, leading to inflammatory disease of the ileocecal region; clostridial superinfection is common	Routine use of antibiotics during this phase causes overgrowth of *Clostridium difficile*; typically pancolitis but could be restricted to right colon or rectosigmoid	CMV infection of the gut (CMV is the leading cause of intraabdominal complications during the early postengraftment period)	Damage to the intestinal mucosa from donor lymphocytes; isolated GI involvement is rare; most commonly there is coexisting involvement of the skin and liver
Clinical features	Triad of abdominal pain or tenderness, fever and neutropenia	Diarrhea, occasionally GI bleeding; diagnosis is made on demonstration of characteristic yellow plaque (pseudomembranes) on endoscopy or demonstration of *C difficle* in feces/biopsy specimen	Diarrhea, occasional GI bleeding; diagnosis is made on biopsy and selective staining of the specimens for CMV	Acute GVHD: maculopapular rash, GI symptoms (odynophagia, nausea, vomiting, diarrhea) and hyperbilirubinemia; chronic GVHD: skin involvement predominates resembling lichen planus or scleroderma; dry oral mucosa
Radiologic features	Paucity of right side gas, mechanical ileus of small bowel owing to thick ileocecal valve; CT shows abnormalities localized to the right side of the colon and terminal ileum (thick IC valve, mucosal enhancement and pericecal fat stranding); ascites; pneumatosis	Significantly thickened submucosa appears as hypoechoic wall thickening on ultrasound causing mucosal apposition (pseudo kidney sign); CT shows diffuse low attenuation wall thickening with trapping of contrast between haustral folds (accordion sign)	Nonspecific bowel wall thickening, ascites and adjacent inflammatory change, especially in the ileocecal region; mimics typhlitis, however unlike typhlitis CMV causes more extensive large and small bowel involvement	Fluid-distended bowel with enhancing granulation tissue replacement of mucosa surrounded by low attenuation outer bowel layers (halo sign); ascites; engorged mesenteric vessels (bowel wall thickening is less compared with typhlitis or PMC but extent of involvement is greater in GVHD)

Abbreviations: CMV, cytomegalovirus; CT, computed tomography; GI, gastrointestinal; GVHD, graft-versus-host disease; IC, ileocecal; PMC, pseudomembranous colitis.

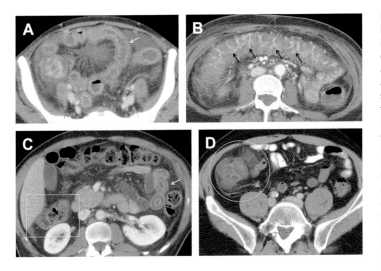

Fig. 13. Bowel involvement after high-resolution computed tomography. (*A*) Acute graft-versus-host disease (GVHD) showing the characteristic mucosal enhancement and hypodense outer wall (Halo sign). (*B*) Pseudomembranous colitis showing the contrast entrapped between the haustral folds (accordion sign) owing to marked diffuse low attenuation wall thickening (*black arrows*). (*C*) Cytomegalovirus enterocolitis shows colonic (*box*) and small bowel involvement (*arrow*). Notice the layered enhancement of the bowel wall in comparison to the predominant mucosal enhancement in GVHD (*white arrows*). (*D*) Neutropenic colitis shows marked cecal and ascending colon wall thickening and stranding of the adjoining fat (*circle*). The rest of the bowel seems to be uninvolved.

cause this problem. Hematuria may occur at any time—from within hours after the administration of these drugs to up to 3 months after treatment—but the peak incidence of hemorrhagic cystitis is within days of chemotherapy administration.[56] On CT and US, focal or diffuse bladder wall thickening may be seen. There may be intraluminal hematoma or sloughed mucosa. Two forms of cystitis have been reported. Preengraftment cystitis, a milder and transient form, is seen in the first few days of transplantation and responds to supportive therapy, whereas postengraftment cystitis that occurs 1 to 2 months after transplantation is protracted, and is associated with severe GVHD and may require operative intervention.[57]

Central Nervous System Diseases

Central nervous system infections
The type of CNS infection depends on the duration and the level of immune impairment after HSCT.

(Fig. 15) provides a detailed timeline of infective and noninfective CNS conditions after HSCT. In the initial posttransplantation period (0–30 days after HSCT), the primary risk is fungal and bacterial infection, mainly owing to the neutropenia encountered in this phase. Factors predisposing to fungemia or bacteremia are long-term use of an indwelling catheter, mucosal damage caused by high-dose chemoradiation therapy, inappropriate use of prophylactic antibiotics, and endemic or hygienic factors.[58] Additionally, if GVHD ensues, then immunosuppressive therapy for acute GVHD can cause profound, catastrophic depression of the immune system.

Bacterial infections are rarely manifested owing to routine prophylaxis. Among the fungal infections, Mucor and aspergillus are common, with aspergillus being the overall most common cause of focal infective brain lesion after HSCT.

During the early (30–100 days) and late (>100 days) post-HSCT period cellular or T-cell–mediated immunity plays an especially

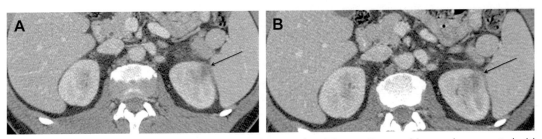

Fig. 14. Axial post contrast computed tomography (CT) images (*A, B*) from a 48-year-old man who presented with flank pain after transplantation. Computed tomography shows formation of a small hypodense renal abscess near the upper pole of the left kidney (*arrows*).

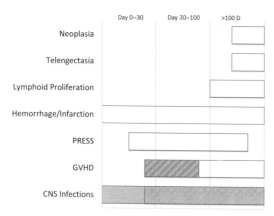

Fig. 15. Timeline of central nervous system (CNS) diseases after hematopoietic stem cell transplantation (HSCT). The x-axis represents the timeline, divided into the preengraftment (days 0–30), early (days 30–100), and late postengraftment (>100 days) periods after HSCT. The zebra striped area indicates acute graft versus-host-disease. The dotted area represents the timeline of the bacterial/fungal infections. The crosshatched area represents viral CNS infections.

important role in the regulation and mediation of the immune response. Viral infections abound during this phase. Most posttransplant infections in this period result from reactivation of latent herpes viruses, Epstein–Barr virus, and varicella zoster virus.[59]

The imaging appearance of the CNS infections also depends on the immune status of the recipient. Abscesses appear as focal lesions. However, owing to immunosuppression, they frequently lack a complete ring, mass effect, or edema. Therefore, brain abscess should be in the differential diagnosis if a focal low-density parenchymal brain lesion is seen after HSCT.

Whereas bacterial and fungal abscesses are seen as single or multiple focal lesions on CT or MR imaging, Mucor is typically an aggressive infection that occludes vessels and can invade the brain parenchyma (**Fig. 16**). Herpes also causes an encephalitis pattern, with characteristic temporal lobe involvement.

Other noninfectious central nervous system conditions

Several other CNS complications can be seen like intra-axial hematomas and infarction that have similar imaging appearance to those seen in the general population. Posterior reversible encephalopathy syndrome is a potentially reversible condition thought to result from pretransplant conditioning and GVHD prophylaxis. It typically occurs within 1 month of the initiation of therapy and is manifested as visual disturbances, cerebellar ataxia, confusion, and seizures. CT and MR imaging reveal abnormalities in the gray and white matter of occipital, parietal, posterior temporal, and frontal lobes (**Fig. 17**).

Post–Hematopoietic Stem Cell Transplantation Neoplasia

Neoplasia after HSCT is categorized into 3 categories: solid tumors, hematologic malignancies, and PTLD. PTLD is one of the most common posttransplant malignancies, occurring usually within the first year after the transplant, whereas solid tumors and hematologic malignancies typically occur late in the posttransplant course (>3 years).[60]

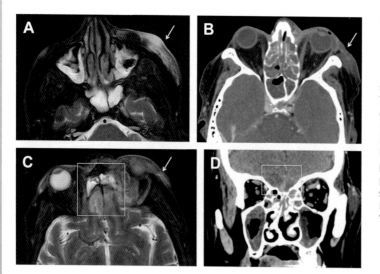

Fig. 16. Axial T2-weighted MR images (A, C) and axial (B) and coronal (D) post contrast computed tomography show invasive fungal rhinosinusitis in a post hematopoietic stem cell transplantation patient. The sinusitis is complicated by intracranial, orbital and facial spread of infection. Inferior frontal cerebritis is seen (box). The left orbital spread is characterized with preseptal and postseptal involvement resulting in proptosis. Left cheek swelling is also seen (arrow). Pathology showed invasive aspergillosis. (Courtesy of Tawnya Rath, MD, Pittsburgh, PA.)

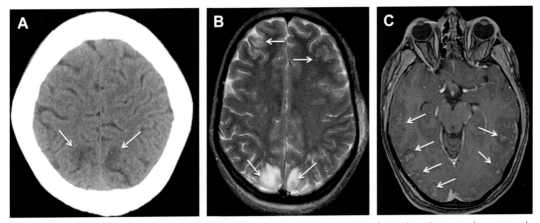

Fig. 17. A 28-year-old patient with seizures after hematopoietic stem cell transplantation. Computed tomography scan shows high parietal hypodensities (*A*). On subsequent MR imaging scan, T2 hyperintensities (*B*) and enhancement (*C*) are noted in the gray and white matter of bilateral occipital, parietal, posterior temporal, and frontal lobes (*arrows*). (*Courtesy of* William Delfyett, MD, Pittsburgh, PA.)

Posttransplant lymphoproliferative disease

After HSCT, PTLD develops mostly as a consequence of reactivation of the Epstein–Barr virus infection of B cells, but may also develop from primary Epstein–Barr virus infection. In cases of primary infection, Epstein–Barr virus may be acquired from the donor graft or, less commonly, from environmental exposure. Overall, PTLD is rare (prevalence 0.5%–1.5%).[61] However, PTLD rates vary greatly depending on the conditioning regimen and the amount of T-cell depletion. Unlike neoplastic lymphoproliferative disorders in immunocompetent patients, the lymphoproliferative process in PTLD may reverse on reduction or withdrawal of immunosuppression. Morphologically and clinically, PTLD has a spectrum of presentations. It can present as a nonmalignant polyclonal B-cell proliferation like infectious mononucleosis-type acute illness or like a malignant polymorphic polyclonal or monoclonal lymphoid infiltrates falling short of criteria for lymphomas, to monomorphic disease consisting of malignant monoclonal lymphoid proliferation meeting all the criteria of B, T, or natural killer cell lymphomas. The clinical spectrum ranges from a rapidly fatal fulminant disease with diffuse involvement to localized involvement that may be indolent and slow growing over months. In general late-onset PTLD tends to be monoclonal, negative for Epstein–Barr virus, and often more refractory to therapy.[62] The most common sites of involvement are lymph nodes, liver, lung, kidney, bone marrow, small intestine, spleen, CNS, large bowel, tonsils, and salivary glands.

PTLD also occurs after solid organ transplantation, but differs from the post-HSCT setting in that it occurs later and is less aggressive.[63] Radiologic features include generalized lymphadenopathy and solid organ involvement either diffusely or as focal masses and nodules like pulmonary nodules and liver masses. PTLD is managed by reducing the degree of immunosuppression, with an obvious tradeoff being graft rejection. Other treatment strategies include use cytotoxic chemotherapy and rituximab, locoregional surgery, or radiation.

SUMMARY

The role of stem cell therapy is treatment of hematologic and nonhematologic conditions is ever increasing. A thorough understanding of the applications of stem cells and transplant physiology is essential in management of these patients. Owing to fluctuations in immunity, these patients are susceptible to a myriad of diseases spanning almost every organ system. Imaging plays an important role in the treatment of these patients. It is possible to make a correct diagnosis on imaging if the findings are interpreted in conjunction with the temporal changes in the immune status of these patients.

REFERENCES

1. Nikolic B, Faintuch S, Goldberg SN, et al. Stem cell therapy: a primer for interventionalists and imagers. J Vasc Interv Radiol 2009;20(8):999–1012.
2. Tuch BE. Stem cells–a clinical update. Aust Fam Physician 2006;35(9):719–21.
3. Hugle T, van Laar JM. Stem cell transplantation for rheumatic autoimmune diseases. Arthritis Res Ther 2008;10(5):217.

4. Mascarenhas S, Avalos B, Ardoin SP. An update on stem cell transplantation in autoimmune rheumatologic disorders. Curr Allergy Asthma Rep 2012; 12(6):530–40.

5. Sullivan KM, Muraro P, Tyndall A. Hematopoietic cell transplantation for autoimmune disease: updates from Europe and the United States. Biol Blood Marrow Transplant 2010;16(1 Suppl):S48–56.

6. Mancardi G, Saccardi R. Autologous haematopoietic stem-cell transplantation in multiple sclerosis. Lancet Neurol 2008;7(7):626–36.

7. Reston JT, Uhl S, Treadwell JR, et al. Autologous hematopoietic cell transplantation for multiple sclerosis: a systematic review. Mult Scler 2011;17(2):204–13.

8. Nash RA, McSweeney PA, Crofford LJ, et al. High-dose immunosuppressive therapy and autologous hematopoietic cell transplantation for severe systemic sclerosis: long-term follow-up of the US multicenter pilot study. Blood 2007;110(4):1388–96.

9. van Laar JM, Naraghi K, Tyndall A. Haematopoietic stem cell transplantation for poor-prognosis systemic sclerosis. Rheumatology (Oxford) 2015. [Epub ahead of print].

10. van Laar JM, Farge D, Sont JK, et al. Autologous hematopoietic stem cell transplantation vs intravenous pulse cyclophosphamide in diffuse cutaneous systemic sclerosis: a randomized clinical trial. JAMA 2014;311(24):2490–8.

11. Illei GG, Cervera R, Burt RK, et al. Current state and future directions of autologous hematopoietic stem cell transplantation in systemic lupus erythematosus. Ann Rheum Dis 2011;70(12):2071–4.

12. Snowden JA, Passweg J, Moore JJ, et al. Autologous hemopoietic stem cell transplantation in severe rheumatoid arthritis: a report from the EBMT and ABMTR. J Rheumatol 2004;31(3):482–8.

13. Young NS, Bacigalupo A, Marsh JC. Aplastic anemia: pathophysiology and treatment. Biol Blood Marrow Transplant 2010;16(1 Suppl):S119–25.

14. Locatelli F, Kabbara N, Ruggeri A, et al. Outcome of patients with hemoglobinopathies given either cord blood or bone marrow transplantation from an HLA-identical sibling. Blood 2013;122(6):1072–8.

15. Gaziev J, Lucarelli G. Hematopoietic stem cell transplantation for thalassemia. Curr Stem Cell Res Ther 2011;6(2):162–9.

16. Lennard AL, Jackson GH. Stem cell transplantation. West J Med 2001;175(1):42–6.

17. Jagannathan JP, Ramaiya N, Gill RR, et al. Imaging of complications of hematopoietic stem cell transplantation. Radiol Clin North Am 2008;46: 397–417.

18. Sable CA, Donowitz GR. Infections in bone marrow transplant recipients. Clin Infect Dis 1994;18:273–84.

19. Soubani AO, Miller KB, Hassoun PM. Pulmonary complications of bone marrow transplantation. Chest 1996;109:1066–77.

20. Afessa B, Abdulai RM, Kremers WK, et al. Risk factors and outcome of pulmonary complications after autologous hematopoietic stem cell transplant. Chest 2012;141(2):442–50.

21. Diab KJ, Yu Z, Wood KL, et al. Comparison of pulmonary complications after nonmyeloablative and conventional allogeneic hematopoietic cell transplant. Biol Blood Marrow Transplant 2012;18(12):1827–34.

22. Escuissato DL, Gasparetto EL, Marchiori E, et al. Pulmonary infections after bone marrow transplantation: High-resolution CT findings in 111 patients. AJR Am J Roentgenol 2005;185:608–15.

23. Kotloff RM, Ahya VN, Crawford SW. Pulmonary complications of solid organ and hematopoietic stem cell transplantation. Am J Respir Crit Care Med 2004; 170(1):22–48.

24. Aronchick JM. Pulmonary infections in cancer and bone marrow transplant patients. Semin Roentgenol 2000;35:140–51.

25. Kontoyiannis DP, Marr KA, Park BJ, et al. Prospective surveillance for invasive fungal infections in hematopoietic stem cell transplant recipients, 2001-2006: overview of the Transplant-Associated Infection Surveillance Network (TRANSNET) Database. Clin Infect Dis 2010;50(8):1091–100.

26. Capizzi SA, Kumar S, Huneke NE, et al. Peri-engraftment respiratory distress syndrome during autologous hematopoietic stem cell transplantation. Bone Marrow Transplant 2001;27(12):1299–303.

27. Spitzer TR. Engraftment syndrome following hematopoietic stem cell transplantation. Bone Marrow Transplant 2001;27:893–8.

28. Wah TM, Moss HA, Robertson RJ, et al. Pulmonary complications following bone marrow transplantation. Br J Radiol 2003;76:373–9.

29. Patz EF Jr, Peters WP, Goodman PC. Pulmonary drug toxicity following highdose chemotherapy with autologous bone marrow transplantation: CT findings in 20 cases. J Thorac Imaging 1994;9:129–34.

30. Ellis SJ, Cleverley JR, Müller NL. Drug-induced lung disease: highresolution CT findings. AJR Am J Roentgenol 2000;175:1019–24.

31. Salmeron G, Porcher R, Bergeron A, et al. Persistent poor long-term prognosis of allogeneic hematopoietic stem cell transplant recipients surviving invasive aspergillosis. Haematologica 2012;97(9):1357–63.

32. Leather HL, Wingard JR. Infections following hematopoietic stem cell transplantation. Infect Dis Clin North Am 2001;15:483–520.

33. Gasparetto EL, Ono SE, Escuissato D, et al. Cytomegalovirus pneumonia after bone marrow transplantation: high resolution CT findings. Br J Radiol 2004;77:724–7.

34. Leung AN, Gosselin MV, Napper CH, et al. Pulmonary infections after bone marrow transplantation: clinical and radiographic findings. Radiology 1999; 210:699–710.

35. Panoskaltsis-Mortari A, Griese M, Madtes DK, et al, American Thoracic Society Committee on Idiopathic Pneumonia Syndrome. An official American Thoracic Society research statement: noninfectious lung injury after hematopoietic stem cell transplantation: idiopathic pneumonia syndrome. Am J Respir Crit Care Med 2011;183(9):1262–79.

36. Kantrow SP, Hackman RC, Boeckh M, et al. Idiopathic pneumonia syndrome: changing spectrum of lung injury after marrow transplantation. Transplantation 1997;63:1079–86.

37. Fukuda T, Hackman RC, Guthrie KA, et al. Risks and outcomes of idiopathic pneumonia syndrome after nonmyeloablative and conventional conditioning regimens for allogeneic hematopoietic stem cell transplantation. Blood 2003;102(8):2777–85.

38. Freudenberger TD, Madtes DK, Curtis JR, et al. Association between acute and chronic graft-versus-host disease and bronchiolitis obliterans organizing pneumonia in recipients of hematopoietic stem cell transplants. Blood 2003;102:3822–8.

39. Majhail NS, Rizzo JD, Lee SJ, et al, Center for International Blood and Marrow Transplant Research (CIBMTR), American Society for Blood and Marrow Transplantation (ASBMT), European Group for Blood and Marrow Transplantation (EBMT), Asia-Pacific Blood and Marrow Transplantation Group (APBMT), Bone Marrow Transplant Society of Australia and New Zealand (BMTSANZ), East Mediterranean Blood and Marrow Transplantation Group (EMBMT); Sociedade Brasileira de Transplante de Medula Ossea (SBTMO). Recommended screening and preventive practices for long-term survivors after hematopoietic cell transplantation. Biol Blood Marrow Transplant 2012;18(3):348–71.

40. Mathew P, Bozeman P, Krance RA, et al. Bronchiolitis obliterans organizing pneumonia (BOOP) in children after allogeneic bone marrow transplantation. Bone Marrow Transplant 1994;13:221–3.

41. Arai S, Lee LA, Vogelsang GB. A systematic approach to hepatic complications in hematopoietic stem cell transplantation. J Hematother Stem Cell Res 2002;11(2):215–29.

42. Coy DL, Ormazabal A, Godwin JD, et al. Imaging evaluation of pulmonary and abdominal complications following hematopoietic stem cell transplantation. Radiographics 2005;25(2):305–17.

43. Ketelsen D, Vogel W, Bethge W, et al. Enlargement of the common bile duct in patients with acute graft-versus-host disease: what does it mean? AJR Am J Roentgenol 2009;193:W181–5.

44. Erturk SM, Mortelé KJ, Binkert CA, et al. CT features of hepatic venoocclusive disease and hepatic graft-versus-host disease in patients after hematopoietic stem cell transplantation. AJR Am J Roentgenol 2006;186(6):1497–501.

45. Semelka RC, Kelekis NL, Sallah S, et al. Hepatosplenic fungal disease: diagnostic accuracy and spectrum of appearances on MR imaging. AJR Am J Roentgenol 1997;169:1311–6.

46. Metser U, Haider MA, Dill-Macky M, et al. Fungal liver infection in immunocompromised patients: depiction with multiphasic contrast-enhanced helical CT. Radiology 2005;235:97–105.

47. Ramasamy K, Lim ZY, Pagliuca A, et al. Incidence and management of hepatic venoocclusive disease in 237 patients undergoing reduced-intensity conditioning (RIC) haematopoietic stem cell transplantation (HSCT). Bone Marrow Transplant 2006;38(12):823–4.

48. McDonald GB, Sharma P, Matthews DE, et al. Venocclusive disease of the liver after bone marrow transplantation: diagnosis, incidence and predisposing factors. Hepatology 1984;4:116–22.

49. Kumar S, DeLeve LD, Kamath PS, et al. Hepatic veno-occlusive disease (sinusoidal obstruction syndrome) after hematopoietic stem cell transplantation. Mayo Clin Proc 2003;78:589–98.

50. McDonald GB, Hinds MS, Fisher LD, et al. Veno-occlusive disease of the liver and multiorgan failure after bone marrow transplantation: a cohort study of 355 patients. Ann Intern Med 1993;118:255–67.

51. Herbetko J, Grigg AP, Buckley AR, et al. Venoocclusive liver disease after bone marrow transplantation: findings at duplex sonography. AJR Am J Roentgenol 1992;158(5):1001–5.

52. Lee JH, Lim GY, Im SA, et al. Gastrointestinal complications following hematopoietic stem cell transplantation in children. Korean J Radiol 2008;9(5):449–57.

53. Ratanatharathorn V, Nash RA, Przepiorka D, et al. Phase III study comparing methotrexate and tacrolimus (Prograf, FK506) with methotrexate and cyclosporine for graft-versus-host disease prophylaxis after HLA-identical sibling bone marrow transplantation. Blood 1998;92:2303–14.

54. Aslanian H, Chander B, Robert M, et al. Prospective evaluation of acute graft-versus-host disease. Dig Dis Sci 2012;57:720–5.

55. Gruss E, Bernis C, Tomas JF, et al. Acute renal failure in patients following bone marrow transplantation: prevalence, risk factors and outcome. Am J Nephrol 1995;15:473–9.

56. Pallera AM, Schwartzberg LS. Managing the toxicity of hematopoietic stem cell transplant. J Support Oncol 2004;2:223–47.

57. Leung AY, Mak R, Lie AK, et al. Clinicopathological features and risk factors of clinically overt haemorrhagic cystitis complicating bone marrow transplantation. Bone Marrow Transplant 2002;29:509–13.

58. Ramphal R. Changes in the etiology of bacteremia in febrile neutropenic patients and the susceptibilities

of the currently isolated pathogens. Clin Infect Dis 2004;39:S25–31.

59. Bjorklund A, Aschan J, Labopin M, et al. Risk factors for fatal infectious complications developing late after allogeneic stem cell transplantation. Bone Marrow Transplant 2007;40: 1055–62.

60. Baker KS, DeFor TE, Burns LJ, et al. New malignancies after blood or marrow stem-cell transplantation in children and adults: incidence and risk factors. J Clin Oncol 2003;21:1352–8.

61. Loren AW, Porter DL, Stadtmauer EA, et al. Posttransplant lymphoproliferative disorder: a review. Bone Marrow Transplant 2003;31:145–55.

62. Knowles DM, Cesarman E, Chadburn A. Correlative morphologic and molecular genetic analysis demonstrates three distinct categories of posttransplantation lymphoproliferative disorders. Blood 1995; 85(2):552–65.

63. Burney K, Bradley M, Buckley A, et al. Posttransplant lymphoproliferative disorder: a pictorial review. Australas Radiol 2006;50:412–8.

Index

Note: Page numbers of article titles are in **boldface** type.

A

Abscess
  and kidney transplantation in children, 284
  and pancreas transplantation, 262
Acute allograft rejection
  and heart transplantation in children, 332
Acute fibrinous and organizing pneumonia
  and lung transplantation, 364
Acute hepatic graft-versus-host disease
  and hematopoietic stem cell transplantation, 386
Acute rejection
  and lung transplantation, 363, 364
  and lung transplantation in children, 325
Acute renal injury
  and hematopoietic stem cell transplantation, 389
ADPKD. See *Autosomal dominant polycystic kidney disease.*
AFOP. See *Acute fibrinous and organizing pneumonia.*
Air trapping
  and lung transplantation, 367, 368
Airspace disease
  and lung transplantation, 362–366
Airspaces
  in lung transplantation, 356, 357
Airways
  in lung transplantation, 356
Anastomotic abscess
  and pancreas transplantation, 263
Anastomotic complications
  and lung transplantation in children, 325–327
Anastomotic leak
  and pancreas transplantation, 263
Anastomotic strictures
  and liver transplantation, 209
Anatomic anomalies
  in lung recipients, 347, 348
Anemia
  and hematopoietic stem cell transplantation, 378
Anogenital cancers
  and immunosuppressive therapy in solid organ
    transplantation, 315, 316
Antibodies
  and immunosuppressive therapy in solid organ
    transplantation, 305
Antimetabolites
  and immunosuppressive therapy in solid organ
    transplantation, 306
Aplastic anemia

  and hematopoietic stem cell transplantation, 378
Arterial anastomosis
  and pancreas transplantation, 259
Arterial stenosis
  and pancreas transplantation, 259
Arterial thrombosis
  and pancreas transplantation, 257–259
Arterioportal fistula
  and liver transplantation, 208
Arteriovenous fistula
  and kidney transplantation, 240, 241
  and pancreas transplantation, 260
Aspergillus infections
  and immunosuppressive therapy in solid organ
    transplantation, 309
Autoimmune diseases
  and hematopoietic stem cell transplantation, 37
Autosomal dominant polycystic kidney disease
  and kidney transplantation, 218, 224, 228
AVF. See *Arteriovenous fistula.*

B

Bacterial infections
  and immunosuppressive therapy in solid organ
    transplantation, 310, 311
Bedside morphometrics
  and lung transplantation, 349
Biliary complications
  and liver transplantation in children, 293–296
Biliary leak
  and liver transplantation, 209
Biliary strictures
  and liver transplantation, 209, 210
Biliary system
  and donor liver imaging, 193
Biopsy
  and kidney transplantation complications, 277
  and pancreas transplantation complications, 264
BO. See *Bronchiolitis obliterans.*
Bone marrow transplantation. See *Hematopoietic
  stem cell transplantation.*
Bowel diseases
  and hematopoietic stem cell transplantation,
    387–389
Brain death
  of lung donors, 340, 341
Bronchial dehiscence
  and lung transplantation, 357, 358

Radiol Clin N Am 54 (2016) 397–407
http://dx.doi.org/10.1016/S0033-8389(16)00013-0
0033-8389/16/$ – see front matter © 2016 Elsevier Inc. All rights reserved.